Resistant Hypertension in Chronic Kidney Disease

Adrian Covic • Mehmet Kanbay
Edgar V. Lerma

Editors

Resistant Hypertension in Chronic Kidney Disease

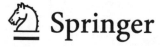 Springer

Editors
Adrian Covic, MD, PhD, FERA, FESC, FRCP
Professor Internal Medicine & Nephrology
Grigore T. Popa University of Medicine
Iași, Romania

Edgar V. Lerma, MD, FACP, FASN,
    FPSN (Hon)
Clinical Professor of Medicine
Section of Nephrology
University of Illinois at Chicago College
    of Medicine/Advocate Christ Medical
    Center
Oak Lawn, IL, USA

Associates in Nephrology
Chicago, IL, USA

Mehmet Kanbay, MD
Professor of Medicine and Nephrology
Department of Medicine, Division of
    Nephrology
University School of Medicine
Istanbul, Turkey

ISBN 978-3-319-86011-4   ISBN 978-3-319-56827-0   (eBook)
DOI 10.1007/978-3-319-56827-0

Printed on acid-free paper

This Springer imprint is published by Springer Nature
The registered company is Springer International Publishing AG
The registered company address is: Gewerbestrasse 11, 6330 Cham, Switzerland

To my family for their unconditional support and to my students for their permanent challenge

Adrian Covic

To all my mentors and friends who encouraged me to become a doctor and eventually decide to pursue nephrology as a career.
To my parents, my two lovely children, Sude and Murat, and my very loving and understanding wife, Asiye, who supported and encouraged me in all steps of my life.

Mehmet Kanbay

To all my mentors and friends at the University of Santo Tomas Faculty of Medicine and Surgery in Manila, Philippines, and Northwestern University Feinberg School of Medicine in Chicago, IL, who have, in one way or another, influenced and guided me to become the physician that I am.

To all the medical students, interns, and residents at Advocate Christ Medical Center whom I have taught or learned from, especially those who eventually decided to pursue nephrology as a career.

To my parents and my brothers, without whose unwavering love and support through the good and bad times, I would not have persevered and reached my goals in life. Most especially, to my two lovely and precious daughters Anastasia Zofia and Isabella Ann, whose smiles and laughter constantly provide me unparalleled joy and happiness, and my very loving and understanding wife, Michelle, who has always been supportive of my endeavors both personally and professionally and who sacrificed a lot of time and exhibited unwavering patience as I devoted a significant amount of time and effort to this project. Truly, they provide me with motivation and inspiration.

Edgar V. Lerma

Foreword

Cardiovascular abnormalities are the major cause accounting for the increased morbidity and mortality in patients with chronic kidney disease. A wide range of factors participate to pathophysiologic mechanisms of cardiovascular complications including diabetes mellitus, vascular nephropathy, general aging of patients, and hypertension. Chronic kidney disease is frequently associated with resistant hypertension defined as blood pressure above optimal goal despite adherence to at least three optimally dosed antihypertensive medications (ideally RAS blocker, CCB), one of which is a diuretic. Recent advances led to increased understanding of causes, pathophysiology, diagnosis, and treatments of resistant hypertension in general populations. The epidemiology, prevalence, clinical characteristics, and outcomes associated with resistant hypertension in chronic kidney disease are less documented, and the aim of this book is to provide comprehensive and detailed review concerning the general workup in CKD-associated resistant hypertension.

The book comprises 22 chapters organized into four parts. The first part comprises six chapters dealing with definitions, epidemiology, characteristics, risk stratification, and outcomes of resistant and apparent treatment-resistant hypertension. The importance of ambulatory and home monitoring of blood pressure for diagnosis and evaluation of hypertension is emphasized in Chap. 4. In the second part, eight chapters cover the pathophysiology and the diagnosis of resistant hypertension, emphasizing the role of ambulatory blood pressure measurement to exclude white coat effect and checking for barriers to antihypertensive treatment (nonadherence or insufficient treatment, salt intake, interfering pressor substances or medications). Four chapters of the second part cover the screening for secondary causes of resistant hypertension, including the role of aging and sleep apnea syndrome. The third part comprises five chapters covering treatment of resistant hypertension in the light of new guidelines, including procedures and devices for neural modulation including renal denervation and barostimulation. The last part of three chapters covers public health approaches to resistant hypertension, excellent teaching program, and resistant hypertension for general practitioners.

This book brings up-to-date informations and is intended to assist nephrologists, internists, cardiologists, and general practitioners taking care of chronic kidney disease patients.

Chair, European Renal and Cardiovascular   Gérard Michel London
Medicine (EURECA-m) Working Group
INSERM U970, Hôpital Européen Georges Pompidou
Paris, France

Preface

This book features practical, referenced information on the care of patients with resistant hypertension and chronic kidney disease. It covers some of the clinical aspects of renal care while also presenting important underlying pathophysiological principles. *Resistant Hypertension in Chronic Kidney Disease* provides a practical guide to diagnosis, understanding, and treatment of all adult patients.

For medical students, it can serve as an excellent resource for reference and review of resistant hypertension. Residents in internal medicine (and other specialties) and most especially, nephrology fellows in training, will appreciate the discussions of diagnostic and therapeutic approaches. General internists, family practitioners, hospitalists, nurses and nurse practitioners, physician assistants, and other allied health-care providers who work with patients with kidney diseases will find this as a very useful reference on management challenges posed by this condition. Moreover, patients and their family members who seek information about the nature of specific diseases and their diagnosis and treatment may also find this book to be a valuable resource.

Striking just the right balance between comprehensiveness and convenience, *Resistant Hypertension in Chronic Kidney Disease* emphasizes the important features of clinical diagnosis and patient management while providing a comprehensive discussion of pathophysiology and relevant basic and clinical science.

This book has been designed to meet the clinician's need for an immediate reference in the clinic as well as to serve as an accessible text for a thorough review of the current published guidelines.

We wish to thank our contributing authors for devoting their precious time and offering their wealth of knowledge in the process of completing this important book. These authors have contributed countless hours of work in regularly reading and reviewing the literature in this specialty, and we have all benefited from their clinical wisdom and commitment.

We would like to thank Elise Paxson for her assistance in managing the flow of manuscripts and materials among the chapter authors, editors, and publisher. This book would not have been possible without the help of Brian Halm, Maria David, Anupradhaa Subramonian, P. Vijay Shanker, and of course, the unwavering support of Gregory Sutorius.

Contents

Contributors

Marcin Adamczak, MD, PhD Department of Nephrology, Transplantation and Internal Medicine, Medical University of Silesia, Katowice, Poland

Ferruh Artunc, MD Department of Internal Medicine, Division of Endocrinology, Diabetology, Vascular Disease, Nephrology and Clinical Chemistry, University Hospital, Tübingen, Germany

Institute of Diabetes Research and Metabolic Diseases (IDM) of the Helmholtz Center Munich at the University of Tübingen, Tübingen, Germany

German Center for Diabetes Research (DZD), Tübingen, Germany

Baris Afsar, MDS Department of Internal Medicine, Division of Nephrology Çünür, Suleyman Demirel University, Doğu yerleşkesi, Isparta Merkez/Isparta, Turkey

Silvia Badarau, MD Department of Nephrology, Gr. T. Popa University of Medicine and Pharmacy, Iaşi, Romania

Maciej Banach Department of Hypertension, Medical University of Lodz, Lodz, Poland

Magdalena Bartmańska, MD Department of Nephrology, Transplantation and Internal Medicine, Medical University of Silesia, Katowice, Poland

Alexandru Burlacu, MD Department of Interventional Cardiology, Cardiovascular Diseases Institute – Iaşi, Iaşi, Romania

Silvio Borrelli, MD Division of Nephrology, Department of Scienze Mediche, Chirurgiche, Neurologiche, Metaboliche e dell'Invecchiamento, University of Campania "Luigi Vanvitelli", Naples, Italy

Mustafa Caliskan, MD Department of Cardiology, Medeniyet University, Goztepe Training and Research Hospital, Istanbul, Turkey

Esmeralda Castillo-Rodríguez, MD IIS-Fundacion Jimenez Diaz, Madrid, Spain

Giuseppe Conte, MD Division of Nephrology, Department of Scienze Mediche, Chirurgiche, Neurologiche, Metaboliche e dell'Invecchiamento, University of Campania "Luigi Vanvitelli", Naples, Italy

Adrian Covic, MD, PhD, FERA, FESC, FRCP Professor Internal Medicine & Nephrology, Grigore T. Popa University of Medicine, Iaşi, Romania

Luca De Nicola, MD Division of Nephrology, Department of Scienze Mediche, Chirurgiche, Neurologiche, Metaboliche e dell'Invecchiamento, University of Campania "Luigi Vanvitelli", Naples, Italy

Raúl Fernández-Prado, MD IIS-Fundación Jiménez Díaz-Universidad Autónoma de Madrid, Madrid, Spain

Charles J. Ferro, BSc, MD, FRCP Department of Nephrology, Queen Elizabeth Hospital, Birmingham, UK

Institute of Cardiovascular Sciences, University of Birmingham, Birmingham, UK

Beata Franczyk, PhD Department of Nephrology, Hypertension and Family Medicine, Medical University of Lodz, Lodz, Poland

Anna Gluba-Brzózka, MD Department of Nephrology, Hypertension and Family Medicine, WAM Teaching Hospital, Lodz, Poland

David Goldsmith, MD Guy's and St Thomas' Hospitals, London, UK

Radu Iliescu, MD, PhD Department of Pharmacology, University of Medicine and Pharmacy "Gr. T. Popa" Iaşi, Iaşi, Romania

Philip A. Kalra, MA, MB, BChir, FRCP, MD Department of Renal Medicine, Salford Royal Hospital, Salford, UK

Asiye Kanbay, MD Istanbul Medeniyet University, Faculty of Medicine, Department of Pulmonary Medicine, Istanbul, Turkey

Mehmet Gungor Kaya, MD Department of Cardiology, Erciyes University, Kayseri, Turkey

Nursen Keles, MD Department of Cardiology, Istanbul Medeniyet University, Goztepe Training and Research Hospital, Istanbul, Turkey

Alper Kirkpantur, MD Department of Nephrology, Acıbadem University Hospital, Ankara, Turkey

Oğuz Köktürk, MD Gazi University, Faculty of Medicine, Department of Pulmonary Medicine, Ankara, Turkey

Edgar V. Lerma, MD, FACP, FASN, FPSN (Hon) Clinical Professor of Medicine, Section of Nephrology, University of Illinois at Chicago College of Medicine/ Advocate Christ Medical Center, Oak Lawn, IL, USA

Associates in Nephrology, Chicago, IL, USA

Roberto Minutolo, MD, PhD Division of Nephrology, Department of Scienze Mediche, Chirurgiche, Neurologiche, Metaboliche e dell'Invecchiamento, University of Campania "Luigi Vanvitelli", Naples, Italy

Aghogho Odudu, MBChB, PhD Division of Cardiovascular Sciences, University of Manchester, Manchester Academic Health Science Centre, Manchester, UK

Department of Renal Medicine, Salford Royal Hospital, Salford, UK

Alberto Ortiz, MD Unidad de Diálisis, IIS-Fundación Jiménez Díaz, Madrid, Spain

Abdullah Özkök, MD Istanbul Medeniyet University, Goztepe Education and Research Hospital, Section of Nephrology, Istanbul, Turkey

Savas Ozturk, MD Nephrology Clinic, Haseki Training and Research Hospital, Istanbul, Turkey

Antoniu Octavian Petriş, MD, PhD, FESC Cardiology Clinic, "St. Spiridon" County Emergency Hospital Iaşi, "Grigore T. Popa" University of Medicine and Pharmacy, Iaşi, Romania

Maharajan Raman, MD Department of Renal Medicine, Salford Royal Hospital, Salford, UK

Francoise Roux, MD, PhD Pulmonary, Critical Care and Sleep Division, Starling Physicians, Hartford, CT, USA

Jacek Rysz Department of Nephrology, Hypertension and Family Medicine, Medical University of Lodz, Lodz, Poland

Liviu Segall, MD Nefrocare MS Dialysis Centre, Iaşi, Romania

Dragomir Nicolae Şerban, MD, PhD Department of Physiology, University of Medicine and Pharmacy "Gr. T. Popa" Iaşi, Iaşi, Romania

Dimitrie Siriopol, MD Nephrology Clinic, Dialysis and Renal Transplant Center, 'C.I. PARHON' University Hospital, 'Grigore T. Popa' University of Medicine, Iaşi, Romania

Yalcin Solak, MD Division of Nephrology, Department of Internal Medicine, Sakarya University Training and Research Hospital, Sakarya, Turkey

Lauren A. Tobias, MD Assistant Professor, Section of Pulmonary, Critical Care and Sleep Medicine, Yale University School of Medicine, New Haven, CT, USA

Faruk Tokmak, MD Department of Nephrology, MVZ Gelsenkirchen-Buer, Gelsenkirchen, Germany

Faruk Turgut, MD Mustafa Kemal University, School of Medicine, Department of Internal Medicine, Division of Nephrology, Antakya, Hatay, Turkey

Luminita Voroneanu, MD Nephrology Clinic, Dialysis and Renal Transplant Center, 'C.I. PARHON' University Hospital, 'Grigore T. Popa' University of Medicine, Iaşi, Romania

Andrzej Więcek, MD, PhD, FRCP (Edin.), FERA Department of Nephrology, Transplantation and Internal Medicine, Medical University of Silesia, Katowice, Poland

Mustafa Yaprak, MD Mustafa Kemal University, School of Medicine, Department of Internal Medicine, Division of Nephrology, Antakya, Hatay, Turkey

Bulent Yardimci, MD Department of Internal Medicine, Nephrology, Istanbul Florence Nightingale Hospital, Istanbul, Turkey

Mikail Yarlioglues, MD Department of Cardiology, Ankara Education and Research Hospital, Ankara, Turkey

Yusuf Yilmaz, MD Department of Cardiology, Istanbul Medeniyet University, Goztepe Training and Research Hospital, Istanbul, Turkey

Chapter 1
Definitions of Resistant Hypertension and Epidemiology of Resistant Hypertension

Charles J. Ferro

Introduction

Hypertension has long been known to be a significant cardiovascular risk factor [1] and remains one of the most preventable causes of premature, especially cardiovascular and renal, morbidity and mortality in both developed and developing countries [2, 3]. Hypertension accounts for, or contributes to, 62% of all strokes and 49% of all cases of heart disease responsible for 7.1 million deaths per year: approximately 13% of total world deaths [2].

Antihypertensive trials consistently demonstrate a significant risk reduction benefit from lowering blood pressure. A reduction of 5 mmHg in diastolic pressure over 5 years is associated with a 42% relative reduction in stroke and a 14% relative reduction in the risk of an ischemic heart disease event [4]. At the start of the millennium, the estimated number of adults with hypertension worldwide was 972 million, with that number expected to rise to 1.56 billion by 2025 [2].

Blood pressure is a continuous variable that is normally distributed [5, 6]. There is no natural "cutoff" above which hypertension definitely exists and one below which it definitely does not. Indeed, the risk of stroke and ischemic heart disease events is continuously associated with blood pressure [7], with no evidence of a threshold value down to at least 115/75 mmHg [5]. Above 115/70 mmHg, the risk of cardiovascular disease doubles for every 20/10 mmHg rise in BP across all the blood pressure ranges for both men and women [5]. Therefore, in the absence of a distinct cutoff value to define hypertension, the threshold blood pressure determining the presence of hypertension is generally defined as the level of blood pressure above which antihypertensive treatment has been shown to reduce the development

C.J. Ferro (✉)
Department of Nephrology, Queen Elizabeth Hospital, Birmingham, UK

Institute of Cardiovascular Sciences, University of Birmingham, Birmingham, UK
e-mail: charles.ferro@uhb.nhs.uk

© Springer International Publishing AG 2017
A. Covic et al. (eds.), *Resistant Hypertension in Chronic Kidney Disease*,
DOI 10.1007/978-3-319-56827-0_1

1

or progression of disease [8]. Most societies and guidelines recommend lowering blood pressure to below 140/90 mmHg [8–13] with some suggesting higher thresholds for the elderly [8, 9, 12] and lower thresholds for those at higher high risk including patients with diabetic mellitus and patients with chronic kidney disease (Table 1.1) [8, 9, 12].

Table 1.1 Guideline comparisons of target blood pressure and definitions of resistant hypertension

	Population	Target blood pressure, mmHg	Definition of resistant hypertension
Report from the panel members of the Eighth Joint National Committee on Prevention, Detection, Evaluation, and Treatment of High Blood Pressure 2014 [10]	General ≥60 years	<150/90	Not specifically defined but no differences highlighted from the Seventh Report of the Joint National Committee (see below)
	General <60 years	<140/90	
	Diabetes mellitus	<140/90	
	Chronic kidney disease	<140/90	
The Seventh Report of the Joint National Committee on Prevention, Detection, Evaluation, and Treatment of High Blood Pressure 2003 [6]	General	<140/90	"Resistant hypertension is defined as the failure to achieve goal BP in patients who are adhering to full doses of an appropriate 3-drug regimen that includes a diuretic"
	Diabetes mellitus	<130/90	
	Chronic kidney disease	<130/90	
American Heart Association/International Society of Hypertension Clinical Practice Guidelines for the management of hypertension in the community [9]	General <80	<140/90	"Blood pressure >140/90 mmHg despite using 3 agents in full or maximally tolerated doses"
	General ≥80 years	<150/90	
	Chronic kidney disease with albuminuria	<130/80	
European Society of Hypertension/European Society of Cardiology guidelines for the management of arterial hypertension 2013 [12]	General nonelderly	<140/90	"Hypertension is defined as resistant to treatment when a therapeutic strategy that includes appropriate lifestyle measures plus a diuretic and two other antihypertensive drugs belonging to different classes at adequate doses (but not necessarily including a mineralocorticoid receptor antagonist) fails to lower blood pressure to <140/90 mmHg"
	General elderly <80 years	<150/90	
	General elderly ≥80 years	<150/90	
	Diabetes mellitus	<140/85	
	Chronic kidney disease: no proteinuria	<140/90	
	Chronic kidney disease with proteinuria	<130/90	

(continued)

Table 1.1 (continued)

	Population	Target blood pressure, mmHg	Definition of resistant hypertension
Kidney Disease: Improving Global Outcomes Blood Pressure Work Group 2012 [13]	Chronic kidney disease: no proteinuria	≤140/90	Not defined
	Chronic kidney disease with proteinuria	≤130/80	
National Institute for Health and Clinical Excellence guideline: clinical management of primary hypertension in adults 2011 [8]	General <80 years	<140/90	"Blood pressure not controlled to <140/90 mmHg despite optimal or best tolerated doses of 3rd line treatment"
	General ≥80 years	<150/90	

Most hypertension can be treated and controlled with lifestyle changes and anti-hypertensive agents [14]. However, there remains a significant subgroup of the hypertensive population that does not achieve optimal control of blood pressure despite adequate hypertension treatment and lifestyle changes [15–19]. The reasons for this are complex and often poorly understood. However, these patients remain at very high cardiovascular and renal risk. It is, therefore, important to use consistent definitions and terminology to accurately characterize these patients, identify risk factors, and elucidate investigation and treatment strategies.

The Term "Resistant Hypertension"

The term *resistant hypertension* appears to have been first used in 1960 [20]. Interestingly, this article examined the effects of iproniazid, an antituberculous agent with antidepressant properties, which had incidentally been observed to lower blood pressure. Twenty hypertensive patients were "carefully selected" and all had a blood pressure of over 200/100 mmHg despite treatment. All had electrocardiographic evidence of hypertensive heart disease and all had hypertensive retinopathy. In this article, the term "intractable" also appears to have been used interchangeably with "resistant" to describe hypertension. The term "refractory hypertension," probably first used in 1958 [21], has also been used interchangeably with "resistant hypertension." Interestingly, patients with refractory hypertension were "defined" in this article as those who had "shown a lack of hypotensive response and an absence of significant symptomatic improvement with various drug therapies." The mean blood pressure in these patients was 236/121 mmHg—eye-watering figures! It is worth remembering, however, that in 1958 these therapies appear to have been limited to drugs such as reserpine [22, 23], hydralazine [24], and autonomic blocking agents including ecolid [25]. No wonder the major cause of therapeutic failure was an intolerance of the antihypertensive agents' side effects.

With an increasing understanding of the critical importance of treating hypertension and blood pressure control, the development of treatment guidelines, and the increasing availability of well-tolerated antihypertensive agents, the need for a clear definition of resistant hypertension became increasingly apparent.

Definitions of Resistant Hypertension

If you cannot measure it you cannot improve it. (Lord Kelvin 1824–1907)

At the most basic level, resistant hypertension can be defined as difficult to control blood pressure in a hypertensive patient. It is not severe hypertension [26]. As with the definition of hypertension itself, any definition of resistant hypertension is to some extent arbitrary. However, any definition also serves to identify patients who might benefit from further investigation or specialist treatment. Indeed, this has been the prime motivator for most efforts to arrive at a workable definition. Several attempts have been made to produce a definition of resistant hypertension that can be consistently applied (Table 1.1).

In 2003, the Seventh Report of the Joint National Committee 7 (JNC7) defined resistant hypertension as "the failure to achieve goal blood pressure in patients who are adhering to full doses of an appropriate 3-drug regimen that includes a diuretic" [6]. Goal blood pressure was defined as less than 140/90 mmHg or less than 130/80 mmHg in patients with diabetes mellitus or chronic kidney disease [6].

In 2008, the American Heart Association further refined the definition of resistant hypertension as "blood pressure that remains above goal in spite of the concurrent use of 3 antihypertensive agents of different classes. Ideally, one of the agents should be a diuretic and all agents should be prescribed at optimal dose amounts" [27]. This definition also includes patients "whose blood pressure is controlled with use of more than 3 medications. That is, patients whose blood pressure is controlled but require 4 or more medications to so should be considered resistant to treatment" [27]. Although an improvement, there remain several ambiguities even in this definition including: "goal" blood pressure is inconsistent across conditions and guidelines; the need for a diuretic to be one of the treatments is not mandatory; and the term "optimal dose amounts" can be considered subjective. Nevertheless, most studies on resistant hypertension since have used different interpretations of this definition [28].

In its recent joint guidelines document, the European Society of Cardiology and European Society of Hypertension further attempted to define resistant hypertension: "Hypertension is defined as resistant to treatment when a therapeutic strategy that includes appropriate lifestyle measures plus a diuretic and two other antihypertensive drugs belonging to different classes at adequate doses (but not necessarily including a mineralocorticoid receptor antagonist) fails to lower systolic and diastolic blood pressure values to less than 140/90 mmHg" [12].

Although not specifically part of the definition, most guidelines recommend the exclusion of apparent or pseudo-resistant hypertension, that is, inadequate blood pressure control in a patient receiving appropriate treatment who does not actually have resistant hypertension. Most often, pseudo-resistance arises from (i) poor clinic blood pressure measurement technique, (ii) the "white coat" effect, (iii) poor patient adherence to prescribed treatment, or (iv) a "suboptimal" antihypertensive regime [29]. Pseudohypertension, or the presence of heavily calcified arteriosclerotic arteries that are poorly compressible giving rise to cuff-related artifact, should also be eliminated before a diagnosis of resistant hypertension is made [29].

Other terms that are being used in the literature include refractory hypertension and controlled resistant hypertension. Refractory hypertension has been defined to include patients who meet the definition but whose blood pressure *IS NOT* controlled on maximally tolerated doses of four or more antihypertensive agents [30]. Controlled resistant hypertension patients are patients who meet the criteria for resistant hypertension but whose blood pressure *IS* controlled on maximal tolerated doses of four or more medications [30]. Although, again arbitrary, these definitions may help to subclassify patients for further investigation or treatment. Perhaps more importantly, they add more clarity when studies reporting findings on resistant hypertension present their results and allow for easier comparison between cohorts.

There is no doubt that any of the definitions, and the accompanying caveats, help in increasing awareness of resistant hypertension as well as focusing on further investigations and treatments. The problems arise, as will be discussed in the next section, when these definitions are interpreted in epidemiological research into the prevalence and impact of this condition, as well as interventional research.

Prevalence of Resistant Hypertension

The reported prevalence of resistant hypertension from population studies with blood pressure control data [31, 32], subpopulations of trials [33–39], retrospective analyses of registry data [15, 40, 41], and population studies specifically identifying patients with resistant hypertension [16, 42, 43] varies widely with estimates ranging from 3% to 34.3%. Pooled prevalence data from North American and European studies, with a combined sample size greater than 600,000 hypertensive patients, suggests the prevalence of resistant hypertension to be 14.8% of treated hypertensive patients [44]. Analysis of randomized controlled trials tends to give higher prevalence estimates than observational studies [29, 45]. This is likely to reflect selection bias with patients at higher cardiovascular risk being included and potentially lacks generalizability to the general hypertensive population. However, at least participation in a clinical trial provides robust data on prescribed doses not normally available from population studies.

In general, most definitions of resistant hypertension do not attempt to distinguish between resistant and pseudo-resistant hypertension: mainly patients with white coat syndrome, improper blood pressure measurements, and nonadherence to prescribed medication [44]. Indeed, one of the main challenges in establishing the prevalence of true resistant hypertension is excluding those patients with pseudo-resistant hypertension [44]. When hypertension is defined as "a properly measured blood pressure > 140/90 mmHg with a mean 24-h ambulatory BP greater than 130/80 mmHg in a patient confirmed to be taking three or more antihypertensive medications," then the prevalence of "true" resistant hypertension is estimated to be lower at 10% of patients with treated hypertension [44].

In order to determine the true prevalence of resistant hypertension would require a prospective cohort study in a large hypertensive population with blood pressure control established by forced titration up to full doses of three different classes of antihypertensive agents, including a diuretic [44, 46]. Such a study would also need to establish adequate medication adherence, appropriate blood pressure measurements, and 24-h ambulatory blood pressure monitoring [44]. Such a study has been performed in a small ($n = 606$) group of young hypertensive patients in Brazil [47]. The initial prevalence of resistant hypertension defined as a blood pressure greater or equal to 140/90 mmHg despite treatment with three antihypertensive agents including a diuretic was 17.5%. However, this figure fell to 4.5% once adherence to medication had been established and 24-h ambulatory blood pressure measurements performed [47].

The American Heart Association definition [27] of resistant hypertension has been the one used by most studies. As discussed, in this definition patients with controlled blood pressure on four or more agents are considered to be the same as those with uncontrolled blood pressure on three or more agents. However, emerging evidence suggests that patients with controlled blood pressure have a "healthier" phenotype with less prevalence of diabetes mellitus and lower LDL-cholesterol than those with controlled blood pressure [28]. These kinds of potential differences need to be taken into account when interpreting the results of studies on patients with resistant hypertension, especially when considering which part of the definition defined the proportions of patients enrolled.

A significant amount of the variability in the prevalence of resistant hypertension may well also arise from inconsistent variations in the interpretation of the American Heart Association 2008 definition. This definition was devised to identify a subset of patients who might benefit from further investigations or treatments and not for research purposes [27]. A study interpreting the American Heart Association definition with different levels of "leniency" on a well-characterized hypertensive population found very different prevalence of resistant hypertension depending on the interpretation used (Fig. 1.1) [48]. After exclusion of patients with documented problems with adherence to medication, the prevalence of resistant hypertension decreased in a stepwise fashion from 30.9% to 3.4% with decreasing "leniency" of the definition interpretation. Interestingly, these figures approximate very closely with the highest (34.3%) and lowest (3.0%) reported prevalence of resistant hypertension, suggesting that differing interpretations of the definition may well explain a significant proportion of the variability.

Further evidence for this comes from another study in which half the patients with resistant hypertension were not receiving "optimal" therapy [42]. The definition of "optimal" in this study was not particularly severe, with patients only having to be on a diuretic and two other antihypertensive agents prescribed at doses greater

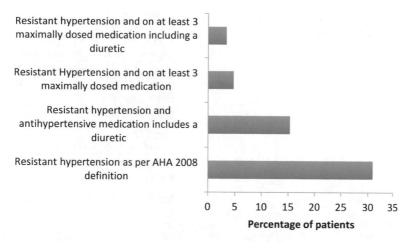

Fig. 1.1 Prevalence of resistant hypertension in a cohort of patients varies depending on the stringency of the definition used (Data from Hayek et al. [48]. The prevalence decreases when the American Heart Association (AHA) 2008 definition is applied at different levels of stringency)

or equal to 50% of the maximum recommended or approved doses for the treatment of hypertension. Indeed, in addition to the prescribing of inadequate doses of antihypertensive agents, other physician-associated factors, including poor office blood pressure measurement technique, inappropriate choice of antihypertensive combinations, clinical inertia, poor communication, and a lack of desire to invest in patient education, are all factors that have been associated with pseudo-resistant hypertension [29].

One of the aims of defining resistant hypertension has been to identify patients for further treatment. Few novel treatments for hypertension have attracted more interest, or indeed controversy, than renal denervation [49–51]. However, caution has to be applied when applying the results of these, and potentially other future studies, as the definitions for eligibility used are often much more stringent than the usual definitions of resistant hypertension [52–54]. Indeed, when the entry criteria to the SYMPLICITY-HTN-3 study [54] were applied to a hypertensive cohort with a reported resistant hypertension prevalence of 30.9%, only 0.8% would have been eligible for the trial [48].

Patient Characteristics Associated with Resistant Hypertension

It has long been recognized that blood pressure is more difficult to control in patients who are older, are diabetic, and have higher baseline blood pressure or longer duration of hypertension, history of cardiovascular disease, black race, obesity, and

Table 1.2 Patient factors associated with resistant hypertension

Older age, especially over 75
Higher baseline blood pressure
Chronicity of uncontrolled hypertension
Presence of target organ damage (left ventricular hypertrophy, albuminuria)
Black race
Diabetes mellitus
Obesity
Atherosclerotic vascular disease
Arteriosclerotic vascular disease
High dietary sodium
Chronic kidney disease

evidence of target organ damage including left ventricular hypertrophy and albuminuria [35]. It is, therefore, perhaps not surprising that all of these factors are consistently overrepresented in patients with resistant hypertension (Table 1.2) [15, 16, 19, 28, 43, 55, 56]. Consistent, and closely linked, with these findings, patients with resistant hypertension have a further clustering of other cardiovascular risk factors including reduced glomerular filtration rate, obstructive sleep apnea, physical inactivity, excess dietary salt, hyperlipidemia, and arteriosclerotic vascular disease [29, 30, 46].

Outcomes in Patients with Resistant Hypertension

The risk of stroke, myocardial infarction, chronic kidney disease, and heart failure rises proportionally with increasing blood pressure, whether treated or not [5, 13]. As discussed above, patients diagnosed with resistant hypertension consistently have an excess of cardiovascular risk factors as well as higher documented cardiovascular events. It is perhaps therefore not surprising that in observational studies, patients with resistant hypertension consistently have worse cardiovascular outcomes and increased mortality compared with other hypertensive patients [29, 30]. A large observational study showed that patients with resistant hypertension are 50% more likely to have an adverse cardiovascular outcome than other hypertensive patients [30]. Intriguingly, this increased risk appeared to be largely explained by the development of chronic kidney disease. What is perhaps less clear is whether having resistant hypertension in itself leads to an increase in cardiovascular risk factors, and consequent higher mortality, or whether an increased prevalence of cardiovascular risk factors leads to a higher prevalence of resistant hypertension. Conceivably these relationships are likely to be very complex and probably bidirectional.

Conclusions

Interest in resistant hypertension has been growing over the last few years with the increasing recognition of its prevalence and associated adverse outcomes. The definitions of resistant hypertension used up until now were derived mainly in response to the clinical need to identify these patients for further investigation, evaluation, and treatment. However, the patients so identified are likely to represent a large, amorphous group. As our understanding of this condition increases, it is likely that subgroups of patients with different characteristics and etiologies are identified. These will require different definitions and probably alternative investigational pathways and treatment strategies. To achieve this, there clearly is a need for further research into resistant hypertension. However, currently used definitions leave some subjectivity in the classification of patients with resistant hypertension. As a consequence, researchers will need to either more clearly define the condition, a move that might make it difficult to use in day-to-day clinical practice, or develop methodologies that create comparable baseline populations. These will need to, at the very least, include pathways or algorithms designed to identify patients with pseudo-resistance and secondary causes of hypertension to standardize the research population.

The adverse impact of resistant hypertension on patients and health economies is likely to increase with time. Its association with factors such as obesity, diabetes mellitus, and advancing age means that even if the prevalence of hypertension remains unchanged, the prevalence of resistant hypertension will continue to increase further. This is likely to occur in parallel, or even synergistically, with the predicted increases in chronic kidney disease worldwide.

References

1. Pickering GW. The natural history of hypertension. Br Med Bull. 1952;8(4):305–9.
2. Kearney PM, Whelton M, Reynolds K, Muntner P, Whelton PK, He J. Global burden of hypertension: analysis of worldwide data. Lancet. 2005;365(9455):217–23.
3. Bromfield S, Muntner P. High blood pressure: the leading global burden of disease risk factor and the need for worldwide prevention programs. Curr Hypertens Rep. 2013;15(3):134–6.
4. Collins R, Peto R, MacMahon S, Hebert P, Fiebach NH, Eberlein KA, et al. Blood pressure, stroke, and coronary heart disease. Part 2, short-term reductions in blood pressure: overview of randomised drug trials in their epidemiological context. Lancet. 1990;335(8693):827–38.
5. Lewington S, Clarke R, Qizilbash N, Peto R, Collins R. Age-specific relevance of usual blood pressure to vascular mortality: a meta-analysis of individual data for one million adults in 61 prospective studies. Lancet. 2002;360(9349):1903–13.
6. Chobanian AV, Bakris GL, Black HR, Cushman WC, Green LA, Izzo JL Jr, et al. Seventh report of the Joint National Committee on prevention, detection, evaluation, and treatment of high blood pressure. Hypertension. 2003;42(6):1206–52.
7. MacMahon S, Peto R, Cutler J, Collins R, Sorlie P, Neaton J, et al. Blood pressure, stroke, and coronary heart disease. Part 1, prolonged differences in blood pressure: prospective observational studies corrected for the regression dilution bias. Lancet. 1990;335(8692):765–74.

8. Clinical management of primary hypertension in adults (NICE guideline 127). National Institute for Health and Clinical Excellence. 2011.
9. Weber MA, Schiffrin EL, White WB, Mann S, Lindholm LH, Kenerson JG, et al. Clinical practice guidelines for the management of hypertension in the community: a statement by the American Society of Hypertension and the International Society of Hypertension. J Clin Hypertens (Greenwich). 2014;16(1):14–26.
10. James PA, Oparil S, Carter BL, Cushman WC, Dennison-Himmelfarb C, Handler J, et al. 2014 evidence-based guideline for the management of high blood pressure in adults: report from the panel members appointed to the Eighth Joint National Committee (JNC 8). JAMA. 2014;311(5):507–20.
11. Board JBS. Joint British Societies' consensus recommendations for the prevention of cardio-vascular disease (JBS3). Heart. 2014;100(Suppl 2):ii1–ii67.
12. Mancia G, Fagard R, Narkiewicz K, Redon J, Zanchetti A, Bohm M, et al. 2013 ESH/ESC guidelines for the management of arterial hypertension: the task force for the management of arterial hypertension of the European Society of Hypertension (ESH) and of the European Society of Cardiology (ESC). J Hypertens. 2013;31(7):1281–357.
13. Kidney Disease: Improving Global Outcomes (KDIGO) Blood Pressure Work Group. KDIGO clinical practice guideline for the management of blood pressure in chronic kidney disease. Kidney Int Suppl. 2012;2(5):337–414.
14. Muxfeldt ES, de Souza F, Margallo VS, Salles GF. Cardiovascular and renal complications in patients with resistant hypertension. Curr Hypertens Rep. 2014;16(9):471.
15. de la Sierra A, Segura J, Banegas JR, Gorostidi M, de la Cruz JJ, Armario P, et al. Clinical features of 8295 patients with resistant hypertension classified on the basis of ambulatory blood pressure monitoring. Hypertension. 2011;57(5):898–902.
16. Persell SD. Prevalence of resistant hypertension in the United States, 2003-2008. Hypertension. 2011;57(6):1076–80.
17. de la Sierra A, Banegas JR, Oliveras A, Gorostidi M, Segura J, de la Cruz JJ, et al. Clinical differences between resistant hypertensives and patients treated and controlled with three or less drugs. J Hypertens. 2012;30(6):1211–6.
18. Acelajado MC, Pisoni R, Dudenbostel T, Dell'Italia LJ, Cartmill F, Zhang B, et al. Refractory hypertension: definition, prevalence, and patient characteristics. J Clin Hypertens (Greenwich). 2012;14(1):7–12.
19. Acharya T, Tringali S, Singh M, Huang J. Resistant hypertension and associated comorbidities in a veterans affairs population. J Clin Hypertens (Greenwich). 2014;16(10):741–5.
20. Vandyne JR. Iproniazid in the treatment of resistant hypertension – a preliminary report on 20 intractable cases. J Am Geriatr Soc. 1960;8(6):454–62.
21. Lee RE, Seligmann AW, Clark MA, Borhani NO, Queenan JT, O'Brien ME. Therapeutically refractory hypertension: causative factors, and medical management with chlorothiazide and other agents. Ann Intern Med. 1958;49(5):1129–37.
22. Krogsgaard AR. Hypotensive effect of reserpine compared with phenobarbital and placebo. Acta Med Scand. 1957;157:379–85.
23. Shapiro AP, Teng HC. Technic of controlled drug assay illustrated by a comparative study of Rauwolfia serpentina, phenobarbital and placebo in the hypertensive patient. N Engl J Med. 1957;256(21):970–5.
24. Khan MA. Effect of hydralazine in hypertension. Br Med J. 1953;1(4800):27–9.
25. Maxwell RD, Howie TJ. Ecolid: a new hypotensive agent. Br Med J. 1955;2(4949):1189–90.
26. Gifford RW Jr, Tarazi RC. Resistant hypertension: diagnosis and management. Ann Intern Med. 1978;88(5):661–5.
27. Calhoun DA, Jones D, Textor S, Goff DC, Murphy TP, Toto RD, et al. Resistant hypertension: diagnosis, evaluation, and treatment: a scientific statement from the American Heart Association Professional Education Committee of the Council for high blood pressure research. Circulation. 2008;117(25):e510–26.

28. Boswell L, Pascual J, Oliveras A. Resistant hypertension: do all definitions describe the same patients? J Hum Hypertens. 2015;29(9):530–4.
29. Myat A, Redwood SR, Qureshi AC, Spertus JA, Williams B. Resistant hypertension. BMJ. 2012;345:e7473.
30. Sarafidis PA, Georgianos P, Bakris GL. Resistant hypertension – its identification and epidemiology. Nat Rev Nephrol. 2013;9(1):51–8.
31. Falaschetti E, Chaudhury M, Mindell J, Poulter N. Continued improvement in hypertension management in England: results from the Health Survey for England 2006. Hypertension. 2009;53(3):480–6.
32. Giannattasio C, Cairo M, Cesana F, Alloni M, Sormani P, Colombo G, et al. Blood pressure control in Italian essential hypertensives treated by general practitioners. Am J Hypertens. 2012;25(11):1182–7.
33. Dahlof B, Devereux RB, Kjeldsen SE, Julius S, Beevers G, de Faire U, et al. Cardiovascular morbidity and mortality in the losartan intervention for endpoint reduction in hypertension study (LIFE): a randomised trial against atenolol. Lancet. 2002;359(9311):995–1003.
34. Pepine CJ, Handberg EM, Cooper-DeHoff RM, Marks RG, Kowey P, Messerli FH, et al. A calcium antagonist vs a non-calcium antagonist hypertension treatment strategy for patients with coronary artery disease. The International Verapamil-Trandolapril Study (INVEST): a randomized controlled trial. JAMA. 2003;290(21):2805–16.
35. Cushman WC, Ford CE, Cutler JA, Margolis KL, Davis BR, Grimm RH, et al. Success and predictors of blood pressure control in diverse north American settings: the antihypertensive and lipid-lowering treatment to prevent heart attack trial (ALLHAT). J Clin Hypertens (Greenwich). 2002;4(6):393–404.
36. Jamerson K, Weber MA, Bakris GL, Dahlof B, Pitt B, Shi V, et al. Benazepril plus amlodipine or hydrochlorothiazide for hypertension in high-risk patients. N Engl J Med. 2008;359(23):2417–28.
37. Gupta AK, Nasothimiou EG, Chang CL, Sever PS, Dahlof B, Poulter NR, et al. Baseline predictors of resistant hypertension in the Anglo-Scandinavian Cardiac Outcome Trial (ASCOT): a risk score to identify those at high-risk. J Hypertens. 2011;29(10):2004–13.
38. Black HR, Elliott WJ, Grandits G, Grambsch P, Lucente T, White WB, et al. Principal results of the Controlled Onset Verapamil Investigation of Cardiovascular End Points (CONVINCE) trial. JAMA. 2003;289(16):2073–82.
39. Julius S, Kjeldsen SE, Brunner H, Hansson L, Platt F, Ekman S, et al. VALUE trial: long-term blood pressure trends in 13,449 patients with hypertension and high cardiovascular risk. Am J Hypertens. 2003;16(7):544–8.
40. McAdam-Marx C, Ye X, Sung JC, Brixner DI, Kahler KH. Results of a retrospective, observational pilot study using electronic medical records to assess the prevalence and characteristics of patients with resistant hypertension in an ambulatory care setting. Clin Ther. 2009;31(5):1116–23.
41. Daugherty SL, Powers JD, Magid DJ, Tavel HM, Masoudi FA, Margolis KL, et al. Incidence and prognosis of resistant hypertension in hypertensive patients. Circulation. 2012;125(13):1635–42.
42. Egan BM, Zhao Y, Li J, Brzezinski WA, Todoran TM, Brook RD, et al. Prevalence of optimal treatment regimens in patients with apparent treatment-resistant hypertension based on office blood pressure in a community-based practice network. Hypertension. 2013;62(4):691–7.
43. Sim JJ, Bhandari SK, Shi J, Liu IL, Calhoun DA, McGlynn EA, et al. Characteristics of resistant hypertension in a large, ethnically diverse hypertension population of an integrated health system. Mayo Clin Proc. 2013;88(10):1099–107.
44. Judd E, Calhoun DA. Apparent and true resistant hypertension: definition, prevalence and outcomes. J Hum Hypertens. 2014;28(8):463–8.
45. Pimenta E, Calhoun DA. Resistant hypertension: incidence, prevalence, and prognosis. Circulation. 2012;125(13):1594–6.

46. Sarafidis PA. Epidemiology of resistant hypertension. J Clin Hypertens (Greenwich). 2011; 13(7):523–8.
47. Massierer D, Oliveira AC, Steinhorst AM, Gus M, Ascoli AM, Goncalves SC, et al. Prevalence of resistant hypertension in non-elderly adults: prospective study in a clinical setting. Arq Bras Cardiol. 2012;99(1):630–5.
48. Hayek SS, Abdou MH, Demoss BD, Legaspi JM, Veledar E, Deka A, et al. Prevalence of resistant hypertension and eligibility for catheter-based renal denervation in hypertensive out-patients. Am J Hypertens. 2013;26(12):1452–8.
49. Schlaich MP, Schmieder RE, Bakris G, Blankestijn PJ, Bohm M, Campese VM, et al. International expert consensus statement: percutaneous transluminal renal denervation for the treatment of resistant hypertension. J Am Coll Cardiol. 2013;62(22):2031–45.
50. Rocha-Singh KJ, Katholi RE. Renal sympathetic denervation for treatment-resistant hyperten-sion...in moderation. J Am Coll Cardiol. 2013;62(20):1887–9.
51. Kandzari DE, Sobotka PA. Ready for a marathon, not a sprint: renal denervation therapy for treatment-resistant hypertension. J Am Coll Cardiol. 2013;62(22):2131–3.
52. Krum H, Schlaich M, Whitbourn R, Sobotka PA, Sadowski J, Bartus K, et al. Catheter-based renal sympathetic denervation for resistant hypertension: a multicentre safety and proof-of-principle cohort study. Lancet. 2009;373(9671):1275–81.
53. Symplicity HTNI, Esler MD, Krum H, Sobotka PA, Schlaich MP, Schmieder RE, et al. Renal sympathetic denervation in patients with treatment-resistant hypertension (The Symplicity HTN-2 Trial): a randomised controlled trial. Lancet. 2010;376(9756):1903–9.
54. Kandzari DE, Bhatt DL, Sobotka PA, O'Neill WW, Esler M, Flack JM, et al. Catheter-based renal denervation for resistant hypertension: rationale and design of the SYMPLICITY HTN-3 trial. Clin Cardiol. 2012;35(9):528–35.
55. Calhoun DA, Booth JN 3rd, Oparil S, Irvin MR, Shimbo D, Lackland DT, et al. Refractory hypertension: determination of prevalence, risk factors, and comorbidities in a large, population-based cohort. Hypertension. 2014;63(3):451–8.
56. Cuspidi C, Macca G, Sampieri L, Michev I, Salerno M, Fusi V, et al. High prevalence of cardiac and extracardiac target organ damage in refractory hypertension. J Hypertens. 2001; 19(11):2063–70.

Chapter 2
Definition and Characteristics of Hypertension Associated with Chronic Kidney Disease: Epidemiological Data

Beata Franczyk, Anna Gluba-Brzózka, Maciej Banach, and Jacek Rysz

Introduction

The prevalence of hypertension appears to be around 30–45% of the general population and it is increasing with age [1]. The kidneys play such a vital role in long-term blood pressure [2]. Chronic kidney disease (CKD) is one of the most common causes of secondary hypertension. The prevalence of hypertension is higher among patients with CKD than in general population, and its frequency increases progressively with the severity of CKD [2–4]. According to US Renal Data System Annual Data Report of 2010, hypertension occurs in 23.3% of individuals without CKD, while in 35.8% of patients with CKD stage 1, in 48.1% with stage 2, in 59.9% with stage 3, and in 84.1% with CKD stages 4–5 [5]. However, the frequency of hypertension may vary in different CKD causes including renal artery stenosis (93%), diabetic nephropathy (87%), and polycystic kidney disease (74%) [2, 6]. The pathogenesis of hypertension associated with chronic kidney disease (CKD) is complex and multifactorial [7, 8]. Numerous studies confirmed the association between renal defects and essential hypertension in humans. As early as in 1983, Curtis et al. [9] demonstrated a remission of essential hypertension after renal transplantation from

B. Franczyk
Department of Nephrology, Hypertension and Family Medicine, Medical University of Lodz, Lodz, Poland

A. Gluba-Brzózka (✉)
Department of Nephrology, Hypertension and Family Medicine, WAM Teaching Hospital, Lodz, Poland
e-mail: aniagluba@yahoo.pl

M. Banach
Department of Hypertension, Medical University of Lodz, Lodz, Poland

J. Rysz
Department of Nephrology, Hypertension and Family Medicine, Medical University of Lodz, Lodz, Poland

© Springer International Publishing AG 2017
A. Covic et al. (eds.), *Resistant Hypertension in Chronic Kidney Disease*,
DOI 10.1007/978-3-319-56827-0_2

normotensive donors. Moreover, Widgren et al. [10] study revealed that salt loading in normotensive individuals with family history of hypertension is associated with lower natriuresis and higher blood pressure than in those with no family history. Additionally, the autopsy of hypertensive victims of fatal accidents demonstrated decreased amount of nephrons [11]. It is estimated that half of patients with chronic kidney disease die of cardiovascular causes before they reach end-stage renal disease.

The pathogenesis of hypertension in chronic kidney disease is multifactorial and can be associated with diabetic nephropathy, glomerulonephritis, nephropathy in the course of connective tissue disorders, vasculitis, pyelonephritis, and obstructive, analgesic, and reflux nephropathy as well as congenital diseases such as polycystic kidney [12]. It is estimated that only 5–10% of all cases of hypertension is associated with secondary causes. Renal parenchymal hypertension is present in 5–6% of cases of secondary hypertension, while renovascular hypertension is diagnosed in 1% of cases. Simple screening for secondary forms of hypertension should comprise the analysis of clinical history (renal disease, urinary tract infection, hematuria, analgesic abuse) and family history of renal disease, physical examination, and routine laboratory tests [13]. The presence of secondary hypertension is suggested by sudden onset of hypertension, severe increase in blood pressure, and problems to lower blood pressure with the use of drug therapy [13]. It has been believed that hypertension in CKD is associated with excessive intravascular volume or excessive activation of the renin–angiotensin system due to sodium/volume imbalance (renin-dependent hypertension) [14–16]. Recently, the role of the following factors has been confirmed: enhanced activity of sympathetic nervous system sodium and potassium retention, disorders of divalent ion metabolism, disturbances in parathyroid hormone (PTH) secretion, decreased amount of endothelium-related dilating factors accompanied by the increase in vasoconstrictive factors (endothelin), baroreceptors dysfunction, oxidative stress, structural changes of the arteries, renal ischemia, and sleep apnea in the development of hypertension in chronic kidney disease [12, 14]. Moreover, it has been suggested that also iatrogenic factors, such as erythropoietin, cyclosporine, steroids, divalent ions, and vitamin D, sympathomimetic agents, and nonsteroidal anti-inflammatory drugs (NSAIDs) may influence the onset and progression of hypertension in CKD [14].

Diagnosis of Hypertension and Chronic Kidney Disease

According to the European Society of Hypertension (ESH) and of the European Society of Cardiology (ESC), the distinction between normotension and hypertension on the basis of cutoff BP values is difficult due to the continuous association between BP and CV and renal events [1]. However, in practice the cutoff BP values are used to simplify the diagnostic approach and to facilitate the decision about treatment. The recommended definition of hypertension remained the same as 2003 and 2007 ESH/ESC guidelines. According to them hypertension is diagnosed when

Table 2.1 Stages of kidney disease

Stage	GFR [mL/min/1.73 m^2]	Description
1	> 90	Normal kidney function; urine tests results, structural abnormalities, or genetic conditioning suggest kidney disease
2	60–89	Mild reduction in kidney function; urine tests results, structural abnormalities, or genetic conditioning suggest kidney disease
3A 3B	45–59 30–44	Moderate reduction in kidney function
4	15–29	Severe reduction in kidney function
5	<15 or on dialysis	Very severe or end-stage renal disease (ESRD)

Adapted from [18]

systolic blood pressure (SBP) values ≥140 mmHg and/or diastolic blood pressure (DPD) values ≥90 mmHg. The same classification is used in young, middle-aged, and elderly subjects [1]. Moreover, according to the Guidelines of Polish Society of Hypertension (2015), the diagnosis of hypertension in patients with BP values below 160/100 mmHg should be confirmed by ambulatory blood pressure monitoring (ABPM) or by home BP measurements. In the case of patients with BP values ≥180/≥ 110 mmHg, the diagnosis of hypertension can be made during the first visit after the exclusion of influence of factors leading to acute BP elevation, such as anxiety, pain, or alcohol intake [17]. 2013 ESH/ESC guidelines for the management of arterial hypertension comprises also the grading of hypertension. High normal blood pressure is diagnosed in patients with a systolic BP of 130–139 mmHg and/or a diastolic BP of 85–89 mmHg, grade 1 hypertension - in persons with a BP of 140–159 and/or 90–99 mmHg, grade 2 hypertension - in those with BP 160–179 and/or 100–109 mmHg, grade 3 hypertension - in persons with BP ≥180 and/or ≥110 mmHg, and isolated systolic hypertension - in individuals with BP ≥140 and <90 mmHg.

Chronic kidney disease is classified using estimated glomerular filtration rate (eGFR) calculated by abbreviated "modification of diet in renal disease" (MDRD) formula, Cockcroft–Gault formula, or Chronic Kidney Disease Epidemiology Collaboration (CKD-EPI) formula [1]. The stages of renal disease are presented in Table 2.1.

Hypertension in Chronic Kidney Disease

Hypertension in chronic kidney disease is primarily associated with sodium retention. Hypervolemia associated with the disturbances with sodium and water excretion with urine results in increase in blood pressure in order to enhance excretion to maintain isovolemia. Kidney ischemia related to renal fibrosis and scarring occurring in CKD patients results in the increase in renin–angiotensin–aldosterone system activity and elevations in blood pressure. Also secondary hyperparathyroidism leading to the increase in intracellular calcium concentration is associated with vasoconstriction and hypertension [12, 19, 20].

Diabetic Nephropathy

Hypertension is common among patients with diabetes mellitus (DM1 and DM2), and its prevalence in these groups of patients is twice as high as in general population. According to studies, high blood pressure correlates with the presence of diabetic nephropathy [12]. Diabetic nephropathy, being one of the chronic complications of diabetes of microangiopathic nature, is defined as a condition characterized by the presence of proteinuria, elevated arterial BP, and diminished GFR. Hypertension is present in 15–25% of patients with microalbuminuria and even in 75–85% with diabetic nephropathy, but the prevalence of HA in diabetes varies across different ethnic, racial, and social groups. Results of other studies demonstrated that the incidence of hypertension in diabetic nephropathy increased with worsening kidney function, reaching 90% in ESRD patients [21].

In patients with diabetic nephropathy, hypertension is defined as systolic blood pressure ≥130 mmHg or a diastolic blood pressure ≥80 mmHg [21]. Diabetic nephropathy, characterized by albuminuria, glomerulosclerosis, and decline in glomerular filtration rate (GFR), is the most common cause of hypertension in patients with type 1 diabetes. According to Lago et al. [22], in patients with type 2 diabetes, hypertension occurs mainly without abnormal renal function and is frequently associated with central obesity. In the early stages of diabetic nephropathy, the increase of mesangium and the thickening of the glomerular basement membrane occur due to the accumulation of extracellular matrix, which in consequence leads to the hypertrophy and glomerulosclerosis [23]. Diabetic nephropathy is diagnosed on the basis of the presence of albuminuria >300 mg/d, coexistence of diabetic retinopathy, and lack of clinical or laboratory evidence of renal and urinary tract disease [23]. The activation of local (renal) RAAS, hyperinsulinemia, overhydration, arterial stiffness as well as obesity, endothelium dysfunction, autonomic nervous system disturbances, oxidative stress, and abnormal NO metabolism are the risk factors for hypertension in diabetic nephropathy. Volume expansion due to increased renal sodium reabsorption and peripheral vasoconstriction are the main reasons for hypertension in diabetes [21]. The activation of RAAS, elevated concentration of endothelin-1, decreased level of nitric oxide, and increased oxidative stress result in the development of hypertension and accelerate kidney disease due to the stimulation of vasoconstriction in vascular smooth muscle cells (VSMC); induction of aldosterone released from the adrenal cortex; enhancement of production of superoxide by activation of NADPH oxidase in the systemic vasculature, heart, and kidney; and augmented sodium reabsorption at the renal proximal tubule

[21]. Increased oxidative stress associated with hyperglycemia and the presence of mediators of both RAAS and endothelial dysfunction contributes to hypertension-enhanced vasoconstriction. As it was mentioned above, also increased activity of sympathetic nervous system (SNS) plays an important role in the pathomechanism of hypertension in patients with diabetic nephropathy. Results of studies suggest that insulin resistance may pose a possible link between SNS activation and hypertension. In diabetic nephropathy, autoregulatory functions of the afferent arteriole responsible for maintaining constant glomerular pressures despite variations in systemic blood pressure are impaired, and thus elevated systemic blood pressure is directly transmitted to the renal microvasculature and glomeruli leading to glomerular hypertension and activation of local mediators that induce inflammation, fibrosis, and further injury [21].

Glomerulonephritis and Vasculitis

Systemic vasculitis is characterized by the presence of inflammatory infiltrates and necrosis within arterial walls. Changes in large and medium renal vessels result in organ ischemia and the development of hypertension [23]. Patients with glomerulonephritis tend to accumulate fluids due to enhanced sodium retention which in consequence results in volume overload and blood pressure increase. In these patients also the suppression of renin–angiotensin system and the increase in atrial natriuretic peptide (ANP) release are observed. The prevalence of hypertension in glomerulonephritis is various and depends on the type of disease [24]. According to studies, hypertension occurs most frequently in patients with membranoproliferative GN (57%), rapidly progressive GN (52%), and endocapillary (acute) GN of poststreptococcal origin (51%), while less frequently in patients with focal sclerosis GN (34%), mesangioproliferative GN (34%), and perimembranous GN (30%). Symptoms of hypertension are aggravated in advanced glomerulonephritis; however, elevated blood pressure is also seen in patients with creatinine concentration within normal range [12]. Mechanisms of hypertension development in acute glomerulonephritis comprise sodium and water retention due to glomerular lesions [24] as well as renin–angiotensin–aldosterone system activation resulting from suppression inadequate to the degree of sodium and water retention. According to studies, in chronic GN with minimal glomerular alterations, the development of hypertension may be preceded by vascular changes [24]. It seems interesting that elevated blood pressure is observed even in patients with confirmed complete recovery from this disease [24].

Clinical symptoms of immunologically caused vasculitis, depending on its severity and type of organ involved, comprise arterial hypertension, hemoptysis, arthralgia, muscle pain, palpable purpura, hematuria, proteinuria, and renal failure [25]. In patients with vasculitis, hypertension is mainly associated with renal ischemia accompanied by the activation of renin–angiotensin–aldosterone system.

Renovascular Hypertension

Ischemia of renal parenchyma associated with renal artery stenosis is the cause of renovascular hypertension. The stenosis of renal artery due to atherosclerosis (75%; mainly elderly population) or fibromuscular dysplasia (25%; most common in young adults) is the cause of 95% of renovascular hypertension. It is believed that atherosclerotic renovascular disease is associated with hastened and more severe target organ injury than essential hypertension [7]. According to Medicare studies in patients with newly identified renovascular disease, the rate of cardiovascular event (including coronary events, myocardial infarction, and heart failure) development is higher than in those without renovascular disease [7].

Characteristic features of renovascular hypertension comprise sudden onset of disease, lack of hypertension risk factors and obesity, lack of family history, high values of blood pressure (>160/100 mmHg) resistant to the treatment with three hypotensive drugs including diuretic, sudden raise in blood pressure in people with well-controlled hypertension, malicious course of disease with signs of organ damage, sudden increase in creatinine level (>30% above the baseline level) following the ACE or sartan treatment, recurrent episodes of pulmonary edema or heart failure with unknown etiology, and the presence of asymmetric or cirrhotic kidney as well as general atherosclerosis. The symptoms of renal artery stenosis include the presence of abdominal bruit with lateralization, hypokalemia, polyglobulia, and progressive decline in renal function [13]. Occlusion in renal artery reducing renal perfusion pressure intensifies sodium retention by slowing blood flow and filtration and increasing peritubular forces resulting in solute reabsorption. Sodium retention is further enhanced by the activation of the renin–angiotensin–aldosterone system. Angiotensin II directly increases sodium transport, while aldosterone stimulates distal sodium retention through the activation of sodium–potassium ATPase resulting in the diminished sodium excretion in the post-stenotic kidney and in consequence to hypertension [7, 26]. Moreover, angiotensin II promotes the hypertrophy of both vascular smooth muscle cells and heart [23]. It also enhances oxidative stress further aggravating imbalance between vasoconstrictive and vasodilatory substances and endothelial dysfunction. Decrease in renal perfusion is also associated with overproduction of renin by juxtaglomerular apparatus, which in consequence leads to the constriction of afferent arteriole and increased sodium reabsorption. High concentration of renin in one kidney hampers its secretion by the second kidney [27].

Renovascular hypertension diagnosis is made on the basis of the demonstration of structural and functional occlusion of the renal vessels. Ultrasound determination of the longitudinal diameter of the kidney is used as a screening procedure. Color Doppler sonography with calculation of peak systolic velocity and resistance indices, MR angiography, CT angiography, or intra-arterial angiography is utilized for the visualization of renovascular lesions. The difference of over 1.5 cm in length between the two kidneys is usually the confirmation of renal artery stenosis. However, this abnormality is present in only 60–70% of such patients, and thus color Doppler sonography or spiral computed tomography with iodine-containing contrast media is used to detect stenoses [13, 28]. According to Vasbinder et al. [29], the analysis of renal vasculature with the use of breath-hold three-dimensional, gadolinium-enhanced magnetic resonance angiography with sensitivity of 95% will be the diagnostic tool of the future.

Polycystic Kidney Disease

Autosomal dominant polycystic kidney disease (ADPKD) is a systemic, hereditary kidney disease. Hypertension occurs early in the course of ADPKD (between the age of 30 and 34) and is associated with increased patient morbidity and mortality and the progression to ESRD [30]. Arterial hypertension is one of the main symptoms of polycystic kidney disease and is observed in 59–79% of patients with various stages of this disease. Results from large ADPKD registry demonstrated that in children with autosomal dominant polycystic kidney disease, blood pressure was higher by 4–6 mmHg in comparison to unaffected age- and gender-matched controls [30, 31]. Moreover, in ADPKD children with hypertension, greater kidney volume and increased number of cysts were observed in comparison to age-matched normotensive ADPKD children [30, 31]. In hypertensive adults with ADPKD, greater LVMI in comparison to matched essential hypertensive men was observed, and it has been found that both LVMI and left ventricular hypertrophy aggravate along with the progression of kidney disease toward renal failure [30]. Early diastolic dysfunction has been demonstrated in this group of patients [32]. Impaired endothelium-dependent relaxation in small resistance vessels was observed in young normotensive patients. Along with the progression of disease, intima–media thickness of carotid arteries increases, and fibromatous areas in carotid walls and important alterations in large arteries appear [32]. Moreover, in hypertensive ADPKD patients, sclerosis of renal arterioles and global glomerulosclerosis is observed. Analysis of renal specimens demonstrated advanced sclerosis of preglomerular vessels, interstitial fibrosis, and tubular atrophy even in patients with normal renal function or early renal failure [33]. The prevalence of target organ damage is also higher in hypertensive ADPKD than in other age-matched hypertensive patients [32]. Greater albuminuria in ADPKD is associated with higher mean blood pressure as well as severe renal cystic development. However, in ADPKD patients, glomerular filtration rate for a long time does not seem to be affected by the progression of renal structural abnormalities due to compensatory hyperfiltration [32]. Numerous studies demonstrated higher rate of increase in kidney volume, enhanced proteinuria, and decreased renal blood flow in hypertensive ADPKD patients with normal renal function in comparison to normotensive patients [30, 34, 35]. Reduced renal blood flow resulting from renal cysts enlargement and concomitant compression of renal vasculature leading to intra renal ischemia, reduction of renal vasculature, and intrarenal activation of the renin–angiotensin–aldosterone system (RAAS) is a characteristic feature of hypertension in ADPKD [30]. It has been suggested that the activation of renin–angiotensin–aldosterone system plays a role in the association between hypertension and increased kidney volume. This hypothesis was confirmed by the observation of the increase in both renin activity and plasma levels of aldosterone in ADPKD patients in comparison to age-, sex-, and kidney function-matched patients with essential hypertensive [32]. Local activation of RAAS leading to hyperplasia of the juxtaglomerular apparatus has also been demonstrated. Results of studies suggest that RAAS inhibition may prove beneficial in the control of blood pressure level, simultaneously limiting renal cyst growth and renal enlargement as well as slowing down the progression to ESRD [32]. Increased concentration of erythropoietin (due to intrarenal ischemia/hypoxia) is another factor involved in the development of hypertension in ADPKD. Moreover, intrarenal ischemia influences renal tubular sodium handling and enhances sympathetic nervous system activity. Hypertension in ADPDK patients may be also associated with the imbalance between vasoconstrictor and vasodilatation factors. High levels of circulating vasopressin and endothelin-1 and diminished activity of nitric oxide synthase are observed in this group of patients [32].

Analgesic Nephropathy

The abuse of painkillers may result in the damage of parenchyma and the development of interstitial nephritis. According to the National Kidney Foundation, analgesic nephropathy (AN) is defined as "a disease resulting from the habitual consumption over several years of a mixture containing at least two anti-pyretic analgesics and usually codeine or caffeine" [36, 37]. Among the main symptoms of analgesic nephropathy, there are arterial hypertension and renal failure. Progressive kidney failure is related to kidney papillary necrosis and chronic interstitial nephritis. Earliest changes in kidneys comprise sclerosis of vasa recta capillaries and patchy tubular necrosis, and they are followed by papillary necrosis and secondary focal segmental glomerulosclerosis, cortical scarring, and interstitial fibrosis [37]. The pathogenesis of hypertension in AN has not been fully elucidated. It seems that the decreased production of vasodilatory substances within renal papilla and sodium and water retention due to the hampering of vasodilatory prostaglandins and bradykinins secretion may play an important role in the development of hypertension [23].

Hypertension in End-Stage Renal Disease Patients

Hypertension is diagnosed in 50–90% of hemodialysis patients and only in 30% of those on peritoneal dialysis. There are no recommendations concerning the optimal blood pressure values for dialysis patients. Among hypertension risk factors in dialysis patients, there are decreased excretion of sodium and water, increased concentration of endothelin, vessel calcification, and overhydration [12]. During hemodialysis, hypertension occurs less frequently due to the better control of volemia than in patients with end-stage renal disease. Among the risks of hypertension in hemodialysis patients, there are overhydration, decreased secretion of sodium and water, increased level of vasoconstrictive endothelin-1, and vessel calcification [38, 39]. Overhydration present in hemodialysis patients negatively influences cardiac output and peripheral resistance. It was shown that lowering of sodium concentration in dialysate, removal of excess water, and the achievement of dry weight can improve interdialytic BP, reduce pulse pressure, and limit hospitalizations. According to the National Kidney Foundation/Disease Outcomes Quality Initiative (NKF/DOQI), optimal blood pressure for dialysis patient should be 135/90 mmHg during day and 120/80 mmHg at night [40].

The use of erythropoietin in end-stage renal disease patients is also associated with the possibility of hypertension development. The exact mechanism of blood pressure increase in response to erythropoietin in patients with chronic uremia is complex and not fully explained. According to studies, increase in systolic and diastolic BP was an average approximately 5–8 mmHg in SBP and 4–6 mmHg in DBP. The incidence of hypertension is Epo dose-dependent. It was demonstrated that the administration of 40, 80, and 120 U/kg of Epo, three times a week for 49 weeks, was associated with hypertension in 28%, 32%, and 56% of treated subjects, respectively [41]. Erythropoietin may increase blood pressure due to its direct vasoconstrictive and mitogenic effects and enhancement of blood viscosity [23]. Clinical studies results suggest that Epo-induced hypertension may be associated with its effect on red blood cell mass and viscosity. Moreover, erythropoietin stimulates both the release of endothelin-1 and enhanced mitogenic response in endothelial cells. Additionally, Epo inhibits extrarenal eNOS/NO production and impairs both NO action and vasodilatory response to endothelial NO. Erythropoietin also enhances adrenergic sensitivity. It has been demonstrated that in hemodialysis patients, angiotensin II infusion during Epo treatment was associated with higher elevation of blood pressure in comparison to pre-Epo condition [41].

Acknowledgments Three authors (AG-B, JR, MB) are (partially) supported by the Healthy Ageing Research Centre project (REGPOT-2012-2013-1, 7FP).

References

1. 2013 ESH/ESC Guidelines for the management of arterial hypertension. The task force for the management of arterial hypertension of the European Society of Hypertension (ESH) and of the European Society of Cardiology (ESC). Eur Heart J. 2013;34:2159–219.
2. Tedla FM, Brar A, Browne R, Brown C. Hypertension in chronic kidney disease: navigating the evidence. Int J Hypertens. 2011;2011:132405.
3. Banach M, Aronow WS, Serban C, Sahabkar A, Rysz J, Voroneanu L, Covic A. Lipids, blood pressure and kidney update 2014. Pharmacol Res. 2015;95-96:111–25.

4. Franczyk-Skóra B, Gluba A, Olszewski R, Banach M, Rysz J. Heart function disturbances in chronic kidney disease: echocardiographic indices. Arch Med Sci. 2014 Dec 22;10(6):1109–16.
5. U S Renal Data System. USRDS 2010 annual data report: Atlas of chronic kidney disease and end-stage renal disease in the United States. Bethesda: National Institutes of Health, National Institute of Diabetes and Digestive and Kidney Diseases. 2010.
6. Ridao N, Luño J, García De Vinuesa S, Gómez F, Tejedor A, Valderrábano F. Prevalence of hypertension in renal disease. Nephrol Dial Transplant. 2001;16(1):70–3.
7. Textor SC. Current approaches to renovascular hypertension. Med Clin North Am. 2009;93(3):717.
8. Banach M, Serban C, Aronow WS, Rysz J, Dragan S, Lerma EV, Apetrii M, Covic A. Lipid, blood pressure and kidney update 2013. Int Urol Nephrol. 2014 May;46(5):947–61.
9. Curtis JJ, Luke RG, Dustan HP. Remission of essential hypertension after renal transplantation. N Engl J Med. 1983;309(17):1009–15.
10. Widgren BR, Herlitz H, Hedner T, et al. Blunted renal sodium excretion during acute saline loading in normotensive men with positive family histories of hypertension. Am J Hypertens. 1991;4(7):570–8.
11. Keller G, Zimmer G, Mall G, Ritz E, Amann K. Nephron number in patients with primary hypertension. N Engl J Med. 2003;348(2):101–8.
12. Malyszko J. Chapter: hypertension and the kidneys. In: Myśliwiec M, editor. Great internal medicine. Nephrology, vol. 1. Warszawa, Poland: Medical Tribune; 2015.
13. Guidelines Committee. 2003 European Society of Hypertension–European Society of Cardiology guidelines for the management of arterial hypertension. J Hypertens. 2003;21:1011–53.
14. Campese VM, Mitra N, Sandee D. Hypertension in renal parenchymal disease: why is it so resistant to treatment? Kidney Int. 2006;69:967–73.
15. Malyszko J, Malyszko JS, Rysz J, Mysliwiec M, Tesar V, Levin-Iaina N, Banach M. Renalase, hypertension, and kidney—the discussion continues. Angiology. 2013;64(3):181–7.
16. Gluba A, Mikhailidis DP, Lip GY, Hannam S, Rysz J, Banach M. Metabolic syndrome and renal disease. Int J Cardiol. 2013;164(2):141–50.
17. Tykarski A, Narkiewicz K, Gaciong Z, Januszewicz A, Litwin M, Kostka-Jeziorny K. 2015 guidelines for the Management of Hypertension. Recommendations of the polish Society of Hypertension. Arterial Hypertens. 2015;19(2):53–83.
18. The Renal Association. CKD stages. Available at: http://www.renal.org/information-resources/the-uk-eckd-guide/ckd-stages#sthash.Ar1Hs9Rh.dpbs.
19. Malyszko J, Banach M. Pre-CKD- do we need another hero? Curr Vasc Pharmacol. 2014;12(4):642–8.
20. Banach M, Rysz J. Current problems in hypertension and nephrology. Expert Opin Pharmacother. 2010;11(16):2575–8.
21. Van Buren PN, Toto R. Hypertension in diabetic nephropathy: epidemiology, mechanisms, and management. Adv Chronic Kidney Dis. 2011;18(1):28–41.
22. Lago RM, Singh PP, Nesto RW. Diabetes and hypertension. Nat Clin Pract Endocrinol Metab. 2007;3:667.
23. Januszewicz A. Arterial hypertension. Outline of pathogenesis, diagnostics and treatment. Kraków: Practical Medicine; 2015.
24. Rosenthal J, editor. Arterial hypertension: pathogenesis, diagnosis, and therapy. Heidelberg: Springer Science & Business Media; 2012.
25. Eicken S, Gugger M, Marti HP. Glomerulonephritis and vasculitis as causes of arterial hypertension. Ther Umsch. 2012;69(5):283–94. [Article in German]
26. Olechnowicz-Tietz S, Gluba A, Paradowska A, Banach M, Rysz J. The risk of atherosclerosis in patients with chronic kidney disease. Int Urol Nephrol. 2013;45(6):1605–12.
27. Rutkowski B. Chronic kidney disease—diagnostics and treatment. Gdańsk: Via Medica; 2012.

28. Krumme W, Blum U, Schwertfeger E, Flügel P, Höllstin F, Schollmeyer P, Rump LC. Diagnosis of renovascular disease by intra- and extrarenal Doppler scanning. Kidney Int. 1996;50:1288–92.
29. Vasbinder BGC, Nelemans PJ, Kessels AGH, Kroon AA, De Leeuw PW, van Engelshoven JMA. Diagnostic tests for renal artery stenosis in patients suspected of having renovascular hypertension: a meta-analysis. Ann Intern Med. 2001;135:401–11.
30. Chapman AB, Stepniakowski K, Rahbari-Oskoui F. Hypertension in autosomal dominant polycystic kidney disease. Adv Chronic Kidney Dis. 2010;17(2):153–63.
31. Fick-Brosnahan GM, Tran ZV, Johnson AM, Strain JD, Gabow PA. Progression of autosomal-dominant polycystic kidney disease in children. Kidney Int. 2001;59:1654–62.
32. Sans-Atxer L, Torra R, Fernández-Llama P. Hypertension in autosomal-dominant polycystic kidney disease (ADPKD). Clin Kidney J. 2013;6:1–7.
33. Zeier M, Fehrenbach P, Geberth S, Mohring K, Waldherr R, Ritz E. Renal histology in polycystic kidney disease with incipient and advanced renal failure. Kidney Int. 1992;42:1259–65.
34. Fick-Brosnahan GM, Belz MM, McFann KK, Johnson AM, Schrier RW. Relationship between renal volume growth and renal function in autosomal dominant polycystic kidney disease: a longitudinal study. Am J Kidney Dis. 2002;39:1127–34.
35. Chapman AB, Johnson AM, Gabow PA, Schrier RW. Overt proteinuria and microalbuminuria in autosomal dominant polycystic kidney disease. J Am Soc Nephrol. 1994;5:1349–54.
36. Henrich WL, Agodoa LE, Barrett B, et al. Analgesics and the kidney: summary and recommendations to the Scientific Advisory Board of the National Kidney Foundation from an Ad Hoc Committee of the National Kidney Foundation. Am J Kidney Dis. 1996;27:162–5.
37. Vadivel N, Trikudanathan S, Singh AK. Analgesic nephropathy. Kidney Int. 2007;72:517–20.
38. Gluba-Brzózka A, Michalska-Kasiczak M, Franczyk-Skóra B, Nocuń M, Banach M, Rysz J. Markers of increased cardiovascular risk in patients with chronic kidney disease. Lipids Health Dis. 2014;13:135.
39. Franczyk-Skóra B, Gluba A, Banach M, Rysz J. Treatment of non-ST-elevation myocardial infarction and ST-elevation myocardial infarction in patients with chronic kidney disease. Arch Med Sci. 2013;30(9):1019–27.
40. NKF/DOQI Workgroup. NKF/DOQI clinical practice guidelines for cardiovascular disease in dialysis patients. Am J Kidney. 2005;45(suppl. 3):S1–53.
41. Krapf R, Hulter HN. Arterial hypertension induced by erythropoietin and erythropoiesis-stimulating agents (ESA). Clin J Am Soc Nephrol. 2009;4(2):470–80.

Chapter 3
Apparent Treatment-Resistant Hypertension and Chronic Kidney Disease: Another Cardiovascular–Renal Syndrome?

Ferruh Artunc

Introduction

Arterial hypertension is the most frequent comorbid condition of chronic kidney disease (CKD) affecting almost 80% of CKD patients [1]. The prevalence of hypertension is higher in patients with kidney damage and preserved glomerular filtration rate and increases further as the glomerular filtration rate declines. Among the participants of the Modification of Diet in Renal Disease Study, the prevalence of hypertension increased from 66 to 95 percent as the glomerular filtration rate fell from 83 to 12 mL/min per 1.73 m^2 [2]. Apparent treatment-resistant hypertension (aTRH) is defined as an office BP $\geq$ 140/90 mmHg despite triple antihypertensive treatment including a diuretic [3] and has become an increasingly recognized subform of arterial hypertension. Among patients with aTRH, true treatment resistance must be discriminated from pseudoresistance that results from inadequate medication, inadherence, white-coat hypertension, or errors/artifacts in correct BP measurement. The prevalence of aTRH was estimated to be 11.8% among hypertensive adults with an increase from 5.5% between 1994 and 1998 to 8.5% between 1998 and 2004 [4]. Ambulatory 24-h blood pressure measurement is an important investigation to identify patients with true treatment-resistant hypertension and to rule out

F. Artunc (✉)
Department of Internal Medicine, Division of Endocrinology, Diabetology, Vascular Disease, Nephrology and Clinical Chemistry, University Hospital Tübingen, Germany
e-mail: ferruh.artunc@med.uni-tuebingen.de

Institute of Diabetes Research and Metabolic Diseases (IDM) of the Helmholtz Center Munich at the University of Tübingen, Otfried-Mueller-Strasse 10, 72076 Tübingen, Germany

German Center for Diabetes Research (DZD), Otfried-Mueller-Strasse 10, 72076 Tübingen, Germany

© Springer International Publishing AG 2017
A. Covic et al. (eds.), *Resistant Hypertension in Chronic Kidney Disease*, DOI 10.1007/978-3-319-56827-0_3

those with white-coat hypertension or incorrect BP measurements in the office setting. A large study that investigated aTRH with the use of ambulatory BP measurement found that one third of the patients had white-coat hypertension leaving a prevalence of true treatment-resistant hypertension of 7.6% [5]. The notorious problem of inadherence to antihypertensive treatment is also one key factor even in patients considered to have true treatment-resistant hypertension. In an elegant study, Jung et al. verified adherence to medical treatment in patients that were judged to have true treatment resistance by measuring antihypertensive drugs or their metabolites in the urine [6]. Surprisingly, inadherence to the prescribed drugs was found in 37% of the patients from whom 30% did not take any of the prescribed drugs.

aTRH increases the cardiovascular risk of the patients substantially as many have a high prevalence of end-organ damage [5, 7]. Particularly, the cardiovascular risk of patients is potentiated when aTRH and CKD convene [8].

Apparent Treatment-Resistant Hypertension in CKD

The prevalence of aTRH is increased among CKD patients [4], and CKD is an important risk factor for the development of treatment-resistant hypertension besides male sex, longer duration of hypertension, current smoking, and diabetes mellitus [5]. A recent population-based cross-sectional study provided more detailed data on the relationship between CKD and aTRH [9]. In that study involving 10,700 hypertensive individuals, the overall prevalence of aTRH based on in-home measurements was 17.9%, the prevalence of CKD 29.2%. Patients with aTRH were treated with an average of 3.6 classes of antihypertensive drugs, mostly diuretics (87%), angiotensin-converting enzyme inhibitors (62%) or angiotensin receptor blockers (40%), beta blockers (73%), and calcium channel antagonists (72%). The main finding of the study was that the prevalence of aTRH was gradually related to both the GFR and albuminuria stages of CKD: in individuals with a GFR ≥ 60, 45–59, and <45 ml/min per 1.73 m^2, aTRH was prevalent in 16%, 25%, and 33%, respectively, and in those with an albumin-to-creatinine ratio (ACR) <10, 10–29, 30–299 in 12%, 21%, 28%, and 48%, and ≥ 300 mg/g, respectively. Both GFR and ACR increased the prevalence of aTRH additively, and patients with a GFR <45 ml/min/1.73m^2 and an ACR ≥ 300 mg/g crea had an almost 60% prevalence of aTRH. The increased prevalence of aTRH in patients with lower GFR and higher ACR stages was still evident after adjustment for other variables including current smoking status, waist circumference, diabetes, history of myocardial infarction or stroke, and patients with GFR <45 ml/min/1.73m^2 and an ACR ≥ 300 mg/g crea had an adjusted prevalence ratio of 3.44 compared to those with GFR ≥ 60 and an ACR <10 mg/g crea (Fig. 3.1). Altogether, the study strongly underscored the close relationship between CKD and aTRH that was incremental with the two dimensions of CKD, namely, GFR and albuminuria that are now part of the CKD classification.

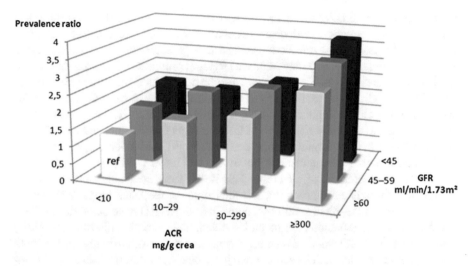

Fig. 3.1 Prevalence ratios for aTRH associated with various GFR and ACR levels after adjustment for demographic and socioeconomic factors, current smoking, alcohol use, waist circumference, diabetes, total cholesterol, HDL cholesterol, statin use, C-reactive protein, history of myocardial infarction, and history of stroke (Data from Tanner et al. [9])

Bidirectional Interaction of CKD and aTRH to Define Cardiovascular–Renal Syndrome

At the heart of the definition of cardiorenal syndrome by Ronco et al. [10] is the interdependence of the heart and the kidney that ensures adequate organ function of each other. When heart failure ensues, there is inevitably kidney dysfunction, and when there is kidney dysfunction, there is also cardiac dysfunction. The classification of Ronco et al. discriminates between cardiorenal syndromes whereby kidney dysfunction is subsequent to cardiac disease (types 1 and 2) and renocardiac syndromes whereby kidney disease comes first and leads to cardiac damage (types 3 and 4). However, in the literature and clinical jargon, the term renocardiac syndrome is not commonly used and cardiorenal syndrome is used as an umbrella term for all types.

Similar to the cardiorenal syndrome, the relationship between CKD and aTRH can also be characterized by a bidirectional interaction and interdependence. Arterial hypertension is on the one hand an important cause of CKD and determinant of CKD progression. This is particularly true for patients with aTRH. On the other hand, advanced CKD and end-stage renal disease lead almost in every instance to the development of de novo arterial hypertension or to exacerbation of preexistent arterial hypertension, possibly resulting in aTRH. Arterial hypertension and aTRH are the most important sequelae of CKD rendering CKD a systemic disease that affects vessels and various organ systems alike. From this perspective, the interaction between CKD and aTRH can be considered as another cardiovascular–renal syndrome that in some cases makes it impossible to determine if CKD and aTRH are cause or consequence. Both diseases have a detrimental effect on each other and are linked by positive feedback loops that are characteristic for a vicious cycle (Fig. 3.2). In practice, CKD may induce aTRH that promotes CKD progression that again exacerbates aTRH. The cycle can also be constructed the other way around: aTRH induces CKD that exacerbates aTRH that in turn exacerbates CKD. It is noteworthy that the bidirectional relationship between aTRH and CKD is related to both the GFR and the albuminuria stages of CKD. Patients with either reduced GFR or high albuminuria have higher prevalence of aTRH [9], and inversely, patients with aTRH have a higher prevalence of albuminuria and lower GFR [5].

Another characteristic of a vicious cycle is that there no steady state or equilibrium unless there is an intervention that interrupts the feedback loops. With regard to the cardiovascular–renal syndrome, both CKD and aTRH have deleterious effects for the patients if left untreated or undertreated. This explains the high morbidity and mortality of CKD and aTRH patients who have extraordinarily high risk of both cardiovascular events such as sudden death, myocardial infarction, stroke, or hemorrhage and cardiovascular diseases such as coronary and peripheral artery disease and heart failure (Fig. 3.2). In a recent study on the outcome of CKD patients with aTRH, de Nicola et al. stratified 436 CKD patients into four groups using ambulatory and office blood pressure measurements [11]. Besides a control group without hypertension (27% of the cohort), patients were classified in those with pseudoresistance (normal 24 h BP, but high office BP; 7%), masked (high 24 h BP, but normal BP; 43%), and true resistant hypertension (high 24 h and office BP; 23%). After a follow-up of 57 months, patients with true hypertension had significantly increased hazard ratios for both cardiovascular and renal events including fatal ones (1.98- and 2.66-fold, respectively). Patients with masked hypertension had also an increased hazard ratio for renal events, whereas patients with pseudoresistance had a favorable outcome without a difference compared to the control group without arterial hypertension. This study again emphasizes that it is highly important to identify those patients within the group of patients with aTRH who have true resistant hypertension with the aid of 24 h ambulatory BP measurements.

Manifestations of the Cardiovascular–Renal Syndrome

Another hallmark of patients with the cardiovascular–renal syndrome is the presence of advanced target-organ damage to the vasculature, heart, and kidney. Hypertensive vasculopathy is characterized by endothelial dysfunction and remodeling of both small and large arteries with the histological findings of hyalinosis, media thickening, and plaque formation. Microangiopathy results from narrowing of the lumen in capillaries and small resistance arteries, whereas macroangiopathy leads to either narrowing of medium conduit arteries due to arterio-/atherosclerosis or aneurysms in large arteries such as the aorta. Hypertensive nephropathy shows similar features of hypertensive vasculopathy leading to ischemia of the glomerulus and tubulus, eventually sclerosis and interstitial fibrosis. Hypertensive

CARDIOVASCULAR RENAL SYNDROME
imposed by aTRH and CKD

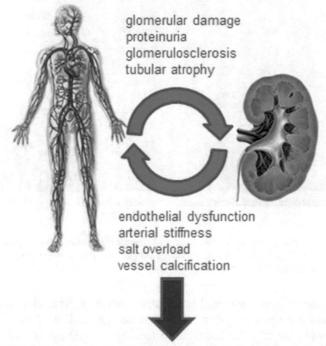

glomerular damage
proteinuria
glomerulosclerosis
tubular atrophy

endothelial dysfunction
arterial stiffness
salt overload
vessel calcification

CARDIOVASCULAR MORBIDITY AND MORTALITY

events	diseases
sudden death	coronary artery disease
myocardial infarction	heart failure
stroke	peripheral artery
hemorrhage	disease

Fig. 3.2 Cardiovascular–renal syndrome imposed by apparent treatment-resistant hypertension (aTRH) and chronic kidney disease (CKD) (Note that only the most prominent interactions between aTRH and CKD are depicted)

heart disease encompasses concentric hypertrophy and diastolic, later systolic dysfunction. On the level of the coronary arteries, both macroangiopathy and microangiopathy can be encountered. Clinical correlates of hypertensive target-organ damage are arterial stiffness, albuminuria, left ventricular hypertrophy, and arterio−/atherosclerosis leading to the known cardiovascular diseases such as coronary and peripheral artery disease, stroke, and heart and renal failure. The identification of hypertension as the major driving risk factor behind these cardiovascular diseases has been, among others, a major success from 50 years of research originating from the Framingham studies [12].

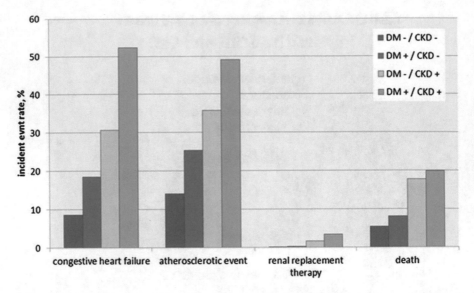

Fig. 3.3 Incident event rates of cardiovascular and renal complications during 2-year time period between 1999 and 2001 in a sample of 1 million Medicare patients. *DM* diabetes mellitus, *CKD* chronic kidney disease (Data from Keith et al. [15])

In the last decade, CKD has emerged as a new and potent cardiovascular risk factor [13, 14] in addition the so-called traditional Framingham-derived risk factors. This is highlighted by the high cardiovascular mortality of CKD patients who have a higher risk to die from cardiovascular disease than to progress to end-stage renal failure [15, 16]. Compared with diabetes mellitus that has been traditionally regarded as a major cardiovascular risk factor, CKD is even a stronger and a more consistent cardiovascular risk factor. In a Medicare sample with approximately 1 million patients, the incidence of congestive heart failure, atherosclerotic event, renal replacement therapy, or death was much higher in CKD patients compared to patients with diabetes mellitus (Fig. 3.3). The presence of CKD in a patient is on one hand a marker that reflects target-organ damage and the burden of cardiovascular disease. On the other hand, CKD and its sequelae directly interfere with the pathogenesis of cardiovascular disease and worsen cardiovascular disease burden. This is similar to the clinical significance of acute kidney injury which is at the same time a risk marker and risk factor for increased mortality among hospitalized patients.

Worsening of cardiovascular disease by CKD can be attributed to mechanisms and sequelae that are unique to advanced CKD. Among these, salt retention and volume expansion, increase of uremic toxins, and deranged calcium–phosphorus balance are major risk factors that not only strikingly aggravate cardiovascular disease but also introduce different pathophysiological pathways. Thus, CKD and its sequelae are now considered as nontraditional cardiovascular risk factors and have opened up an intensely studied area of current research.

Altered Pathophysiology of Arteriosclerosis in Cardiovascular–Renal Syndrome

The vasculopathy of CKD is characterized by media calcification that is unique to CKD patients in contrast to intimal calcification of cholesterol-rich plaques in patients with common atherosclerosis [17]. Media calcification in CKD is considered not to be merely a passive process resulting from elevated calcium x phosphorus product but also an active process involving induction of an osteoblast-like phenotype of smooth muscle cells of the media (also termed osteoblastic transdifferentiation; [18]). Key molecule triggering these events is phosphate that enters the cells via transporters such as the sodium-dependent phosphate transporter (PiT-1). The complex derangements encompassing chronic kidney disease–mineral bone disorder (CKD–MBD) include also increases in the fibroblast growth factor 23, decreases in the FGF23 coreceptor klotho, and eventually increased parathyroid hormone. CKD–MBD is associated with widespread vascular calcification (Fig. 3.4) and arterial stiffness. Clinically, this translates to increased pulse wave velocity and high blood pressure amplitude (pulse pressure). Arterial stiffness leads to pulse wave reflections that increases cardiac afterload and promotes development of left ventricular hypertrophy. The hemodynamic consequences of arterial stiffness are dramatic, and the perfusion in these stiff vessels without vasomotor function becomes dependent on cardiac output (CO) and cannot be regulated adequately, particularly when there is a drop in CO. This gives rise to sudden ischemic events

Fig. 3.4 Completely calcified aorta of a 65-year-old female patient with long-standing CKD (>20 years; current stage CKD 4 T)

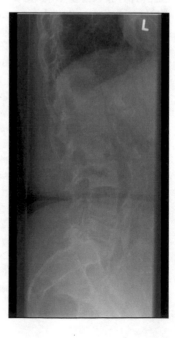

and even sudden death that is the leading cause of death in patients with ESRD and thought to result from myocardial ischemia and ventricular fibrillation.

In CKD-associated vasculopathy, cholesterol-rich plaque formation seems to be less relevant and statin therapy which is undoubtedly protective in atherosclerosis of the non-CKD population is losing its efficacy as CKD progresses to ESRD. In the Study of Heart and Renal Protection (SHARP), risk reduction of cholesterol-lowering was confined to CKD patients with stages 3–4, but not observed in ESRD patients [19]. In this regard, acute myocardial infarction resulting from plaque rupture and thrombosis of a coronary artery (type I infarction according to the third universal classification [20]) is in ESRD patients less common compared to myocardial damage and infarction resulting from relative ischemia (type II) due to reduced perfusion and drop in CO. In the 4D trial that investigated the effects of 20 mg simvastatin versus placebo in ESRD patients, fatal acute myocardial infarction occurred only in 15% of the patients compared to a 50% of fatalities due to sudden death [21].

Salt Retention and Overhydration in Cardiovascular–Renal Syndrome

Another important determinant of CKD-related cardiovascular disease burden is salt retention and volume overload that is common in CKD patients. In a study using bioimpedance spectroscopy, overhydration as defined by an excess of 7% or more of the extracellular volume was found in 52% of the patients with predialysis CKD [22] and strongly correlated with systolic blood pressure. Our group similarly found that overhydration was common in CKD patients and correlated to both the GFR and albuminuria stages of CKD (Fig. 3.5; [23]). Multiple regression analysis revealed that proteinuria was the strongest independent predictor of overhydration pointing to a causative role of proteinuria in the genesis of overhydration and salt retention. In CKD patients, salt retention might occur due to the activation of the epithelial sodium channel ENaC which is an important determinant of sodium homeostasis in both health and disease. Although sodium reabsorption by ENaC accounts for only a few percent of the filtered sodium load, ENaC activity determines the final concentration of sodium in the urine. Serine proteases are powerful regulators of ENaC activity by cleaving its gamma subunit and increasing the open probability of the channel. Under physiological conditions serine proteases such as prostasin or tissue kallikreins are involved in this process; however, under the pathophysiological conditions of proteinuria, ENaC might be illicitly activated by the serine protease plasmin that is generated from aberrantly filtered plasminogen [24]. Plasminogen is a large protein (91 kDa) that is normally withheld by the intact glomerulus. However, after glomerular injury, larger amounts of plasminogen can be filtered and converted to plasmin in the tubulus lumen by the urokinase-type

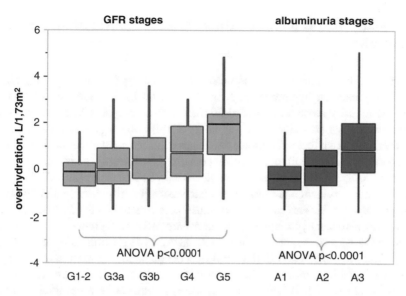

Fig. 3.5 Relationship between overhydration and GFR and albuminuria stages of CKD [23]

plasminogen activator (uPA) that is expressed in the tubular epithelium. Urinary excretion of plasmin has been found to strongly correlate with both proteinuria and albuminuria ($r > 0.8$ [23]) and more importantly with overhydration in proteinuric diabetic patients and CKD patients. The relationship between proteinuria and over-hydration seems to be linear and extends to patients with proteinuria in the non-nephrotic range as well [25].

ENaC activation by proteinuria and/or plasminuria is an attractive mechanism explaining the high prevalence of overhydration and edema in CKD patients and a link to aTRH. Indeed, in the study of de la Sierra et al. [5], higher albuminuria stages were an independent factor associated with an increased prevalence of aTRH. The link between proteinuria and salt retention in CKD patients could also explain the finding that arterial hypertension of CKD patients is particularly salt-sensitive and that high salt intake exacerbates blood pressure control and associates with adverse renal outcomes in CKD patients [26]. Altogether, these findings under-score the detrimental role of salt in patients with cardiovascular–renal syndrome and the importance of a salt restriction in the diet. A number of studies have shown reductions in blood pressure during salt restriction in CKD patients. Salt restriction also improves the response to the antihypertensive effects of angiotensin-converting enzyme inhibitors. In a randomized study with proteinuric CKD patients (mean proteinuria 1.5 g/24 h) and a relatively preserved GFR (mean creatinine clearance 70 ml/min), moderate salt restriction resulting in a reduction in urinary sodium excretion from 186 mmol to 106 mmol per day markedly enhanced the blood pressure lowering effect of lisinopril [27]. Similarly, salt restriction also augmented the antiproteinuric effect of lisinopril.

Diagnostic Workup and Evaluation of Cardiovascular–Renal Syndrome

Twenty-four hours ambulatory BP measurement is the gold standard for the diagnosis of true resistant hypertension. It is an essential investigation in patients with aTRH to identify those with normal 24 h BP that corresponds to pseudoresistance or white-coat hypertension. The prognosis of this subgroup is more benign [11]; however, it is a risk factor for future development of resistant hypertension [28]. The utilization of 24 h ambulatory BP measurement differs from country to country, but in general utilization seems to be low and should be increased [29]. Obstacles to a more frequent utilization are probably related to availability, costs, patient participation, and logistical issues as the device must be returned the next day. Besides diagnosing true resistant hypertension, 24 h ambulatory BP measurement is also essential in the follow-up of patients with true resistant hypertension to ensure adequate blood pressure control and to decide if new drugs including reserve drugs such as minoxidil must be introduced. In addition, demonstration of a treatment refractory state using ambulatory BP measurement is the prerequisite to warrant interventional therapies such as renal denervation or baroreceptor stimulation. The use and interval of ambulatory BP measurement during follow-up must be decided individually and can be monthly, 6-monthly, or annually. Although the correlation of home BP measurement to ambulatory BP measurement is fair to moderate, patients with cardiovascular renal syndrome should implement home BP measurement to help the physicians in their assessment of adequate BP control at a visit.

During the initial workup of patients with cardiovascular renal syndrome, the most common secondary causes of hypertension should be ruled out. These are in descending order of frequency [30]: obstructive sleep apnea syndrome (60–70% of the patients with true resistant hypertension), hyperaldosteronism (7–20%), renal artery stenosis (2–24%), renoparenchymal disease (1–2%), drug or alcohol-induced (2–4%), and thyroid disorder (1%). These entities can be investigated in an outpatient setting by careful history taking, duplex sonography, and laboratory analyses. Polygraphy to screen for sleep apnea syndrome should be available when a patient reports daytime sleepiness or snoring. When a new patient is referred, results of the diagnostic workup should be reviewed and new tests or retests ordered when there is a gap or equivocal results. Once completely done, retesting is usually not necessary unless there is clinical suspicion of newly developed disease, e.g., arteriosclerotic renal artery stenosis after long-standing aTRH.

Another important aspect of the diagnostic workup of patients with cardiovascular–renal syndrome is the thorough evaluation of target end-organ damage to estimate the burden of disease and to identify established cardiovascular or renal disease (stroke, coronary artery disease, heart failure, peripheral artery disease, nephropathy, advanced retinopathy). From patient to patient, differences in end-organ damage may be present depending on the presence of microangiopathy or macroangiopathy or nephropathy or cardiac disease. These lead to differences in vulnerability of the individual patient and help to stratify the future risk, e.g., development of heart failure or end-stage renal disease. After broad testing for end-organ damage initially, physicians can confine to follow those parameters reflecting the present end-organ damage more regularly than those which were negative. Established markers of end-organ damage that can be controlled during follow-up are albuminuria, estimated GFR, pulse wave velocity, pulse pressure, carotid wall thickening, ankle–brachial index, and left ventricular hypertrophy. The latter can be best investigated using echocardiography that provides further important information on cardiac status; however, the availability of echocardiography is sometimes limited, and echocardiographic parameters change only slowly so that the interval of repeat echocardiography may be two or more years unless there is clinical suspicion of newly developed cardiac disease, e.g., development of congestive heart failure.

Implications of Cardiovascular–Renal Syndrome for Treatment

To account for the bidirectional interaction of CKD and aTRH in cardiovascular–renal syndrome, it is necessary to pursue a bidirectional or multilayered treatment approach that ultimately stops the vicious cycle of the cardiovascular renal syndrome. Treating physicians must analyze the pathophysiological interaction of CKD and aTRH and identify the triggering factors individually since these are numerous and can vary from patient to patient. Some factors will be not modifiable as they represent end-organ damage such as arterial stiffness or glomerulosclerosis. However, others can be identified and are amenable to specific treatment, e.g., inadequate blood pressure control due to unidentified secondary causes of aTRH, volume expansion, or identification of renoparenchymal disease. In the next step, physicians must implement rigorous treatment goals aimed to correct for the triggering factors. This could be the rigorous correction of salt overload and volume expansion in a patient with aTRH that is triggered by proteinuric CKD using antiproteinuric and diuretic drugs. Disappearance of edema and achievement of dry weight could be taken as surrogate treatment goals to control aTRH in such a patient. Even without visible edema, saluretic medication should be considered in any patients with aTRH and CKD to guarantee salt excretion. In this context, spironolactone deserves special attention as its addition to a multiple drug regimen often dramatically improves blood pressure control in aTRH. This was first seen in the ASCOT trial [31] and most recently in the PATHWAY-2 Study [32]. The high efficacy of spironolactone as an add-on treatment challenges the current definition of aTRH that is defined by treatment resistance on a triple antihypertensive regimen including a diuretic. According to these results, the diagnosis of true resistance should only be reserved for those patients with persistent high blood pressure after add-on treatment with spironolactone.

In another patient with aTRH, progression of hypertensive nephropathy rescue treatment with minoxidil may be warranted (after add-on treatment with spironolactone had no effect) and sometimes needed since this potent drug is often the last remedy in patients with otherwise refractory hypertension [33]. However, it has side effects that preclude its widespread use and requires experience. Generally, the physician should be familiar with the pharmacological armamentarium to treat cardiovascular–renal syndrome including second- and third-line drugs or regimens including interventional therapies such as renal denervation or baroreceptor stimulation.

Aggressive and rigorous pharmacological therapies in patients with CKD and aTRH have the high potential of side effects due to the presence of end-organ damage and organ dysfunction. Hence, many contacts and revisits are required to ensure safety while cautiously targeting the treatment goals. These serve to monitor the adequacy of treatment and to identify side effects, some of which can be serious and lead to hospitalization or patient death. During treatment with minoxidil, for example, edema formation is a serious side effect that in some cases can progress to life-threatening pericardial effusion. Monitoring of weight, the development of edema, and adjustment of concomitant diuretic therapy are of great importance with this drug. Other pharmacological treatments involving renin–angiotensin blockade and diuretics often result in deterioration of renal function and development of electrolyte derangements that can only be diagnosed in the early stages by laboratory checks. Pharmacotherapy with these substances often needs careful titration to find out tolerated doses without side effects. However, changes in salt and water balance either by seasonal variation (hot summer) or by disease (e.g., diarrhea) can quickly lead to derangements. Altogether, therapeutic rigor as much as patient motivation is needed to achieve treatment goals in patients with cardiovascular renal syndrome.

Conclusions

The coincidence of CKD and aTRH can indeed be coined as another cardiovascular renal syndrome that is characterized by a bidirectional interaction. Patients with cardiovascular renal syndrome have a high burden of end-organ damage and are at a very high risk for mortality. Multifaceted treatment adopted for the individual patients and therapeutic rigor is necessary to break the vicious cycle of cardiovascular renal syndrome and to ultimately improve patient outcome.

Disclosure There are no relationships with companies that may have a financial interest in the information contained in this manuscript.

References

1. Whaley-Connell AT, Sowers JR, Stevens LA, McFarlane SI, Shlipak MG, Norris KC, et al. CKD in the United States: Kidney Early Evaluation Program (KEEP) and National Health and Nutrition Examination Survey (NHANES) 1999–2004. Am J Kidney Dis. 2008;51(4 Suppl 2):S13–20.
2. Buckalew VM, Berg RL, Wang SR, Porush JG, Rauch S, Schulman G. Prevalence of hypertension in 1,795 subjects with chronic renal disease: the modification of diet in renal disease study baseline cohort. Modification of Diet in Renal Disease Study Group. Am J Kidney Dis. 1996;28(6):811–21.
3. Calhoun DA, Jones D, Textor S, Goff DC, Murphy TP, Toto RD, et al. Resistant hypertension: diagnosis, evaluation, and treatment. A scientific statement from the American Heart Association Professional Education Committee of the Council for High Blood Pressure Research. Hypertension. 2008;51(6):1403–19.
4. Egan BM, Zhao Y, Axon RN, Brzezinski WA, Ferdinand KC. Uncontrolled and apparent treatment resistant hypertension in the United States, 1988 to 2008. Circulation. 2011;124(9):1046–58.
5. de la Sierra A, Segura J, Banegas JR, Gorostidi M, de la Cruz JJ, Armario P, et al. Clinical features of 8295 patients with resistant hypertension classified on the basis of ambulatory blood pressure monitoring. Hypertension. 2011;57(5):898–902.
6. Jung O, Gechter JL, Wunder C, Paulke A, Bartel C, Geiger H, Toennes SW. Resistant hypertension? Assessment of adherence by toxicological urine analysis. J Hypertens. 2013;31(4):766–74.
7. Daugherty SL, Powers JD, Magid DJ, Tavel HM, Masoudi FA, Margolis KL, et al. Incidence and prognosis of resistant hypertension in hypertensive patients. Circulation. 2012;125(13):1635–42.
8. De Nicola L, Borrelli S, Gabbai FB, Chiodini P, Zamboli P, Iodice C, et al. Burden of resistant hypertension in hypertensive patients with non-dialysis chronic kidney disease. Kidney Blood Press Res. 2011;34(1):58–67.
9. Tanner RM, Calhoun DA, Bell EK, Bowling CB, Gutiérrez OM, Irvin MR, et al. Prevalence of apparent treatment-resistant hypertension among individuals with CKD. Clin J Am Soc Nephrol. 2013;8(9):1583–90.
10. Ronco C, Haapio M, House AA, Anavekar N, Bellomo R. Cardiorenal syndrome. J Am Coll Cardiol. 2008;52(19):1527–39.
11. De Nicola L, Gabbai FB, Agarwal R, Chiodini P, Borrelli S, Bellizzi V, et al. Prevalence and prognostic role of resistant hypertension in chronic kidney disease patients. J Am Coll Cardiol. 2013;61(24):2461–7.
12. Kannel WB. Fifty years of Framingham study contributions to understanding hypertension. J Hum Hypertens. 2000;14(2):83–90.
13. Sarnak MJ, Levey AS. Cardiovascular disease and chronic renal disease: a new paradigm. Am J Kidney Dis. 2000;35(4 Suppl 1):S117–31.
14. Wali RK, Henrich WL. Chronic kidney disease: a risk factor for cardiovascular disease. Cardiol Clin. 2005;23(3):343–62.
15. Keith DS, Nichols GA, Gullion CM, Brown JB, Smith DH. Longitudinal follow-up and outcomes among a population with chronic kidney disease in a large managed care organization. Arch Intern Med. 2004;164(6):659–63.
16. Foley RN, Murray AM, Li S, Herzog CA, McBean AM, Eggers PW, Collins AJ. Chronic kidney disease and the risk for cardiovascular disease, renal replacement, and death in the United States Medicare population, 1998 to 1999. J Am Soc Nephrol. 2005;16(2):489–95.
17. Amann K. Media calcification and intima calcification are distinct entities in chronic kidney disease. Clin J Am Soc Nephrol. 2008;3(6):1599–605.
18. Mizobuchi M, Towler T, Slatopolsky E. Vascular calcification: the killer of patients with chronic kidney disease. J Am Soc Nephrol. 2009;20(7):1453–64.

19. Baigent C, Landray MJ, Reith C, Emberson J, Wheeler DC, Tomson C, et al. The effects of lowering LDL cholesterol with simvastatin plus ezetimibe in patients with chronic kidney disease (study of heart and renal protection): a randomised placebo-controlled trial. Lancet. 2011;377(9784):2181–92.
20. Thygesen K, Alpert JS, Jaffe AS, Simoons ML, Chaitman BR, White HD, Writing Group on behalf of the Joint ESC/ACCF/AHA/WHF Task Force for the Universal Definition of Myocardial Infarction. Third universal definition of myocardial infarction. J Am Coll Cardiol. 2012;60(16):1581–98.
21. Wanner C, Krane V, März W, Olschewski M, Mann JF, Ruf G, et al. Atorvastatin in patients with type 2 diabetes mellitus undergoing hemodialysis. N Engl J Med. 2005;353(3):238–48.
22. Hung SC, Kuo KL, Peng CH, Wu CH, Lien YC, Wang YC, Tarng DC. Volume overload correlates with cardiovascular risk factors in patients with chronic kidney disease. Kidney Int. 2014;85(3):703–9.
23. Schork A, Woern M, Kalbacher H, Voelter W, Nacken R, Bertog M, et al. Association of plasminuria with overhydration in CKD patients. Clin J Am Soc Nephrol. 2016;11(5):761–9.
24. Passero CJ, Hughey RP, Kleyman TR. New role for plasmin in sodium homeostasis. Curr Opin Nephrol Hypertens. 2010;19(1):13–9.
25. Andersen H, Friis UG, Hansen PB, Svenningsen P, Henriksen JE, Jensen BL. Diabetic nephropathy is associated with increased urine excretion of proteases plasmin, prostasin and urokinase and activation of amiloride-sensitive current in collecting duct cells. Nephrol Dial Transplant. 2015;30(5):781–9.
26. Smyth A, O'Donnell MJ, Yusuf S, Clase CM, Teo KK, Canavan M, Reddan DN, Mann JF. Sodium intake and renal outcomes: a systematic review. Am J Hypertens. 2014;27(10):1277–84.
27. Slagman MC, Waanders F, Hemmelder MH, Woittiez AJ, Janssen WM, Lambers Heerspink HJ, et al. Moderate dietary sodium restriction added to angiotensin converting enzyme inhibition compared with dual blockade in lowering proteinuria and blood pressure: randomised controlled trial. BMJ. 2011;343:d4366.
28. Mancia G, Bombelli M, Brambilla G, Facchetti R, Sega R, Toso E, Grassi G. Long-term prognostic value of white coat hypertension: an insight from diagnostic use of both ambulatory and home blood pressure measurements. Hypertension. 2013;62(1):168–74.
29. Shimbo D, Kent ST, Diaz KM, Huang L, Viera AJ, Kilgore M, et al. The use of ambulatory blood pressure monitoring among Medicare beneficiaries in 2007-2010. J Am Soc Hypertens. 2014;8(12):891–7.
30. Vongpatanasin W. Resistant hypertension: a review of diagnosis and management. JAMA. 2014;311(21):2216–24.
31. Chapman N, Dobson J, Wilson S, Dahlöf B, Sever PS, Wedel H, et al. Effect of spironolactone on blood pressure in subjects with resistant hypertension. Hypertension. 2007;49(4):839–45.
32. Williams B, MacDonald TM, Morant S, Webb DJ, Sever P, McInnes G, et al. Spironolactone versus placebo, bisoprolol, and doxazosin to determine the optimal treatment for drug-resistant hypertension (PATHWAY-2): a randomised, double-blind, crossover trial. Lancet. 2015;386(1008):2059–68.
33. Sica DA. Minoxidil: an underused vasodilator for resistant or severe hypertension. J Clin Hypertens (Greenwich). 2004;6(5):283–7.

Chapter 4

The Importance of Ambulatory and Home Monitoring Blood Pressure in Resistant Hypertension Associated with Chronic Kidney Disease

Silvio Borrelli, Luca De Nicola, Giuseppe Conte, and Roberto Minutolo

Introduction to Out-of-Office BP Monitoring

Out-of-office blood pressure (BP) measurements include ambulatory blood pressure monitoring (ABPM) lasting 24 h and home BP monitoring (HBPM) obtained with patient at home, seated and resting. ABPM provides a more precise assessment of BP profiles and a description of circadian rhythm of BP (dipping status), whereas HBPM only discloses abnormal BP profiles [1].

ABP monitors are compact, typically worn on a belt or in a pouch, and connected to a sphygmomanometer cuff on the upper arm by a tube. The monitors are usually programmed to obtain readings every 15–30 min throughout the day and night, and it is obtained while patients perform their normal daily activities. At the end of the recording period, the readings are downloaded into a computer for processing. Patients must fill out a diary during the monitoring period to document any symptoms, awakening and sleeping times, naps, periods of stress, timing of meals, and medication ingestion [1].

Based on the goal proposed by current guidelines [1, 2], combining clinical BP and ABPM allows disclosing four pressor profiles (Table 4.1). This assessment is not a "semantic exercise," because it optimizes refining the risk profile of hypertensive patients [3–5].

Alternatively, for the detection of white coat hypertension (WCH) and masked hypertension (MH), HBP monitoring may be suitable, by means of self-reporting of BP values. This approach for measuring BP outside of the clinic provides a great

S. Borrelli • L. De Nicola • G. Conte • R. Minutolo (✉)
Division of Nephrology, Department of Scienze Mediche, Chirurgiche, Neurologiche, Metaboliche e dell'Invecchiamento, University of Campania "Luigi Vanvitelli", Naples, Italy
e-mail: roberto.minutolo@unicampania.it

© Springer International Publishing AG 2017
A. Covic et al. (eds.), *Resistant Hypertension in Chronic Kidney Disease*,
DOI 10.1007/978-3-319-56827-0_4

Table 4.1 Main information derived from ambulatory blood pressure monitoring (ABPM) and office blood pressure (BP)

	ABPM	Office BP
Recommended target[a]	24 h ABP <130/80 Daytime ABP <135/85 Nighttime ABP <120/70	≤140/90 (Ualb < 30 mg/d) ≤130/80 (Ualb 30–300 mg/d) ≤130/80 (Ualb >300 mg/d)
Pressor profiles		
Controlled hypertension	At goal	At goal
White coat hypertension	At goal	Not at goal
Masked hypertension	Not at goal	At goal
Sustained hypertension	Not at goal	Not at goal
Circadian profiles		
Dipper	Nighttime BP < daytime BP by 10–20%	–
Extreme dipper	Nighttime BP < daytime BP by >20%	–
Non-dipper	Nighttime BP < daytime BP by 0–10%	–
Inverse dipper	Nighttime BP greater than daytime BP	–

[a]Recommendations on BP targets are based on Refs. [1, 2]

advantage that is well accepted and cheaper than ABPM. In order to obtain an accurate HBPM, the measurements must be performed by the patient two times in the morning and two times in the evening. A minimum of three consecutive days and a preferred period of 7 consecutive days of HBPM is a reasonable approach for clinical practice. HBPM results are obtained by averaging all values recorded after excluding the readings obtained on the first day of HBPM [1]. The recommended BP threshold for optimal HBPM is <135/85 mmHg [1].

A major shortcoming of HBPM is the lack of data on nocturnal BP that makes this technique less accurate for an optimal evaluation of cardiovascular risk in CKD. Conversely, ABPM provides an accurate picture of circadian rhythm of BP and the detection of nocturnal hypertension. Indeed, BP is physiologically lower during sleep by 10–20% as compared to daytime values. Therefore, a night/day ratio of BP ranging between 0.8 and 0.9 is considered normal, and patients are defined as "dipper," while the lack of nighttime BP reduction by at least 10% identifies individuals as "non-dipper." In particular, as described in Table 4.1, a decline of nocturnal BP between 0 and 10% with respect to diurnal BP (night/day BP ratio: 0.9:1.0) defines the "non-dipper" condition, whereas if nocturnal BP is higher than diurnal BP (night/day BP ratio > 1.0), the patient is defined as "reverse dipper." Some patients may experience a marked reduction of night BP, greater than 20% (night/day BP ratio < 0.8); this infrequent condition is defined as "extreme dipping" [1]. This classification is relevant for prognosis of hypertensive patients since several studies and meta-analyses have reported that non-dipping status and nocturnal hypertension are associated with increased risk for cardiovascular (CV) events and all-cause mortality, independent of clinical and daytime blood pressure levels [6, 7].

Importance of Ambulatory/Home BP Monitoring in CKD Patients

ABPM and HBPM as Continuous Variables

The inconclusive results on the prognostic role of the BP target in patients with CKD [8–10] might relate to the limited ability of clinical BP readings to adequately stratify the global risk in this high-risk population [11, 12]. Three large prospective cohort studies provided clear evidence that HBPM and ABPM are superior to clinical BP readings in predicting all-cause mortality, CV events, and end-stage renal disease (ESRD) [13–16]. Agarwal and Andersen demonstrated in a cohort study of 217 veterans with CKD who were followed for a median of 3.5 years the superiority of ABPM over clinical BP for predicting a composite endpoint of death or ESRD [16]. Similar results were obtained when considering HBPM versus office BP in the same cohort [13]. Furthermore, an analysis of 617 CKD patients in the African American Study of Kidney Disease and Hypertension (AASK) study found ABPM to be superior to office BP for predicting both CV events and a composite of death, ESRD, or doubling of serum creatinine over a median follow-up of 5 years [14]. Finally, Minutolo et al. [15] reported that in a cohort study of 436 CKD patients followed for a median of 4.2 years, office BP did not predict CV events or composite of death and ESRD, while ABPM, and in particular nighttime BP, increased the risk of either adverse outcome. In that study, the cardio-renal risk increased significantly when daytime or nighttime BP exceeded 135/85 or 120/70 mmHg, respectively. These data confirmed that normality thresholds for daytime and nighttime BP proposed for essential hypertension may also confidently apply to hypertension CKD [15].

All the previous studies on ABPM have used a single set of measurements, which represents a potential source of inaccuracy in properly classifying patients with BP at goal for daytime and nighttime ABPM that potentially leads to imprecise risk estimation. To address this issue, we recently tested whether an additional assessment of ABPM after 1 year provides incremental estimate of the renal risk beyond the initial evaluation [17]. We found that patients not reaching the goal for daytime and nighttime systolic BP at the two ABPM had the worst renal prognosis, while patients not at goal at baseline but reaching the goal at second ABPM were not exposed to a greater renal risk. The use of a second ambulatory monitoring after 1 year allows to correctly reclassify risk profile in 15–22% of patients based on daytime or nighttime systolic BP [17]. Therefore, in routine clinical practice, physicians may perform ABPM in order to identify patients with nocturnal hypertension, which constitutes a major predictor of CV events and progression to ESRD. Reassessment of ABPM at 1 year further refines renal prognosis and it should specifically be considered in patients with uncontrolled BP at baseline.

Altered BP Profiles

ABPM or HBPM allows for better assessment of hypertension control by identifying patients with altered BP pattern (Table 4.1). The identification of inconsistent achievement of clinical and ambulatory BP goals is helpful at refining prognosis. Three recent meta-analyses in the setting of essential hypertension have shown that WCH does not associate with increased CV risk, whereas MH heralds a higher risk of CV events [3–5]. This assessment is particularly important in CKD because the prevalence of WCH and MH appears to differ from that reported in patients with essential hypertension where the prevalence of WCH and MH is 13% and 11%, respectively [18, 19]. Indeed, a meta-analysis, including six studies and 980 CKD patients with out-of-office BP measures, reported that WCH was more frequent in patients with CKD (18%), whereas MH seems to be less common in CKD (8%) [20]. However, these estimates were strongly influenced by the BP thresholds used for classifying WCH and MH and the use of antihypertensive drugs [20]. Of note, when considering more recent studies not included in the meta-analysis, a further source of bias emerges. Indeed, the prevalence of WCH is higher than that of MH in Caucasian patients [21–23], while the opposite was found in studies enrolling Afro-American or Asian patients [24, 25] (Table 4.2).

A critical question is when to perform an out-of-office measurement of BP to detect altered pressor profiles or, alternatively, what clinical and demographic

Table 4.2 Prevalence of white coat hypertension (WCH), masked hypertension (MH), and non-dipping status in cohorts of CKD patients

Cohort	Ethnicity	Thresholds for defining BP profiles (mmHg)		WCH (%)	MH (%)	Non-dipper definition	Non-dipper (%)
		Office BP	ABPM				
Italian cohort [23]	Caucasian 100%	<140/90	Day/night <135/85/<120/70	22.1	14.5	N/D ratio SBP > 0.9	62.4
Spanish registry [21]	Caucasian 100%	<140/90	24-h BP <130/80	28.8	7.0	NA	NA
Veterans cohort [22]	Caucasian 80%	<130/80	Awake BP <130/80	24.6	4.7	N/D ratio SBP > 0.9	80.2
AASK study [28]	Afro-American 100%	<140/90	Daytime BP <135/85	5.3	25.1	N/D change SBP <10%	80.2
JAC-CKD cohort [24]	Asian 100%	<140/90	24-h BP <130/80	5.6	30.9	N/D change SBP <10%	53.5
Chinese cohort [25]	Asian 100%	≤140/90	24-h BP ≤130/80	9.7	18.2	N/D change SBP <10%	75.5

WCH white coat hypertension, *MH* masked hypertension, *ABPM* ambulatory blood pressure monitoring, *CBP* clinical blood pressure, *BP* blood pressure, *NA* not available conditions may predict the presence of WCH or MH and, consequently, require ABPM or HBP. Two studies addressed this issue in CKD patients, separately for WCH [26] and MH [27]. Minutolo et al. [26] reported that, among 228 CKD patients stages 2–5 with high office BP, 40% of patients had WCH, and this condition was significantly associated with proteinuria >1 g/day (odds ratio [OR], 3.12), left ventricular hypertrophy (OR, 1.94), and higher office BP (OR, 1.61 for each 10 mmHg). Agarwal et al. [27], in a cohort of 295 CKD patients (stages 2–4) with normal clinical BP (<140/90 mmHg), found that MH was a common condition whose prevalence varied from 27% (using daytime BP) to 33% (using 24 h BP) up to 56% when both daytime and nighttime BP were considered. The authors suggested that a confirmatory ABPM can be avoided in patients with office systolic BP <110 mmHg, that, however, represent the large minority of patients seen in nephrology clinics. Conversely, ABPM should be mandatory in patients with office BP values in the range of prehypertension (130–139 mmHg) by considering that two out of three of these patients have MH and also considered when office BP is in the 120–129 range, that is, a condition associated with MH in 34% of cases [27].

This more accurate estimate of hypertensive status offered by ABPM with respect to clinical BP translates into better risk stratification in CKD patients. Indeed, while the global prognosis of patients with sustained hypertension (either target not at goal) is worse than for normotensive patients (both BP targets at goal), the risk for renal death (composite of ESRD and all-cause mortality) and fatal and nonfatal CV events markedly differ between WCH and MH (Fig. 4.1). Patients with MH showed

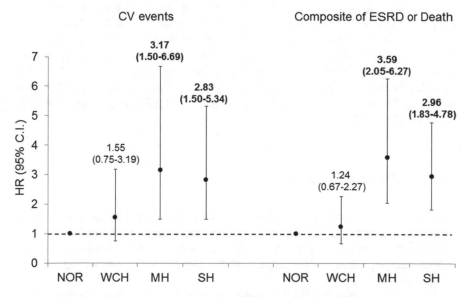

Fig. 4.1 Risk of fatal and nonfatal CV events and dialysis therapy initiation or all-cause death associated with pressor profiles identified by ABPM. In bold are indicated significant hazards. Model is adjusted for age, sex, body mass index, diabetes, history of CV disease, hemoglobin level, estimated glomerular filtration rate, 24-h proteinuria, non-dipping status, and use of angiotensin-converting enzyme inhibitor/angiotensin receptor blocker and stratified for center [23]

similar cardio-renal risk as those with sustained hypertension, whereas having WCH was not associated with a higher risk for any event, therefore suggesting that the different prognosis can be ascribed reasonably to poor achievement of the ABPM target rather than office BP target [23]. Interestingly, the cardio-renal prognosis associated with WCH and MH was independent from the office and ABPM thresholds used to define BP profiles [23]. Indeed, the poor cardio-renal survival in MH patients, as well as the lack of increased risk in WCH, was consistently detected assuming the cutoff values of office BP and ABPM adopted in Spanish Registry, AASK study, Japanese study, and in a veterans cohort [15, 21, 24, 28].

It is important to note that classifying patients based on both clinical and out-of-office BP has relevant therapeutic implications by helping physicians to select the most appropriate therapeutic decision algorithm for their hypertensive patients. BP management merely driven by clinical BP may leave MH patients at higher risk due to uncontrolled ambulatory BP. On the other hand, tailoring antihypertensive treatment based only on office BP values can expose WCH patients to excessive lowering of BP, especially at night [26] and in elderly patients [29], with consequent ischemic episodes affecting renal, cerebral, and cardiac function. In this regard, it is interesting to note that in hypertensive patients with clinical BP not at goal but ambulatory BP at goal, starting antihypertensive therapy is not effective in preventing CV events compared to placebo treatment [30]. Very recently, the randomized Systolic Blood Pressure Intervention Trial (SPRINT) study has shown that lower BP (goal systolic <120 mmHg), as compared to standard control (<140 mmHg), is less effective in reducing the CV and not effective at all in preventing renal endpoints in the subgroup of patients with CKD with respect to those without CKD [31]. Indeed, driving the intensity of treatment on the basis of office BP only has led to higher rates of hypotensive episodes and acute renal injury. In this trial, it is therefore possible to hypothesize that lack of protective effect in CKD subgroup could be associated with the presence of a large prevalence of WCH, that is, a condition exposing patients at high risk of ischemic episodes. This hypothesis will be tested by the ancillary study of SPRINT trial enrolling 600 patients performing ABPM will be available [32].

Altered Circadian Profile

The distinctive characteristic of ABPM is mainly represented by the possibility of obtaining information on nighttime BP, now considered the ABPM component more strictly linked to adverse outcome [33]. Indeed, even when daytime BP is well controlled, the presence of nocturnal hypertension portends a greater risk of renal progression [15].

The lack of physiological BP decline during nighttime (non-dipping status) occurs frequently in CKD patients, being consistently above 53% in all the studies available (Table 4.2). Prevalence increases with aging [29] and in more advanced CKD stages. In a group of 459 CKD patients regularly followed in renal clinics, the risk of being non-dipper was significantly associated with older age, diabetes, left ventricular hypertrophy, and anemia [29]. In a large Japanese cohort of CKD patients, non-dipping status was associated also with more advanced CKD, seasonal variation, and, as expected, nocturia [24].

Altered circadian profiles are strongly associated with adverse clinical outcomes in CKD [15, 16], similar to general population and essential hypertension [6, 7, 34]. In particular, in CKD patients, non-dippers and reverse dippers displayed a twofold greater CV risk and a 60–70% higher risk of renal events [15]. Agarwal and Andersen reported similar results in a cohort of veterans with CKD and highlighted that a similar risk of CV outcomes occurred by using day or night versus awake or sleep BP and that dipping status defined as the night/day ratio confers higher CV risk as compared to dipping defined as an absolute change [35]. Therefore, an adjunctive reason to perform an ABP recording in patients with CKD is to identify patients with nocturnal hypertension, which constitutes a major predictor of CV events and progression to ESRD and represents a potential target for therapy. Indeed, it has been suggested that non-dippers may benefit of antihypertensive treatment based on "chronotherapeutic" approach. This consists in the administration of one or more drugs at bedtime in order to restore the physiological nighttime BP decline. This approach has been tested in a pilot uncontrolled study, in which one antihypertensive drug was switched to bedtime in 32 CKD non-dipper patients [36]. ABPM was repeated at 8 weeks, and 28 of the 32 subjects became dippers. Noteworthy, restoring the normal nocturnal dip allowed a significant reduction of proteinuria [36]. More recently, a randomized controlled open-label crossover trial was performed in 147 former subjects from the AASK study with average GFR of 45 mL/min/1.73 m^2 with 76% patients being non-dipper. This study did not confirm a significant BP reduction at night when either one antihypertensive drug or all drugs were administered bedtime as compared with administration of therapy in the morning [37]; these results suggest that effectiveness of chronotherapy may not apply to all ethnic groups. Finally, a randomized trial tested effectiveness of chronotherapy in 661 CKD patients (66% non-dippers at baseline) and reported a surprising 65% reduction in the relative risk of the composite endpoint of death or CV events [38]. The strongly positive outcomes of this study are encouraging, but caution must be exercised. Indeed, some methodological aspects of this study (the open-label treatment for practitioners and the lack of specific algorithm used to manage BP during the follow-up) raise concerns that the positive outcomes associated with the bedtime dosing were not because of the intervention itself but because of a bias in treatment.

These issues assume greater importance in CKD with RH that represent a cluster of patients where cardio-renal risk is particularly high.

Resistant Hypertension: Definition, Cause, and Epidemiology

Hypertension is defined "resistant" (RH) when BP levels persist above the therapeutic target, despite the use of at least three antihypertensive drugs at full dose, including the diuretic, or when BP is at target, but four or more antihypertensive agents are prescribed [39, 40]. Although the exact prevalence is unknown, several observational studies suggest that RH is a common clinical problem in general population [41–46], accounting for about 9% of hypertensive patients, and this prevalence increases to 13% when only treated patients are considered [41].

RH may be caused by biological-behavioral factors (such as smoking and obesity), drugs (NSAIDs, sympathomimetics, steroids, and cyclosporine) or exogenous substances (cocaine, amphetamines, oral contraceptive hormones, liquorice, ginseng, etc.), and secondary causes of hypertension (parenchymal and vascular renal disease, primary hyperaldosteronism, sleep apnea, pheochromocytoma, Cushing's syndrome, thyroid diseases, etc.).

Pseudoresistance

Before defining the hypertensive patient as resistant, it is mandatory to exclude the so-called pseudoresistance [39, 40]. This condition, which refers to the "apparent" failure to reach BP target despite the prescription of an appropriate antihypertensive treatment, can be dependent on factors influencing either drug therapy or BP measurement, the two essential parameters required for RH diagnosis. Poor adherence of patients to antihypertensive therapy is a critical aspect to ascertain when diagnosing RH, as suggested by several studies reporting very high discontinuation rate of drugs in hypertensive patients [47, 48]. A further critical aspect is the "therapeutic inertia," that is, the provider's failure to modify therapy despite recognition that treatment goals are unmet [49, 50]. Despite guidelines for patients with CKD having repeatedly highlighted the importance of lowering BP [2, 51, 52], control rates of hypertension remain largely unsatisfactory, in nephrology as non-nephrology setting [53–58]. Poor achievement of BP goal in CKD patients may be due to resistance to antihypertensive treatment, but it is important to underline that uncontrolled hypertension is not equivalent of RH; indeed, a patient cannot be classified as having RH if he/she is not challenged with an adequate number of drugs including a diuretic at a dose correctly up-titrated with GFR worsening. On this regard, a retrospective study in hypertensive CKD patients newly referred to one renal clinic reported that the increment in full-dose antihypertensive medications and diuretic therapy increased the diagnosis of RH from 26% on referral to 38% at month 6 [59]. Therefore, reducing clinical inertia allows to properly reveal the frequency of RH whose identification is clinically meaningful being associated with adverse outcome (see below).

Inadequate assessment of BP represents the second determinant of pseudoresistance. Improper office BP measurement technique contributes to the occurrence of pseudoresistance by producing falsely high BP readings as it occurs when some recommended rules are not followed (leave the patient in a quiet room for at least 5 min; avoid smoking, caffeine, and exercise in the 30 min before measurement; obtain 2–3 readings; use appropriate cuff size). Furthermore, the presence of arteriosclerotic and calcified arteries, usually occurring in elderly individuals, can also result in office BP overestimation leading in turn to a false diagnosis of RH [39, 40]. More important, the presence of WCH is a further cause of pseudoresistance. In the large Spanish ABP registry, among the 68,045 patients examined, 12% were diagnosed as RH; however, after ABP monitoring, as many as 37% of RH patients were identified as pseudoresistant [60]. A multivariable analysis identified older age, female gender, shorter duration of hypertension, non-smoking, absence of diabetes, more preserved renal function, and negative history of previous CV disease as significant demographic and clinical conditions in which it is more likely to detect pseudoresistance [60]. This issue holds even more true in CKD where WCH is common [20, 21, 26, 29, 35]. With this background, we recently explored the phenomenon of pseudoresistance and true (ABPM verified) resistance in a cohort of 436 hypertensive patients with nondialysis CKD under regular nephrology care. Patients were classified according to 24-h ABP normal (<125/75 mmHg) or high (≥125 mmHg and/or ≥75 mmHg) and the absence or presence of RH (office BP ≥ 130/80 mmHg on 3 full-dose drugs including a diuretic agent or any office BP if the patient was taking four drugs) [61]. In this CKD cohort, 30% of patients (131/436) were diagnosed as resistant on the basis of only clinical BP measurements; however, combining the information derived from ABP with RH status, we found that among patients classified as RH, pseudoresistance (WCH in RH patients) involved about one patient out of four (31/131, 24%). This prevalence is lower than that reported in hypertensive patients (39%) [62].

Notably, the assessment of ABP monitoring allows disclosing a prevalence of "true" RH in about a quarter of CKD patients (100/436) that corresponds to a prevalence three times greater than that reported in essential hypertension (~8%) [60]. As illustrated in Fig. 4.2, the prevalence of true RH increased in the

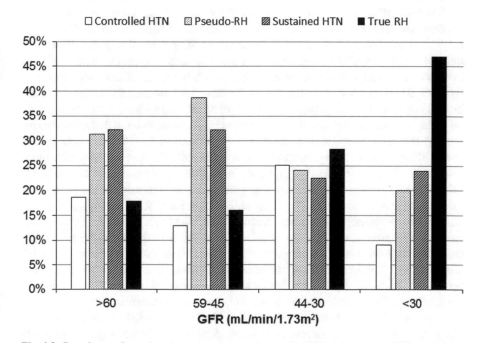

Fig. 4.2 Prevalence of pseudoresistance and true resistance in CKD patients over CKD stages [61]

more advanced CKD stages, whereas pseudoresistance is typically encountered in early stages of CKD and virtually disappeared in advanced CKD [61].

Resistant Hypertension in CKD

Keeping in mind that CKD is at the same time cause [53, 54, 63, 64] and complication [65] of poorly controlled hypertension, the evaluation of RH in CKD patients is highly relevant. In this population, in fact, RH is a common finding as testified by several studies reporting a prevalence ranging from 30% to 42% (Table 4.3) [41, 59, 61, 66–69]. Interestingly, based on these studies, we can state that CKD is one cause of RH in the general hypertensive population but, at the same time, that not all CKD patients have RH. Prevalence of RH progressively increases with worsening of renal function and with increasing urinary excretion of albumin [66]. However, these estimates are partially confounded by the phenomenon of pseudoresistance (which overestimates the prevalence of RH) and by the occurrence of clinical inertia, which underestimates the RH frequency. The large prevalence among CKD patients may be explained not only by the large burden of hypertension in this population but also by the coexistence of pathogenetic factors, such as sodium retention, overexpression of the renin-angiotensin-aldosterone system (RAAS), and enhanced activity of the sympathetic nervous system, that may explain the poor response to the treatment [70]. The main disorder in CKD is the salt and water retention, occurring in the majority of patients with low glomerular filtration rate (GFR). The resulting increase of the extracellular volume (ECV), which allows preserving the external balance of sodium, has the harmful trade-off of the development of persistent (and often refractory) hypertension. In these patients, the entity of ECV expansion is directly dependent on the degree of GFR impairment and corresponds to approximately 5–10% of body weight, even in the absence of peripheral edema [71]. Of note, the salt sensitivity of BP is not a feature limited to the advanced stages of renal disease, but begins before the development of clear hypertension and severe GFR decline [72, 73]. The fact that sodium excretion is commonly impaired in renal patients may also explain the large prevalence of nocturnal hypertension in CKD as compared to essential hypertension [74]. Furthermore, in CKD patients, systemic hypertension is also in part sustained by the RAAS, which is inappropriately activated when considering the ECV expansion. The ensuing glomerular hypertension leads to the progressive kidney damage in the long term. Therefore, RAAS inhibition is the cornerstone of the nephroprotective treatment in CKD [71]. The evaluation of clinical features associated with the presence of true RH allows physicians to identify patients who may benefit from intensive BP monitoring including out-of-office BP assessment and early therapeutic. Clinical correlates of true RH in CKD are diabetes, left ventricular hypertrophy, proteinuria, and poor adherence to low-salt diet. Each of these factors independently increases by two- to threefold the probability of having true RH [61]. Among individuals with CKD enrolled in the Reasons for Geographic and Racial Differences in Stroke (REGARDS) study, higher prevalence

Table 4.3 Prevalence of apparent resistant hypertension (aRH) in CKD patients

Authors [ref.]	Data collection (years)	Patients	Participants (N)	CKD patients	aRH (%)
Persell [41]	2003–2008	General population	3710	3710 (19.9%)	24.7
Tanner [66]	2003–2009	General population	10,700	3134 (29.3%)	28.1
Hung [69]	2000–2010	Hypertensives from insurance database	111,986	2894 (2.6%)	24.8
Sim [68]	2006–2010	Hypertensives from insurance database	470,386	122,300 (26%)	22.0
De Nicola [59]	2002–2006	CKD	300	300 (100%)	38.0
De Nicola [61]	2003–2005	CKD	436	436 (100%)	30.0*
Muntner [67]	2003–2007	CKD	3612	3612 (100%)	42.3
De Beus [77]	2004–2010	CKD	788	788 (100%)	34.1

*After excluding patients with pseudoresistance by detecting white coat hypertension through ABPM, the prevalence of RH ("true RH") declined to 22.9%

of RH was detected in men, blacks, individuals with large waist circumferences, diabetes, and individuals with a history of stroke or myocardial infarction [66].

Prognostic Meaning of RH in CKD

RH increases the risk of renal damage in the general population and worsens the cardio-renal prognosis of patient with overt renal damage [68]. In the setting of essential hypertension, the presence of mild-to-moderate GFR reduction and/or microalbuminuria amplifies the cardiovascular risk correlated to RH [68, 75, 76].

In the first study exploring the prognostic role of RH in CKD patients, we reported that RH (diagnosis not verified by means of ABPM) was associated with greater risk of renal death (HR, 1.85, 95% CI, 1.13–3.03), independently from main clinical features and degree of BP control [59]. More recently, in a cohort of 788 CKD patients, de Beus et al. confirmed the increase of risk of renal and CV outcomes associated with RH [77]. However, the main limitation of these studies targeting the role of RH in CKD patients is the lack of out-of-office BP measurement, which does not allow an accurate estimate of BP load and cannot exclude the white coat effect (pseudoresistance).

This issue has been addressed in a cohort study including 436 CKD patients in which BP was assessed concurrently by ABPM and office measurement in order to correctly classify resistant patients as having pseudoresistance and true RH [61].

During 57 months of follow-up, we recorded 165 renal events (death, ESRD, or transplantation) and 109 fatal and nonfatal CV events. Patients with normal ABP had the best prognosis for either outcome independently from the RH status, whereas the highest risk for cardio-renal events was observed only in true resistance. After adjustment for confounders, true resistance predicted CV and renal risk, while sustained hypertension (ABP above the goal without RH) associated only with renal outcome (Fig. 4.3). Of note, pseudoresistant patients were not exposed to higher cardio-renal risk [61]. These findings are clinically relevant as these highlight the need to identify pseudoresistant CKD patients by ABPM to avoid aggressive and potentially harmful antihypertensive therapy. Indeed, these patients were characterized by systolic BP levels during daytime, and especially at nighttime, close to the threshold limit of hypoperfusion (100 mmHg). Under these circumstances, a tighter control of BP merely based on the detection of elevated BP in office may expose patients to ischemia-induced worsening of cardio-renal damage [78] and eventually convert their prognosis from favorable to unfavorable.

The mechanisms underlying the different prognostic value of RH are not readily apparent; however, we can hypothesize that persistence of hypertension despite optimal antihypertensive treatment specifically identifies patients with more severe vascular damage. The abovementioned correlates of true resistance (diabetes, left ventricular hypertrophy, higher proteinuria, and high salt intake) are in fact all associated with endothelial dysfunction and arterial stiffness [79–82]. In particular, proteinuria, rather than GFR, relates to the severity of hypertension [83]. Indeed,

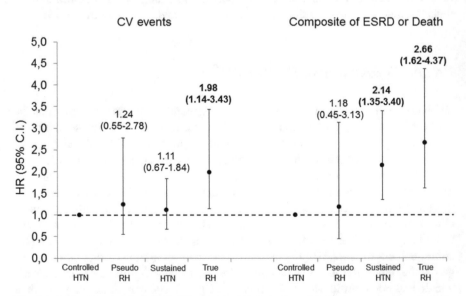

Fig. 4.3 Risk of fatal and nonfatal CV events and dialysis therapy initiation or all-cause death for each of four groups identified by ABPM and RH: true normotension (controlled HTN), pseudoresistance (pseudo RH), sustained hypertension (sustained HTN), and true resistance (true RH) [61]. Model is adjusted for age, sex, BMI, diabetes, history of cardiovascular disease, natural log-transformed 24-h proteinuria, and GFR [61]

although low GFR is recognized as a CV risk factor [84], proteinuria is considered a better marker of the presence of vascular disease in CKD patients [85].

Treatment of RH in CKD Patients

In CKD patients with RH, the cornerstone of therapy is certainly represented by the restriction of sodium intake [86]. However, this dietary measure is implemented only in about 20% of the CKD population at large regularly followed in nephrology clinics [87–89]. Interestingly, we found higher levels of sodium intake in RH patients (164 ± 68 mmol/day) compared to controls (141 ± 49 mmol/day), and consequently the adherence to low-salt diet resulted poorer in RH (14.1%) as compared to patients without RH (26.3%; $P = 0.026$) [61, 90]. This is a paradoxical condition if one considers that CKD is typically characterized by high salt sensitivity [91]. More important, a small randomized crossover trial of dietary salt restriction in patients with RH but without CKD has demonstrated that low-salt diet remarkably decreased office systolic and diastolic BP (by 23 and 9 mmHg, respectively) and 24-h BP from 150/82 to 130/72 mmHg [92]. This antihypertensive effect of dietary sodium restriction may occur directly through a correction of volume expansion and indirectly by enhancing the antihypertensive effects of RAAS inhibitors [93]. Table 4.4 reports some practical suggestions to help patients in reducing their dietary sodium intake. These recommendations should be implemented by patients over a period of 2–4 months in order to give them the time to adapt their taste receptor cells to the lower saltiness.

RH definition is based on the presence of a diuretic, while type and dose of these agents are not mentioned. While this is not a major issue in essential hypertension, selecting the class of diuretic and the correct dose becomes critical in CKD patients. Indeed, if patients with mild renal impairment (GFR >40 mL/min/1.73 m²) may respond to thiazide diuretics, those with more advanced CKD require the use of loop diuretics and doses must be titrated to the reduced GFR [86, 94]. In a clinical

Table 4.4 Practical recommendations to restrict sodium intake

1. Look for the amount of sodium on food labels
2. Abolish salt-containing condiments (e.g., ketchup, mayonnaise, mustard, barbecue sauce)
3. Move the salt shaker away from the table
4. Cook pasta, rice, and cereals without salt (add in smaller amount directly on cooked food)
5. In cooking and at the table, increase the use of spices (e.g., herbs, lemon, vinegar, hot pepper)
6. Look for low-salt bread
7. Look for fresh or plain frozen foods
8. Avoid frozen dinners, canned soups, packaged mixes, cured meat and fish (e.g., ham, bacon, salami, anchovies, salmon)
9. Choose fresh rather than seasoned cheese
10. Rinse canned foods (e.g., tuna, legumes) to remove some sodium contained as additives
11. Abolish salty snack foods (e.g., chips, nuts, crackers)

trial performed in patients with GFR in the range 10–40 mL/min, correction of volume expansion (evidenced by body weight reduction of 2.0 kg coupled with a marked reduction in BP) was safely induced by oral administration of furosemide at doses inversely proportional to GFR level (1.0, 2.5, and 4.0 mg/kg body weight per day in patients with GFRs of 40–31, 30–20, and 19–10 mL/min, respectively) [95]. Therefore, to improve the modalities of treatment, it is helpful to start diuretic treatment with a low dose that can be progressively increased if body weight does not decrease (the goal is weight loss of 0.5 kg/day). The lack of a significant body weight reduction with increasing diuretic doses likely suggests the presence of diuretic resistance that can be overcome by adding other agents (such as metolazone) in order to limit the breaking phenomenon (sodium over-reabsorption in the distal tubule) [96]. Disappointingly enough, nephrologists are today still reluctant to use adequately loop diuretics in their hypertensive CKD patients. This erroneous attitude cannot be justified by the fear of side effects, which are infrequent, usually reversible and predictable when the patient is regularly followed [97].

A further diuretic agent successfully tested in RH patients is spironolactone based on the finding that plasma aldosterone levels are higher in patients with RH than in those with controlled hypertension [98]. Efficacy of spironolactone has been evidenced in 175 patients with true RH and normal renal function when treated with doses of 25–100 mg/day and prospectively followed for 1 year [99]. The main finding of the study was a significant and marked reduction of 24-h systolic and diastolic BP (16 and 9 mmHg, respectively) persisting up to 15 months, without difference in the entity of daytime and nighttime decline. More important, the antihypertensive effects of spironolactone have been evaluated in a randomized, controlled, double-blind study carried out in 117 patients with RH. Spironolactone was administered at doses of 25 mg/day for 8 weeks in addition to the preexisting therapy. At the end of 8 weeks of the study, systolic BP (measured in and out office) was significantly reduced in treated patients in the absence of adverse effects [100]. However, assessment of spironolactone efficacy has not been tested in patients with CKD that is a condition associated with higher risk of hyperkalemia.

Conclusions

RH is a common condition in CKD due to a combination of factors including sodium retention and enhanced neurohumoral activity. However, the higher prevalence of WCH in CKD patients likely makes mandatory out-of-office monitoring in order to distinguish between pseudoresistance and true RH. Therefore, a greater use of ABPM in CKD patients is desirable in the attempt of limiting the misclassification of hypertensive status and thus avoiding unnecessary aggressive antihypertensive medication. Catheter-based radiofrequency ablation of the renal sympathetic nerves has been proposed, but the inconclusive results provided so far and the lack of long-term data on its efficacy and safety do not recommend the use of renal denervation for treatment of RH in routine clinical practice [101]. More efforts are required to nephrologists to improve adherence to pharmacological therapy, expand the use of low-salt diet, and correctly prescribe diuretic therapy. These strategies, being probably more effective than renal denervation [102], must be considered as the first-choice therapeutic approach for controlling RH in CKD patients.

References

1. O'Brien E, Parati G, Stergiou G, et al.; for the European Society of Hypertension Working Group on Blood Pressure Monitoring. European Society of Hypertension position paper on ambulatory blood pressure monitoring. J Hypertens. 2013;31(9):1731–68.
2. Kidney Disease: Improving Global Outcomes (KDIGO) Blood Pressure Work Group. KDIGO clinical practice guideline for the management of blood pressure in chronic kidney disease. Kidney Int Suppl. 2012;2:337–414.
3. Fagard RH, Cornelissen VA. Incidence of cardiovascular events in white-coat, masked and sustained hypertension versus true normotension: a meta-analysis. J Hypertens. 2007; 25(11):2193–8.
4. Hansen TW, Kikuya M, Thijs L, Björklund-Bodegård K, Kuznetsova T, Ohkubo T, et al. Prognostic superiority of daytime ambulatory over conventional blood pressure in four populations: a meta-analysis of 7030 individuals. J Hypertens. 2007;25(8):1554–64.
5. Pierdomenico SD, Cuccurullo F. Prognostic value of white-coat and masked hypertension diagnosed by ambulatory monitoring in initially untreated subjects: an updated meta analysis. Am J Hypertens. 2011;24(1):52–8.
6. Boggia J, Li Y, Thijs L, Hansen TW, Kikuya M, Björklund-Bodegård K, et al. International database on ambulatory blood pressure monitoring in relation to cardiovascular outcomes (IDACO) investigators. Prognostic accuracy of day versus night ambulatory blood pressure: a cohort study. Lancet. 2007;370:1219–29.
7. Hansen TW, Li Y, Boggia J, Thijs L, Richart T, Staessen JA. Predictive role of the nighttime blood pressure. Hypertension. 2011;57:3–10.
8. Upadhyay A, Earley A, Haynes SM, Uhlig K. Systematic review: blood pressure target in chronic kidney disease and proteinuria as an effect modifier. Ann Intern Med. 2011; 154:541–8.
9. Lv J, Ehteshami P, Sarnak MJ, et al. Effects of intensive blood pressure lowering on the progression of chronic kidney disease: a systematic review and meta-analysis. CMAJ. 2013;185:949–57.
10. Lv J, Neal B, Ehteshami P, Ninomiya T, Woodward M, Rodgers A, et al. Effects of intensive blood pressure lowering on cardiovascular and renal outcomes: a systematic review and meta-analysis. PLoS Med. 2012;9:e1001293.
11. Borrelli S, De Nicola L, Minutolo R, Sagliocca A, Garofalo C, Liberti ME, et al. Limitations of blood pressure target in non-dialysis chronic kidney disease: a question of method? G Ital Nefrol. 2012;29(4):418–24.
12. Lewis JB. Blood pressure control in chronic kidney disease. Is less really more? J Am Soc Nephrol. 2010;21:1086–92.
13. Agarwal R, Andersen MJ. Prognostic importance of clinic and home blood pressure recordings in patients with chronic kidney disease. Kidney Int. 2006;69:406–11.
14. Gabbai FB, Rahman M, Hu B, Appel LJ, Charleston J, Contreras G, et al. Relationship between ambulatory BP and clinical outcomes in patients with hypertensive CKD. Clin J Am Soc Nephrol. 2012;7(11):1770–6.
15. Minutolo R, Agarwal R, Borrelli S, Chiodini P, Bellizzi V, Nappi F, et al. Prognostic role of ambulatory blood pressure monitoring in patients with nondialysis CKD. Arch Intern Med. 2011;171(12):1090–8.

54   S. Borrelli et al.

16. Agarwal R, Andersen MJ. Prognostic importance of ambulatory blood pressure recordings in patients with chronic kidney disease. Kidney Int. 2006;69(7):1175–80.
17. Minutolo R, Gabbai FB, Chiodini P, Garofalo C, Stanzione G, Liberti ME, et al. Reassessment of ambulatory blood pressure improves renal risk stratification in nondialysis chronic kidney disease: long-term cohort study. Hypertension. 2015;66(3):557–62.
18. Pickering TG, James GD, Boddie C, Harshfield GA, Blank S, Laragh JH. How common is white coat hypertension? JAMA. 1988;259(2):225–8.
19. Pickering TG, Davidson K, Gerin W, Schwartz JE. Masked hypertension. Hypertension. 2002;40(6):795–6.
20. Bangash F, Agarwal R. Masked hypertension and white coat hypertension in chronic kidney disease: a meta-analysis. Clin J Am Soc Nephrol. 2009;4(3):656–64.
21. Gorostidi M, Sarafidis PA, de la Sierra A, Segura J, de la Cruz JJ, Banegas JR, et al.; for Spanish ABPM Registry Investigators. Differences between office and 24-hour blood pressure control in hypertensive patients with CKD: a 5,693-patient cross-sectional analysis from Spain. Am J Kidney Dis. 2013;62(2):285–94.
22. Andersen MJ, Khawandi W, Agarwal R. Home blood pressure monitoring in CKD. Am J Kidney Dis. 2005;45(6):994–1001.
23. Minutolo R, Gabbai FB, Agarwal R, Chiodini P, Borrelli S, Bellizzi V, et al. Assessment of achieved clinic and ambulatory blood pressure recordings and outcomes during treatment in hypertensive patients with CKD: a multicenter prospective cohort study. Am J Kidney Dis. 2014;64(5):744–52.
24. Iimuro S, Imai E, Watanabe T, et al.; for the Chronic Kidney Disease Japan Cohort Study Group. Clinical correlates of ambulatory BP monitoring among patients with CKD. Clin J Am Soc Nephrol. 2013;8(5):721–30.
25. Wang C, Gong WY, Zhang J, Peng H, Tang H, Liu X, Ye ZC, Lou T. Disparate assessment of clinic blood pressure and ambulatory blood pressure in differently aged patients with chronic kidney disease. Int J Cardiol. 2015;183:54–62.
26. Minutolo R, Borrelli S, Scigliano R, Bellizzi V, Chiodini P, Cianciaruso B, et al. Prevalence and clinical correlates of white coat hypertension in chronic kidney disease. Nephrol Dial Transplant. 2007;22:2217–23.
27. Agarwal R, Pappas MK, Sinha AD. Masked uncontrolled hypertension in CKD. J Am Soc Nephrol. 2016;27:924–32.
28. Pogue VA, Rahman M, Lipkowitz M, et al.; for African American Study of Kidney Disease and Hypertension Collaborative Research Group. Disparate estimates of hypertension control from ambulatory and clinic blood pressure measurements in hypertensive kidney disease. Hypertension. 2009;53(1):20–7.
29. Minutolo R, Borrelli S, Chiodini P, Scigliano R, Bellizzi V, Cianciaruso B, et al. Effects of age on hypertensive status in patients with chronic kidney disease. J Hypertens. 2007;11:2325–33.
30. Fagard RH, Staessen JA, Thijs L, Gasowski J, Bulpitt CJ, Clement D, et al.; for the Systolic Hypertension in Europe (Syst-Eur) Trial Investigators. Response to antihypertensive therapy in older patients with sustained and nonsustained systolic hypertension. Circulation. 2000;102(10):1139–44.
31. The SPRINT Research Group. A randomized trial of intensive versus standard blood-pressure control. N Engl J Med. 2015;373:2103–16.
32. Effect of Intense vs. Standard Hypertension Management on Nighttime Blood Pressure – an Ancillary Study to SPRINT. ClinicalTrials.gov. Identifier: NCT01835249.
33. Sinha AD, Agarwal R. The complex relationship between CKD and ambulatory blood pressure patterns. Adv Chronic Kidney Dis. 2015;22:102–7.
34. Fagard RH, Celis H, Thijs L, Staessen JA, Clement DL, De Buyzere ML, De Bacquer DA, et al. Daytime and nighttime blood pressure as predictors of death and cause-specific cardiovascular events in hypertension. Hypertension. 2008;51(1):55–61.
35. Agarwal R, Andersen MJ. Blood pressure recordings within and outside the clinic and cardiovascular events in chronic kidney disease. Am J Nephrol. 2006;26(5):503–10.

36. Minutolo R, Borrelli S, Chiodini P, Scigliano R, Trucillo P, Baldanza D, et al. Changing the timing of antihypertensive therapy to reduce nocturnal blood pressure in CKD: an 8-week uncontrolled trial. Am J Kidney Dis. 2007;50(6):908–17.
37. Rahman M, Greene T, Phillips RA, Agodoa LY, Bakris GL, Charleston J, et al. A trial of 2 strategies to reduce nocturnal blood pressure in blacks with chronic kidney disease. Hypertension. 2013;61(1):82–8.
38. Hermida RC, Ayala DE, Mojon A, Fernandez JR. Bedtime dosing of antihypertensive medications reduces cardiovascular risk in CKD. J Am Soc Nephrol. 2011;22(12):2313–21.
39. Calhoun DA, Jones D, Textor S, et al.; American Heart Association Professional Education Committee. Resistant hypertension: diagnosis, evaluation, and treatment: a scientific statement from the American Heart Association Professional Education Committee of the Council for High Blood Pressure Research. Circulation. 2008;117:510–526.
40. Sarafidis PA, Bakris GL. Resistant hypertension: an overview of evaluation and treatment. J Am Coll Cardiol. 2008;52:1749–57.
41. Persell SD. Prevalence of resistant hypertension in the United States, 2003–08. Hypertension. 2011;57:1076–80.
42. Pimenta E, Calhoun DA. Resistant hypertension: incidence, prevalence, and prognosis. Circulation. 2012;125(13):1594–6.
43. Hajjar I, Kotchen TA. Trends in prevalence, awareness, treatment, and control of hypertension in the United States, 1988-2000. JAMA. 2003;290:199–206.
44. ALLHAT Officers and Coordinators for the ALLHAT Collaborative Research Group. The Antihypertensive and Lipid- Lowering Treatment to Prevent Heart Attack Trial. Major outcomes in high-risk hypertensive patients randomized to angiotensin-converting enzyme inhibitor or calcium channel blocker vs diuretic: The Antihypertensive and Lipid-Lowering Treatment to Prevent Heart Attack Trial (ALLHAT). JAMA. 2002;288:2981–97.
45. Sarafidis PA, Georgianos P, Bakris GL. Resistant hypertension its identification and epidemiology. Nat Rev Nephrol. 2012;9(1):51–8.
46. Moser M, Setaro JF. Clinical practice. Resistant or difficult to control hypertension. N Engl J Med. 2006;355:385–92.
47. Mazzaglia G, Mantovani LG, Sturkenboom MC, Filippi A, Trifirò G, Cricelli C, et al. Patterns of persistence with antihypertensive medications in newly diagnosed hypertensive patients in Italy: a retrospective cohort study in primary care. J Hypertens. 2005;23:2093–100.
48. Vrijens B, Vincze G, Kristanto P, Urquhart J, Burnier M. Adherence to prescribed antihypertensive drug treatments: longitudinal study of electronically compiled dosing histories. BMJ. 2008;336:1114–7.
49. Phillips LS, Branch WT, Cook CB, Doyle JP, El-Kebbi IM, Gallina DL, Miller CD, Ziemer DC, Barnes CS. Clinical inertia. Ann Intern Med. 2001;135:825–34.
50. Berlowitz DR, Ash AS, Hickey EC, Friedman RH, Glickman M, Kader B, Moskowitz MA. Inadequate management of blood pressure in a hypertensive population. N Engl J Med. 1998;339:1957–63.
51. James PA, Oparil S, Carter BL, Cushman WC, Dennison-Himmelfarb C, Handler J, et al. 2014 evidence-based guideline for the management of high blood pressure in adults: report from the panel members appointed to the Eighth Joint National Committee (JNC 8). JAMA. 2014;311(5):507–20.
52. ESH/ESC Task Force for the Management of Arterial Hypertension. 2013 practice guidelines for the management of arterial hypertension of the European Society of Hypertension (ESH) and the European Society of Cardiology (ESC): ESH/ESC task force for the Management of Arterial Hypertension. J Hypertens. 2013;31(10):1925–38.
53. De Nicola L, Chiodini P, Zoccali C, Borrelli S, Cianciaruso B, Di Iorio B, et al. Prognosis of CKD patients receiving outpatient nephrology care in Italy. Clin J Am Soc Nephrol. 2011;6(10):2421–8.
54. De Nicola L, Borrelli S, Chiodini P, Zamboli P, Iodice C, Gabbai FB, et al. Hypertension management in chronic kidney disease: translating guidelines into daily practice. J Nephrol. 2011;24(6):733–41.

55. Marín R, Fernández-Vega F, Gorostidi M, et al. COPARENAL (COntrol de la hiPertensión Arterial en Pacientes con Insuficiencia RENAL) study investigators. Blood pressure control in patients with chronic renal insufficiency in Spain: a cross-sectional study. J Hypertens. 2006;24:395–402.
56. Stevens PE, O'Donoghue DJ, de Lusignans S, Van Vlymen J, Klebe B, Middleton R, et al. Chronic kidney disease management in the United Kingdom: NEOERICA project results. Kidney Int. 2007;72:92–9.
57. Minutolo R, De Nicola L, Zamboli P, Chiodini P, Signoriello G, Toderico C, et al. Management of hypertension in patients with CKD: differences between primary and tertiary care settings. Am J Kidney Dis. 2005;46:18–25.
58. Minutolo R, Sasso FC, Chiodini P, Cianciaruso B, Carbonara O, Zamboli P, et al. Management of cardiovascular risk factors in advanced type 2 diabetic nephropathy: a comparative analysis in nephrology, diabetology and primary care settings. J Hypertens. 2006;24:1655–61.
59. De Nicola L, Borrelli S, Gabbai FB, Chiodini P, Zamboli P, Iodice C, et al. Burden of resistant hypertension in hypertensive patients with non-dialysis chronic kidney disease. Kidney Blood Press Res. 2011;34(1):58–67.
60. de la Sierra A, Segura J, Banegas JR, Gorostidi M, de la Cruz JJ, Armario P, et al. Clinical features of 8295 patients with resistant hypertension classified on the basis of ambulatory blood pressure monitoring. Hypertension. 2011;57:898–902.
61. De Nicola L, Gabbai FB, Agarwal R, Chiodini P, Borrelli S, Bellizzi V, et al. Prevalence and prognostic role of resistant hypertension in Chronic Kidney Disease. J Am Coll Cardiol. 2013;61(24):2461–7.
62. Salles GF, Cardoso CR, Muxfeldt ES. Prognostic influence of office and ambulatory blood pressures in resistant hypertension. Arch Intern Med. 2008;168(21):2340–6.
63. Jha V, Garcia-Garcia G, Iseki K, Li Z, Naicker S, Plattner B, et al. Chronic kidney disease: global dimension and perspectives. Lancet. 2013;382(9888):260–72.
64. Klag MJ, Whelton PK, Randall BL, Neaton JD, Brancati FL, Ford CE, et al. Blood pressure and end-stage renal disease in men. N Engl J Med. 1996;334(1):13–8.
65. Garofalo C, Borrelli S, Pacilio M, Minutolo R, Chiodini P, De Nicola L, Conte G. Hypertension and prehypertension and prediction of development of decreased estimated GFR in the general population: a meta-analysis of cohort studies. Am J Kidney Dis. 2016;67:89–97.
66. Tanner RM, Calhoun DA, Bell EK, et al. Prevalence of apparent treatment-resistant hypertension among individuals with CKD. Clin J Am Soc Nephrol. 2013;8:1583–90.
67. Muntner P, Anderson A, Charleston J, Chen Z, Ford V, Makos G, et al.; the Chronic Renal Insufficiency Cohort (CRIC) Study Investigators. Hypertension awareness, treatment, and control in adults with CKD: results from the Chronic Renal Insufficiency Cohort (CRIC) Study. Am J Kidney Dis. 2010; 55:441–451.
68. Sim JJ, Bhandari SK, Shi J. Reynolds K2, Calhoun DA3, Kalantar-Zadeh K4, Jacobsen SJ. Comparative risk of renal, cardiovascular, and mortality outcomes in controlled, uncontrolled resistant, and nonresistant hypertension. Kidney Int. 2015;88(3):622–32.
69. Hung CY, Wang KY, Wu TJ, Hsieh YC, Huang JL, Loh EW, Lin CH. Resistant hypertension, patient characteristics, and risk of stroke. PLoS One. 2014;9(8):e104362.
70. Campese VM, Mitra N, Sandee D. Hypertension in renal parenchymal disease: why is it so resistant to treatment? Kidney Int. 2006;69:967–73.
71. De Nicola L, Minutolo R, Bellizzi V, Zoccali C, Cianciaruso B, Andreucci VE, et al. Investigators of the Target Blood Pressure Levels in Chronic Kidney Disease (TABLE in CKD) Study Group. Achievement of target blood pressure levels in chronic kidney disease: a salty question? Am J Kidney Dis. 2004;43:782–95.
72. Cianciaruso B, Bellizzi V, Minutolo R, Colucci G, Bisesti V, Russo D, et al. Renal adaptation to dietary sodium restriction in moderate renal failure resulting from chronic glomerular disease. J Am Soc Nephrol. 1996;7(2):306–13.
73. Konishi Y, Okada N, Okamura M, Morikawa T, Okumura M, Yoshioka K, Imanishi M. Sodium sensitivity of blood pressure appearing before hypertension and related to histological damage in IgA nephropathy. Hypertension. 2001;38(1):81–5.

74. Sachdeva A. WederAB: nocturnal sodium excretion, blood pressure dipping and sodium sensitivity. Hypertension. 2006;48:527–33.
75. Salles GF, Cardoso CR, Pereira VS, Fiszman R, Muxfeldt ES. Prognostic significance of a reduced glomerular filtration rate and interaction with microalbuminuria in resistant hypertension: a cohort study. J Hypertens. 2011;29:2014–23.
76. Salles G, Cardoso C, Fiszman R, Muxfeldt E. Prognostic importance of baseline and serial changes in microalbuminuria in patients with resistant hypertension. Atherosclerosis. 2011;216:199–204.
77. de Beus E, Bots ML, van Zuilen AD, Wetzels JF, Blankestijn PJ, MASTERPLAN Study Group. Prevalence of apparent therapy-resistant hypertension and its effect on outcome in patients with chronic kidney disease. Hypertension. 2015;66(5):998–1005.
78. Palmer BF. Renal dysfunction complicating the treatment of hypertension. N Engl J Med. 2002;347(16):1256–61.
79. Christen AI, Armentano RL, Miranda A, Graf S, Santana DB, Zócalo Y, et al. Arterial wall structure and dynamics in type 2 diabetes mellitus methodological aspects and pathophysiological findings. Curr Diabetes Rev. 2010;6:367–77.
80. Weir MR, Townsend RR, Fink JC, Teal V, Anderson C, Appel L, et al. Hemodynamic correlates of proteinuria in chronic kidney disease. Clin J Am Soc Nephrol. 2011;6:2403–10.
81. Sanders PW. Vascular consequences of dietary salt intake. Am J Physiol Renal Physiol. 2009;297:F237–43.
82. Sarnak MJ, Levey AS, Schoolwerth AC, Coresh J, Culleton B, Hamm LL, et al. Kidney disease as a risk factor for development of cardiovascular disease: a statement from the American Heart Association Councils on Kidney in Cardiovascular Disease, High Blood Pressure Research, Clinical Cardiology, and Epidemiology and Prevention. Hypertension. 2003; 42(5):1050–65.
83. Agarwal R, Light RP. GFR, proteinuria and circadian blood pressure. Nephrol Dial Transplant. 2009;24(8):2400–6.
84. De Zeeuw D, Remuzzi G, Parving HH, Keane WF, Zhang Z, Shahinfar S, et al. Albuminuria, a therapeutic target for cardiovascular protection in type 2 diabetic patients with nephropathy. Circulation. 2004;110(8):921–7.
85. Hemmelgarn BR, Manns BJ, Lloyd A, James MT, Klarenbach S, Quinn RR, Wiebe N, Tonelli M. Alberta kidney disease network. Relation between kidney function, proteinuria, and adverse outcomes. JAMA. 2010;303(5):423–9.
86. De Nicola L, Minutolo R, Bellizzi V, Zoccali C, Cianciaruso B, Andreucci VE, et al. Achievement of target blood pressure levels in chronic kidney disease: a salty question? Am J Kidney Dis. 2004;43(5):782–95.
87. De Nicola L, Minutolo R, Gallo C, Zoccali C, Cianciaruso B, Conte M, et al. Management of hypertension in chronic kidney disease: the Italian multicentric study. J Nephrol. 2005; 18(4):397–404.
88. De Nicola L, Conte G, Chiodini P, D'Angiò P, Donnarumma G, Minutolo R. Interaction between phosphorus and parathyroid hormone in non-dialysis CKD patients under nephrology care. J Nephrol. 2014;27(1):57–63.
89. De Nicola L, Provenzano M, Chiodini P, Borrelli S, Garofalo C, Pacilio M, et al. Independent role of underlying kidney disease on renal prognosis of patients with chronic kidney disease under nephrology care. PLoS One. 2015;10(5):e0127071.
90. Borrelli S, De Nicola L, Stanzione G, Conte G, Minutolo R. Resistant hypertension in non-dialysis chronic kidney disease. Int J Hypertens. 2013;2013:929183.
91. Koomans HA, Roose JC, Mees EJD, Delawi IMK. Sodium balance in renal failure: a comparison with normal subjects under extremes of sodium intake. Hypertension. 1985; 7(5):714–21.
92. Pimenta E, Gaddam KK, Oparil S, Aban I, Husain S, Dell'Italia LJ, Calhoun DA. Effects of dietary sodium reduction on blood pressure in subjects with resistant hypertension: results from a randomized trial. Hypertension. 2009;54(3):475–81.

93. Slagman MCJ, Waanders F, Hemmelder MH, Woittiez AJ, Janssen WM, Lambers Heerspink HJ, et al. Moderate dietary sodium restriction added to angiotensin converting enzyme inhibition compared with dual blockade in lowering proteinuria and blood pressure: randomised controlled trial. BMJ. 2011;343:d4366.
94. Rose BD. Diuretics. Kidney Int. 1991;39(2):336–52.
95. Dal Canton A, Fuiano G, Conte G, Terribile M, Sabbatini M, Cianciaruso B, Andreucci VE. Mechanism of increased plasma urea after diuretic therapy in uraemic patients. Clin Sci. 1985;68(3):255–61.
96. Fliser D, Schröter M, Neubeck M, Ritz E. Coadministration of thiazides increases the efficacy of loop diuretics even in patients with advanced renal failure. Kidney Int. 1994; 46(2):482–8.
97. Moser M. Why are physicians not prescribing diuretics more frequently in the management of hypertension? JAMA. 1998;279(22):1813–6.
98. Gaddam KK, Nishizaka MK, Pratt-Ubunama MN, Pimenta E, Aban I, Oparil S, Calhoun DA. Characterization of resistant hypertension: association between resistant hypertension, aldosterone, and persistent intravascular volume expansion. Arch Intern Med. 2008;168(11): 1159–64.
99. de Souza F, Muxfeldt E, Fiszman R, Salles G. Efficacy of spironolactone therapy in patients with true resistant hypertension. Hypertension. 2010;55:147–52.
100. Vaclavík J, Sedlak R, Plachy M, Navrátil K, Plásek J, Jarkovsky J, et al. Addition of spironolactone in patients with resistant arterial hypertension (ASPIRANT): a randomized, double-blind, placebo-controlled trial. Hypertension. 2011;57:1069–75.
101. Lobo MD, de Belder MA, Cleveland T, Collier D, Dasgupta I, Deanfield J, et al.; British Hypertension Society; British Cardiovascular Society; British Cardiovascular Intervention Society; Renal Association. Joint UK societie' 2014 consensus statement on renal denervation for resistant hypertension. Heart. 2015;101:10–16.
102. Fadl Elmula FE, Hoffmann P, Larstorp AC, Fossum E, Brekke M, Kjeldsen SE, et al. Adjusted drug treatment is superior to renal sympathetic denervation in patients with true treatment-resistant hypertension. Hypertension. 2014;63(5):991–9.

Chapter 5
Resistant Hypertension and Outcomes in Patients with and Without Chronic Kidney Disease

Aghogho Odudu, Maharajan Raman, and Philip A. Kalra

Introduction

The definitions of aTRH is expanded in other chapters, but we briefly summarize the terminology in Fig. 5.1 and Table 5.1. The American Heart Association reached a consensus to define apparent treatment-resistant hypertension (aTRH) as uncontrolled BP with three or more antihypertensive drugs or requiring four antihypertensive drugs irrespective of BP [5]. Uncontrolled BP is defined as >140/90 mmHg in average-risk populations and >130/80 mmHg in higher-risk populations such as those with chronic kidney disease (CKD) or diabetes. This dual definition of aTRH may describe two overlapping but distinct phenotypes. A recent study reported patients with non-controlled BP had more frequent diabetes (72% vs 49%), higher plasma glucose, and worse lipid profile [6]. Reported prevalence of aTRH varies widely from 3% to 30% of generally hypertensive populations largely due to the extent that pseudoresistance is excluded to define only "true" resistant hypertension (RH). There is also inconsistency in whether the lower BP threshold of 130/80 mmHg that is recommended by some guidelines but not others is used [7, 8]. The prevalence of aTRH has a stepwise increase with declining stages of CKD or degree of albuminuria and has typically double the prevalence compared to matched non-CKD groups [9, 10]. The Chronic Renal Insufficiency Cohort recently reported overall prevalence of ATRH of 40%, rising from 22% to 54% between CKD stages 2 to 4 [11]. Incidence data confirm that CKD is likely a consequence as well as a

A. Odudu
Division of Cardiovascular Sciences, University of Manchester,
Manchester Academic Health Science Centre, Manchester, UK

Department of Renal Medicine, Salford Royal Hospital, Salford, UK

M. Raman • P.A. Kalra (✉)
Department of Renal Medicine, Salford Royal Hospital, Salford, UK
e-mail: Philip.Kalra@srft.nhs.uk

© Springer International Publishing AG 2017
A. Covic et al. (eds.), *Resistant Hypertension in Chronic Kidney Disease*,
DOI 10.1007/978-3-319-56827-0_5

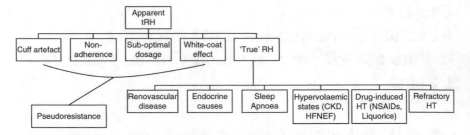

Fig. 5.1 Classification and causes of resistant hypertension. Abbreviations: *CKD* chronic kidney disease, *HT* hypertension, *HFNEF* heart failure with normal ejection fraction, *NSAIDs* nonsteroidal anti-inflammatory drugs, *RH* resistant hypertension, *tRH* treatment-resistant hypertension

cause of aTRH [12]. Table 5.2 summarizes contemporary clinical outcome data for aTRH with and without CKD, and we will describe these studies below.

Clinical Outcomes in Observational Studies of Non-CKD Populations

A prospective observational study of [14] evaluated the prognostic importance of office versus ambulatory BP monitoring (ABPM) in 556 mainly Caucasian patients with aTRH using the previously stated definition. Patients with a mean age of 66 years were enrolled between 1999 and 2004 with a median follow-up of 4.9 years. Drug adherence was assessed as moderate by a standard questionnaire. Patients were also divided into "true" RH or white coat hypertension based on ABPM. One hundred and nine patients (19.6%) reached a composite primary outcome of all-cause mortality, major cardiovascular events, and major renal events (all-cause death, stroke, acute myocardial infarction, myocardial revascularization, new-onset heart failure, sudden death, limb amputation, or initiation of dialysis). When compared to the 447 patients who did not reach the primary outcome, this group had a higher mean serum creatinine of 1.3 ± 0.8 mg/dl ($P < 0.001$), higher ABPM and greater prevalence of true RH (77% vs 57%). Unadjusted survival analysis showed significantly greater cardiovascular events and cardiovascular mortality for true RH compared to white coat hypertension. Multivariable-adjusted survival models showed no prognostic value for any office BP, while higher mean ambulatory BPs were independent predictors of the composite outcome. Ambulatory systolic and diastolic BP were equivalent predictors, and both were better than pulse pressure. Nocturnal BP was superior to daytime BP. The only independent predictor of all-cause mortality was an ABPM diagnosis of true RH. The only significant interaction found was that the prognostic value of true RH was stronger in those with diabetes (hazard ratio [HR], 5.5; 95% confidence interval [CI], 2.3–13.2) compared to those without diabetes (HR, 1.5; 95% CI, 0.8–2.5). In total, the study demonstrated the value of performing ABPM in patients with aTRH to identify the

Table 5.1 Definition of terms associated with resistant hypertension adapted from Judd and Calhoun [1]; with permission

Term	Definition	Comments
Resistant hypertension (RH)	Uncontrolled BP despite maximal effective dosing of ≥3 medications of different classes including a diuretic or controlled BP on ≥4 medications	Includes all patients controlled on ≥4 medications irrespective of BP
True resistant hypertension	Same definition as resistant hypertension emphasizing that pseudoresistance was excluded by ambulatory monitoring, optimal dosing, and assessing drug-adherence	The term is often necessary to differentiate from published data where the term resistant hypertension is used despite not excluding pseudoresistance
Apparent treatment resistant hypertension (aTRH)	Meeting criteria for resistant hypertension but unable to exclude pseudoresistance	Typically used in large observational studies of office BP. Many published studies of resistant hypertension neither excluded pseudoresistance nor used this term
Pseudoresistance	Uncontrolled office BP while receiving ≥3 medications in the setting of white coat hypertension, medication nonadherence, improper BP measurement technique, cuff artifact, and suboptimal dosing	Presumed to contribute to as much as 50% of resistant hypertension
White coat hypertension	A major cause of pseudoresistance defined as uncontrolled office BP with average BP by 24-h ambulatory monitoring <130/80 mmHg or home BP <135/85 mmHg	
Masked uncontrolled hypertension	Controlled office BP (<140/90 mmHg) with an elevated average BP by 24-h ambulatory monitoring >130/80 mmHg or home BP >135/85 mmHg	Seen in up to 30–60% of patients with CKD and hypertension due mainly to nocturnal hypertension [2, 3]
Refractory hypertension	Uncontrolled BP despite maximal medical therapy (≥5 antihypertensive medications at maximal effective dosing and of different class)	The differences in characteristics between resistant and refractory hypertension were recently reviewed [4]

Abbreviations: *BP* blood pressure, *CKD* chronic kidney disease

higher-risk group with true RH. In a separate report, the authors of the latter study analyzed largely the same cohort to determine the prognostic effect of baseline and serial changes in albuminuria among 531 patients with aTRH [16]. Urinary albumin was measured by 24-h urine collections at baseline and 2 years. Participants were divided into normal or microalbuminuric groups using a threshold of >30 mg/24 h

Table 5.2 Contemporary longitudinal studies reporting renal, cardiovascular, or mortality events for resistant hypertension with and without CKD

1st author [Ref]	Year	Country	Number	Age (years)[a]	eGFR[a]	ABPM	RH definition	Mean/median follow-up (years)	Adjusted hazard ratios (95% CI) for resistant hypertension compared to nonresistant hypertension			Note
									Renal events	CV events	All-cause mortality	
Pierdomenico [13]	2005	Italy	742	61 ± 12	1.04 ± 0.4[b]	Yes	1	4.9	NR	2.94(1.02–8.41)	NR	1
Salles [14]	2008	Brazil	556	65.8 ± 11.2	1.1 ± 0.5[b]	Yes	1	4.8	NR	1.88(0.93–3.80)	2.00(1.12–3.55)	2
De Nicola [15]	2011	Italy	300	67.3 ± 11.3	41 ± 16.6	Yes	2	3.1	1.85(1.13–3.03)	NR	NR	3,4
Salles [16]	2011	Brazil	531	68.5 ± 12	106(82–133)[c]	Yes	1	4.9	NR	4.64(2.15–10.02)	2.90(1.52–5.52)	5,6
Daugherty [12]	2012	United States	18,036	60.6(60.2–60.9)	NR	No	1	3.8	NR	1.47(1.32–1.62)	NR	7,8
De Nicola [17]	2013	Italy	436	68.2 ± 10.9	30.2 ± 5.9	Yes	2	4.8	2.66(1.62–4.37)	1.98(1.14–3.43)	NR	3,9
Irvin [18]	2013	United States	14,522	67.6 ± 8.6	NR	No	1	6	NR	1.69(1.27–2.24)	1.29(1.14–1.46)	10,11
Muntner [19]	2014	North America	14,684	66.6 ± 7.5	72.5 ± 18.9	No	1	4.9	1.95(1.11–3.41)	1.46(1.29–1.64)	1.30(1.11–1.52)	12,2
Sim [20]	2015	United States	470,386	64(56–73)	74(59–88)	No	1	<5	1.32(1.27–1.37)	1.24(1.20–1.28)	1.06(1.03–1.08)	11,13
Thomas [11]	2016	United States	3367	60.6 ± 9.2	38.9 ± 13.7	No	3	<5	1.28(1.11–1.46)	1.48(1.28–1.72)	1.24(1.06–1.45)	12
Kaboré [21]	2016	France	1629	75.1 ± 5.6	74 ± 17.0	No	1	4	2.78(1.33–5.81) 2.91(1.49–5.70)	NR	NR	14

RH Definitions: (1) Office BP ≥140/90 mmHg despite ≥3 anti-hypertensive medications (2) Office BP ≥130/80 mmHg despite ≥3 antihypertensive drugs including a diuretic in full dosages or <130/80 mmHg requiring ≥4 antihypertensive drugs in full doses (3) Office BP ≥140/90 mmHg despite ≥3 antihypertensive drugs including a diuretic in full dosages or requiring ≥4 antihypertensive medications regardless of BP

Notes: *1*. Relative risk reported. *2*. CV event was composite outcome of fatal and nonfatal CV events *3*. Renal event is composite outcome of all-cause death, dialysis, or transplantation. *4*. CV event is CV mortality *5*. Hazard Ratios compare RH in the presence or absence of microalbuminuria. Adjusted Hazard Ratios for eGFR <60 mL/min/1.73 m² with microalbuminuria (§2.90; 95% CI, 1.52–5.52) were greater than for those without microalbuminuria (1.38; 95% CI, 0.73–2.63). *6*. CV event was composite of nonfatal MI, CCF, stroke and new-onset CKD by diagnostic coding or MDRD-eGFR <60 mL/min/1.73 m² on 2 occasions after follow-up. New-onset CKD was the predominant CV event. *8*. Unadjusted renal outcomes of new-onset CKD were 14.5% for RH versus 10.4% for non-RH. *8*. CV event was composite of fatal and non-fatal CV events *10*. Renal event was composite of death due to renal disease or requiring dialysis or renal transplantation *10*. CV event was composite of nonfatal myocardial infarction or death due to coronary heart disease. *11*. Renal event was requiring dialysis or renal disease or requiring dialysis or renal transplantation *12*. Renal event defined as 50% decrease in eGFR, dialysis, or renal transplantation *13*. CV event was by incident diagnostic coding for coronary events comprising myocardial infarction, angina, percutaneous coronary intervention, or coronary bypass grafting *14*. Renal event was rapid CKD progression as defined by MDRD-eGFR decline >5 mL/min/year with separate Hazard Ratios reported for RH versus non-RH that was controlled 2.78 (1.33–5.81) or uncontrolled 2.91(1.49–5.70)

Abbreviations: *ABPM* ambulatory blood pressure monitoring, *CKD* chronic kidney disease, *eGFR* estimated glomerular filtration rate in mL/min/1.73 m², *HR* hazard ratio, *NR* not reported, *RCT* randomized controlled trial, *RH* resistant hypertension

[a]Age and eGFR are ±SD or (25th–75th centile)
[b]Serum creatinine in mg/dl
[c]Serum creatinine in µmol/l

urinary albumin. After a median follow-up of 4.9 years, 72 patients (13.6%) died, and there were 96 cardiovascular events. After adjustment for several cardiovascular risk factors, baseline albuminuria, either as a continuous variable or categorized at different cutoff values, was an independent predictor of the composite outcome of all-cause and cardiovascular mortality, strokes, and coronary events. Each ten-fold increase in 24-h urinary albumin conferred a 1.5- to twofold higher risk of each component of the composite outcome. Serial changes in microalbuminuria status during follow-up reflected changes in cardiovascular risk. Reduction of microalbuminuria was associated with a 27% lower risk of cardiovascular events compared to a 65% increased risk associated with increased microalbuminuria. This study demonstrated the prognostic effect of microalbuminuria in a cohort with RH. The authors suggested that microalbuminuria reduction may be an important surrogate target in treatment of RH.

It has been recognized that 10–20% of a population with normal office BP have isolated ambulatory hypertension (masked hypertension). Recent meta-analyses report a prevalence of masked hypertension of 17% in a general hypertensive population of 25,629 patients [22] and 8% in 980 patients with CKD stages 2 to 4 [2]. More recent data in 333 predominantly male veterans with a mean age of 70 and CKD stages 2 to 4, suggested higher prevalence of masked hypertension in CKD of between 27% and 56% depending on whether daytime, nighttime, or average ambulatory BP was used as a diagnostic criterion [23]. The Uppsala Longitudinal Study of Adult Men was the first major study to describe clinical outcomes in masked hypertension in 578 men aged 70 years that did not take antihypertensive drugs [24]. Of these, 188 (33%) were normotensive by both office and ambulatory BP. Eighty-two (14%) showed masked hypertension, whereas 308 (53%) subjects had sustained hypertension by both office and ambulatory BP. Plasma glucose levels, measures of abdominal obesity, and left ventricular wall thickness were increased at baseline in subjects with isolated ambulatory hypertension. Seventy-two cardiovascular morbid events occurred over 8.4 years of follow-up. The prognostic value of isolated ambulatory and sustained hypertension was assessed with Cox proportional hazard regression adjusting for serum cholesterol, smoking, and diabetes. Isolated ambulatory hypertension was associated with a nearly threefold increased risk of cardiovascular morbidity compared to the normotensive group (HR, 2.8; 95% CI, 1.3–6.7) with a similar prognosis to sustained hypertension (HR, 2.9; 95% CI, 1.5–5.8). While the latter study described clinical outcomes in elderly men with untreated hypertension, a subsequent prospective study described prognosis of masked hypertension in 742 treated hypertensives [13]. The groups were classified by ABPM into responder (normal clinic and ambulatory BP, $n = 340$), masked (normal clinic but high ambulatory BP, $n = 126$), pseudoresistant (high clinic but normal ambulatory BP, $n = 146$), and true RH (high clinic and ambulatory BP, $n = 130$). In this study, a clinic BP of <140/90 mmHg and daytime ambulatory BP <135/85 mmHg was considered normal. No assessment of drug compliance was reported, and it was not specified whether the minimum of three antihypertensive drugs in the group with true RH included diuretics. Compared to the responder group, the true RH group had greater baseline end-organ damage with more prevalent left ventricular hypertrophy (50% vs 13.5%), diabetes (13.8 versus 3.2%), and higher serum creatinine (1.0 ± 0.4 vs 0.8 ± 0.2 mg/dl). The masked hypertensive group had a greater prevalence of left ventricular hypertrophy (23% versus 13.5%). After a mean of 5 years of follow-up, 63 cardiovascular events occurred (myocardial infarction, coronary or peripheral revascularization, hospitalization for heart failure, fatal and nonfatal strokes, and renal failure requiring dialysis). Multivariable Cox regression showed age, smoking, LDL cholesterol, left ventricular hypertrophy, diabetes, masked hypertension, and true RH were independent predictors of cardiovascular events. Compared to the normotensive responder group, pseudoresistance had equivalent prognosis for cardiovascular events (relative risk, 1.2; 95% CI, 0.5–3.3). Masked hypertension doubled the relative risk of cardiovascular events (2.3; 95% CI, 1.1–4.7). True RH nearly trebled the relative risk of cardiovascular events (2.9; 95% CI, 1.0–8.4). This study emphasized the high cardiovascular risk associated with masked hypertension and true RH and the relatively benign prognosis of pseudoresistance. This underlines the practical and prognostic importance of ABPM in reclassifying patients to avoid overtreating those with white coat hypertension and undertreating those with masked hypertension. To date, there are no clinical outcome data describing clinical outcomes of masked hypertension relative to RH in the setting of CKD.

Most observational studies of aTRH describe clinical outcomes based on baseline prevalence in cross-sectional studies. Daugherty and coworkers used longitudinal healthcare insurance registry data to report the first estimate of new-onset aTRH from 205,750 patients with incident hypertension [12]. Definition of incident aTRH was an increase from using 1 to 3 or more antihypertensive drugs with BP >140/90 mmHg or >130/80 mmHg for those with diabetes mellitus or chronic kidney disease. Pseudoresistance was determined by nonadherence to therapy using pharmacy data but could not exclude white coat or masked hypertension as only office BP was available. Incident aTRH developed in 1.9% ($n = 3960$) of the entire cohort during a median follow up of 1.5 years. Resistant patients were more often older, male, with higher rates of diabetes mellitus, CKD, and other comorbidities. After a median follow-up of 3.8 years and exclusion of 5876 (25%) patients with prior cardiovascular events, a total of 18,036 patients remained. There were 344 (1.9%) deaths and 2206 (12.2%) incident cardiovascular events. Univariate analyses showed more frequent cardiovascular events in the aTRH group compared to nonresistant hypertension group (18% vs 13.5%, respectively). In unadjusted and adjusted survival analyses, patients with aTRH were significantly more likely to experience the combined outcomes of death, myocardial infarction, congestive heart failure, stroke, or CKD, (unadjusted HR, 1.5; 95% CI, 1.4–1.7; adjusted HR, 1.5; 95% CI, 1.3–1.6). Sensitivity analyses excluding 269 patients with pseudoresistance due to nonadherence did not alter the findings. This study showed that among patients with incident hypertension newly starting treatment, 1 in 50 will go on to develop resistant hypertension within 1.5 years. In addition, one in six patients taking three hypertension medications will continue to meet criteria for resistant hypertension over follow-up. Adverse cardiovascular outcomes were 50% higher in those with incident aTRH hypertension than in those without.

Few studies describe clinical outcomes of hypertension phenotypes in unselected cohorts including those who never achieve controlled BP and few separately describe renal outcomes. A recent retrospective study used electronic health records in a large, ethnically diverse population to evaluate and compare the risk of renal, cardiovascular, and mortality outcomes among individuals with controlled resistant hypertension (cRH), uncontrolled resistant hypertension (uRH), and nonresistant hypertension (non-RH) [20]. Data were derived using office BP among 470,386 individuals enrolled to a prepaid integrated health plan in the USA, of which 60,327 (12.8%) were identified as having aTRH. With the exception of sleep apnea, individuals with diagnosed secondary causes of hypertension were excluded. Definition of aTRH was office BP $\geq$140/90 mmHg with three different antihypertensive medications or needing four or more antihypertensive medications irrespective of BP. There was no ABPM available and pseudoresistance was partly excluded by assessing medication adherence from pharmacy dispensation data. A subset of patients intolerant of diuretics were included in the aTRH cohort; however, 97% of the aTRH population were using a diuretic. When compared to the non-RH group, the aTRH group had greater prevalence of diabetes (48% vs 30%), CKD defined as eGFR <60 mL/min/1.73 m^2 (45% vs 24%), ischemic heart disease (41% vs 22%), and cerebrovascular disease (16% vs 9%). There was no significant difference in comorbidities between controlled and uncontrolled aTRH groups. A total of 114,364 events occurred comprising all-cause death, ischemic heart disease events, congestive heart failure, stroke, and incident end-stage renal disease. Both unadjusted and adjusted event rates were greater in the aTRH group for all measured outcomes. Uncontrolled aTRH was associated with a greater stroke risk (HR, 1.23; 95% CI, 1.14–1.31) and greater end-stage renal disease risk (HR, 1.25; 95% CI, 1.18–1.33). This study concluded that compared to non-RH, aTRH had greater risks of incident ischemic heart disease, heart failure, stroke, and end-stage renal disease. Among those with aTRH, there was a further increased risk of stroke and end-stage renal disease for uncontrolled versus controlled BP.

Clinical Outcomes in Observational Studies of CKD Populations

A retrospective Italian study evaluated the burden of RH in 300 patients referred for management of CKD stages 2 to 5 [15]. Staging of CKD used Kidney Disease: Improving Global Outcomes (KDIGO) guidelines [25] and eGFR was calculated by serum creatinine in the 4-variable Modified Diet in Renal Disease equation [26]. Home BP or ABPM were used to exclude pseudoresistance by white coat hypertension. Adherence to medication and dietary salt restriction were assessed by questionnaire, pill counts, and 24-h urinary sodium. True RH was diagnosed as office BP $\geq$130/80 mmHg despite three antihypertensive drugs at optimal dose including a diuretic, or as controlled BP using four or more drugs. Five hundred and fifty patients were screened, and 250 were excluded for pseudoresistance due to white coat hypertension or nonadherence. The remaining 300 patients with true RH had a mean age of 67 years with frequent comorbidities including obesity (body mass index, 30 ± 6 kg/m^2), diabetes (38%), left ventricular hypertrophy (65%), and 24-h urinary protein >1 g (23%). In the first 6 months, the prevalence of those achieving controlled BP increased from 12% to 19% while incidence of true RH increased from 26% to 38%, largely driven by intensified drug therapy. Predictors of persistent RH included proteinuria and diabetes. A composite outcome of renal death was defined as all-cause mortality or requiring dialysis or renal transplantation. After a median follow-up of 3 years, 79 renal deaths occurred with significantly more events in the group with RH at 6 months. Compared to the non-RH group, the adjusted risk of renal death for true RH was approximately doubled (HR, 1.9; 95% CI, 1.1–3.0). The authors speculated that the characteristics of RH in CKD might be different with proteinuria rather than GFR being a better predictor. However, their findings largely reflect non-CKD studies in that baseline evidence of cardiovascular end-organ damage predicts RH. There are further difficulties when statistically regarding the competing risks of renal transplantation, dialysis, and death as having equally adverse outcomes when renal transplantation might well improve survival compared to advanced CKD.

In a prospective cohort study, the same authors reported prognosis of 436 CKD patients [17]. The diagnosis of aTRH was office BP $\geq$130/80 mmHg, despite adherence to three full-dose antihypertensive drugs including a diuretic or use of $\geq$4 antihypertensives irrespective of BP. Patients were asked the number of times they had missed taking their prescribed medication in the last 2 weeks and were excluded from analysis if the missing rate for medication was $\geq$ 20%. The cohort was phenotyped into controlled (ambulatory BP <125/75 mmHg without aTRH); pseudoresistant (aTRH and ambulatory BP <125/75 mmHg); sustained hypertension (ambulatory BP $\geq$125/75 mmHg without aTRH); and true RH (ambulatory BP $\geq$125/75 mmHg with aTRH). Compared to the controlled BP group, those with true RH had greater body mass index, more frequent diabetes, proteinuria, left ventricular hypertrophy, prior cardiovascular disease, and lower eGFR. After a median of 4.8 years of follow-up, there were 165 renal events (end-stage renal disease or death due to renal failure) and 109 cardiovascular events (fatal and nonfatal myocardial infarction, heart failure, stroke, peripheral or coronary revascularization, amputation for peripheral vascular disease). Patients with true RH showed worse renal and cardiovascular event-free survival in unadjusted analyses (Fig. 5.2). In multivariable-adjusted event analyses, true RH was associated with double the risk of renal events and 2.7-fold increased risk of cardiovascular events (renal event HR, 2.0; 95% CI, 1.1–3.4; cardiovascular event HR, 2.7; 95% CI, 1.6–4.4). Notably pseudoresistance was not associated with increased cardiorenal risk and sustained hypertension had intermediate risk being predictive of renal but not cardiovascular events. This study exemplifies the incremental risk for phenotypes of RH in CKD that can only be parsed using ABPM. Use of ABPM identified 43% of subjects with suboptimal BP for whom office BP control was adequate. The risk for cardiorenal events was highest in patients with "true" RH. Those with sustained and pseudoresistant hypertension were not at increased cardiovascular risk compared to control subjects. Those with

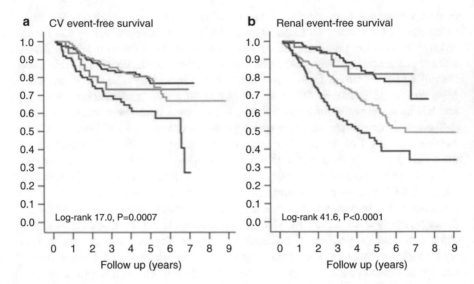

Fig. 5.2 Cardiovascular and renal survival by hypertensive status phenotyped by ambulatory blood pressure monitoring in 436 patients. Control subjects are in *green*, pseudoresistance in *blue*, sustained hypertension in *orange*, and true resistance in *red* (Reproduced with permission from study with Ref. [17])

sustained hypertension had a greater risk of renal events. This gradient of risk across ABPM-based phenotypes suggest a need to have greater use of ABPM in order to better utilize resources, improve clinical outcomes, and avoid harms in hypertensive CKD populations. Future studies are needed to determine whether treatment decisions based on accurate phenotyping of hypertension in CKD improves outcomes.

A recent study reported clinical outcomes of aTRH in 3367 hypertensive participants with non-dialysis CKD from the Chronic Renal Insufficiency Cohort (CRIC) [11]. Pseudoresistance was partly excluded by assessing medication adherence but only office BP was available. Compared to those without aTRH, those with aTRH were older (61 vs 58 years) with more prevalent evidence of end-organ damage. Age, male sex, black race, presence of diabetes, and greater body mass index were independently associated with the presence of aTRH. Doubling of proteinuria was associated with 28% greater odds of aTRH, and each 5 mL/min/1.73 m² decline in eGFR was associated with 14% greater odds of aTRH. In unadjusted survival analyses aTRH was associated with increased cardiovascular and renal events (Fig. 5.3). In multivariable-adjusted survival analysis, aTRH had hazard ratios of 1.5 (95% CI, 1.3–1.7) for cardiovascular outcomes, 1.3 (95% CI, 1.1–1.5) for renal events, and 1.2 (95% CI, 1.1–1.5) for all-cause mortality. While ABPM is clearly preferred to phenotype hypertensive CKD populations, this study emphasizes that even an office BP diagnosis of aTRH identifies a high-risk group.

A recent report from the REasons for Geographic And Racial Difference in Stroke (REGARDS) observational cohort compared cardiovascular outcomes in 2043 participants with aTRH to 12,479 without TRH [18]. Diagnosis of aTRH used

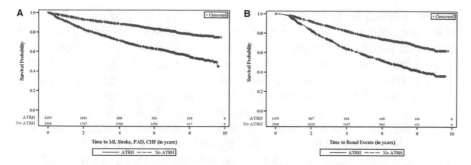

Fig. 5.3 (a) Cumulative incidence of composite cardiovascular outcomes (composite of myocardial infarction [*MI*], stroke, peripheral arterial disease [*PAD*], and congestive heart failure [*CHF*]) between patients with and without apparent treatment resistant hypertension (*ATRH*). (b) Cumulative incidence of renal outcomes between patients with and without ATRH. (**a, b**), *Top line*, No ATRH; *bottom line*, ATRH (Reused with permission from Thomas et al. [11])

the American Heart Association definition of uncontrolled hypertension (>140/90 mmHg) on three or more antihypertensive medication classes (uncontrolled aTRH) or controlled hypertension (<140/90 mmHg) on four or more antihypertensive medications (controlled aTRH) [5]. Absence of aTRH was defined as controlled hypertension on three or less antihypertensive medications or uncontrolled hypertension on one or two classes of antihypertensive medication. Sensitivity analyses explored the subgroup who were intolerant of diuretics. The Morisky Medication Adherence Scale was used [27]. Compared to those without aTRH, the aTRH group had a higher prevalence of diabetes (46% vs 29%), coronary artery disease (35% vs 21%), and prior stroke (14% vs 9%). The aTRH group also had predominantly black ethnicity (60%) with higher waist circumference, greater baseline prevalence of CKD (28% vs 15%), and greater baseline albuminuria (34% vs 18%). Over around 5 years of follow-up, the multivariable-adjusted hazard ratio associated with aTRH versus no aTRH was 1.7 (95% CI, 1.3–2.2) for coronary heart disease and 1.3 (95% CI, 1.1–1.5) for all-cause mortality. The hazard ratio for stroke was not statistically significant (1.3; 95% CI, 0.9–1.7). Comparing uncontrolled aTRH to controlled aTRH showed a hazard ratio of 2.3 (95% CI, 1.2–4.5) for coronary heart disease that was not seen for stroke or all-cause mortality. This study shows the association of aTRH with an increased risk of coronary heart disease and all-cause mortality but not stroke. Within the aTRH group uncontrolled aTRH had greater risks of coronary heart disease compared with controlled aTRH. The study emphasizes the stepwise increase in cardiovascular risk from nonresistant hypertension, to controlled aTRH and uncontrolled aTRH among a group defined only by office BP.

Cross-sectional studies consistently show a strong incremental association between stage of CKD and prevalence of aTRH, but little is known about the longitudinal effect of aTRH on CKD progression in terms of the rate of decline in eGFR, particularly in the elderly. Recent insights were provided by a population-based study in a community-dwelling elderly population [21]. The Three-City study is a population-based prospective cohort that included 9294 non-institutionalized individuals aged 65 years or older randomly selected from electoral rolls of three French cities from March 1999 to March 2001. Both office BP and kidney function were measured in a standardized manner at baseline in 8695 participants of which 4265 were had treated hypertension. Hypertension groups were defined as controlled if office BP was <140/90 mmHg with ≤3 antihypertensive drug classes, and as uncontrolled nonresistant, if it was ≥140/90 mmHg with ≤2 drugs; aTRH was defined as uncontrolled BP ≥140/90 mmHg in patients receiving ≥3 antihypertensive drug classes or ≥4, regardless of BP. Baseline prevalence of aTRH, controlled nonresistant hypertension and uncontrolled nonresistant hypertension was 6.5%, 62.3%, and 31.2%, respectively. The overall mean MDRD-eGFR was 74 ± 17.0 mL/min/1.73 m^2. Participants with aTRH were significantly older with greater prevalence of obesity, diabetes, and history of cardiovascular disease. Prevalence of CKD as defined by eGFR <60 mL/min/1.73 m^2 was 35% in the aTRH group compared to 19% and 17% in the controlled and uncontrolled hypertension groups, respectively. Around 75% of the participants with aTRH reported taking diuretics and renin-angiotensin system inhibitors, while less than 66% reported calcium channel blockers and beta-blockers. At the 4-year follow-up, 1629 of 3865 participants with treated hypertension had a second creatinine measurement; 739 also had urine protein or albumin creatinine ratio. Progression of CKD was determined by a calculated slope using the difference between the baseline and 4-year eGFR divided by the follow-up time. Multinomial regression was used to estimate odds ratios for the association of aTRH at the 4-year follow-up with an eGFR decline rate ≥3 mL/min/1.73 m^2 per year adjusted for age, gender, smoking, obesity, diabetes, history of cardiovascular disease, and study site. This cutoff was selected due to being roughly three times greater than the annual physiological kidney function decline due to aging. At baseline, lower MDRD-eGFR values were independently associated with higher odds of aTRH, compared to both reference groups (odds ratio for eGFR decline of 15 mL/min/1.73 m^2 of 1.29 [95% CI, 1.16–1.48] relative to controlled hypertension or 1.33 [95% CI, 1.19–1.48] relative to uncontrolled nonresistant hypertension. At 4 years, 6.4% were classified with aTRH, 50% with controlled hypertension, and 43.5% with uncontrolled nonresistant hypertension. Among those without aTRH at baseline, 149 participants developed new-onset aTRH with a calculated incidence of 3.5% over 4 years (0.5 per 100 person-years). Baseline MDRD-eGFR level was not related to new-onset aTRH. In contrast, a rapid MDRD-eGFR decline ≥3 mL/min/1.73 m^2 per year was significantly associated with greater risk of new-onset aTRH, regardless of the reference group and independent of mean MDRD-eGFR over the period and other covariates (Table 5.3). International guidelines define progression of CKD as an eGFR decline rate ≥5 mL/min/1.73 m^2 per year. Use of this eGFR cutoff tended to higher odds ratios. Use of the Chronic Kidney Disease Epidemiology Collaboration (CKD-EPI) equation for eGFR did not change these associations. This study provides a rare estimate of incidence of aTRH reporting 7 in 50 hypertensive participants on ≤2 drugs developed aTRH over 4 years. The standardized incidence of 0.7 new cases per 100 person-years compares to the only previous estimate of 0.5 per 100 person-years [12]. The low prevalence of aTRH in

Table 5.3 Significant associations of kidney function at baseline and kidney function decline rate with new-onset apparent treatment-resistant hypertension in the Three-City Study [21]

| | Adjusted ORs | |
	aTRH vs persistent cHT	aTRH vs persistent ucHT
All participants at baseline	$n = 162$ vs 620	$n = 162$ vs 1054
Male	2.44 [1.67–3.55]	0.98 [0.69–1.38]
Body mass index $\geq$30 Kg/m^2	1.57 [1.02–2.40]	1.69 [1.14–2.52]
Diabetes	3.31 [2.12–5.16]	2.26 [1.53–3.35]
History of CVD	0.75 [0.44–1.28]	1.86 [1.12–3.09]
Participants with eGFR measured at 4 years	$n = 74$ vs 269	$n = 74$ vs 433
Male sex	2.24 [1.29–3.91]	1.11 [0.66–1.86]
Diabetes	3.15 [1.60–6.21]	1.93 [1.06–3.51]
eGFR decline $\geq$3 mL/min/1.73 m^2 per year	1.89 [1.09–3.29]	1.99 [1.19–3.35]
eGFR decline $\geq$5 mL/min/1.73 m^2 per year	2.78 [1.33–5.81]	2.91[1.49–5.70]

All analyses were adjusted for center
Abbreviations: *aTRH* incident apparent treatment-resistant hypertension, *cHT* controlled hypertension, *ucHT* uncontrolled hypertension with two antihypertensive drugs, *OR* odds ratios, *CI* 95% confidence interval, *eGFR* glomerular filtration rate estimated using the MDRD equation, *MDRD* Modification of Diet in Renal Disease, *CVD* cardiovascular disease

this cohort is likely due to selection of a healthier community-dwelling population with high rates of undertreatment exemplified by about 40% of the cohort still having uncontrolled hypertension on $\leq$2 drug after 4 years. Consistent with several other studies, the authors found a prevalence of aTRH about twice as high in participants with than without CKD. The novelty of this study lies in the finding that a rapid decline in kidney function was associated with a greater risk of new-onset aTRH independent of eGFR level and other major risk factors for RH. This reinforces the likelihood that CKD is both a cause and consequence of RH.

Clinical Outcomes from Primary or Post Hoc Analyses of Randomized Clinical Trials

A post hoc analysis of the Antihypertensive and Lipid-Lowering Treatment to Prevent Heart Attack Trial (ALLHAT) evaluated the impact of baseline aTRH on incidence of cardiovascular and renal outcomes [19]. Trial participants were randomly allocated to treatment with amlodipine, chlortalidone, or lisinopril with dose titration and addition of further antihypertensive drugs using a prespecified protocol. Based on the year 2 study visit (1996–2000), 13% ($n = 1870$) of 14,684 trial participants were characterized as having aTRH defined by office BP greater than 140/90 mmHg despite three or more antihypertensive medications or requiring four or more antihypertensive medications irrespective of BP. No ABPM were available to exclude pseudoresistance due to white coat hypertension. The aTRH group were more commonly of black ethnicity (43% vs 31%), higher body mass index (31 vs 30), more frequent ECG criteria for left ventricular hypertrophy (21% vs 15%), and lower eGFR (72.5 vs 75.4 mL/min/1.73 m^2). The multivariable-adjusted hazard ratios comparing participants with versus without aTRH were reported for several outcomes: Coronary heart disease (1.4; 95% CI, 1.2–1.8), stroke (1.6; 95% CI, 1.2–2.1), all-cause mortality (1.3; 95% CI, 1.1–1.5), heart failure (1.9; 95% CI, 1.5–2.3), and end-stage renal disease (2.0; 95% CI, 1.1–3.4). These results demonstrate that aTRH increases the risk for cardiovascular disease and end-stage renal disease. Studies are needed to identify approaches to prevent aTRH and reduce risk for adverse outcomes among individuals with aTRH.

Conclusions

Among patients newly starting treatment for hypertension, 1 in 50 will go on to develop resistant hypertension within 1.5 years. In addition, one in six patients taking three hypertension medications will continue to meet criteria for resistant hypertension over follow-up. Observational studies of RH have reported higher rates of vascular disease and end-organ damage at baseline. Those with RH have a greater risk for cardiovascular events, renal events, and mortality under follow-up even when restricted to those with no prior events at baseline. The prevalence of RH has a stepwise increase with declining stages of CKD and is typically two to three times greater than a matched non-CKD group. Study comparisons are hampered by variation in the definitions of RH used in the studies and the extent to which pseudoresistance has been excluded. For example, many studies use the term RH without reporting whether there was optimal dosing, exclusion of nonadherence or use of diuretics. The preferred use of the term apparent resistance to emphasize that pseudoresistance has not been excluded has been inconsistent. Normotension, responder hypertension, nonresistant hypertension, and controlled RH have all been used to describe the same groups. Despite the presence of CKD being the greatest risk factor for developing RH, there is a particular lack of robust evidence to guide the clinical care of patients with RH in the setting of CKD. It is disappointing that both past and recent well-designed trials of hypertension and RH have routinely excluded those with CKD, despite this group having the greatest potential benefit. For example, the recently reported Prevention And Treatment of resistant Hypertension With Algorithm based therapY (PATHWAY-2) trial is the first randomized controlled trial to directly compare spironolactone with other active BP-lowering treatments (alpha-blockers and beta-blockers) in 335 patients with well-characterized RH [28]. The trial showed that RH could be controlled in the majority of patients and that spironolactone was a superior fourth line treatment to other drug classes in terms of home BP reduction. These early results are important as they suggest that in some participants, true RH is driven by subclinical hyperaldosteronism or fluid retention despite optimal dosing of

Table 5.4 Unmet needs for research in resistant hypertension with and without CKD

Improve epidemiology data by phenotyping of resistant hypertension at all stages of CKD with greater use of ambulatory or home BP monitoring and assessment of drug adherence
Large-scale randomized outcome trials in resistant hypertension across all stages of CKD to determine: 1. Optimum blood pressure targets 2. Preferred fourth line drug combinations through networked trials such as those pursued by the British Hypertension Society PATHWAY project 3. The efficacy of procedures and device-based therapies.
More epidemiology reporting the psychosocial and socioeconomic effect of resistant hypertension in CKD
Integrating patient-important outcomes and patient-reported experience measures to traditional clinical outcomes in observational and intervention studies. Clinicians and researchers must acknowledge that a key factor in drug nonadherence is reduced quality of life from taking multiple drugs that is a competing risk to the quality of life impact of cardiovascular and renal events. Patients and clinicians make these tradeoffs when choosing to stop a drug or limit a dose. Integrating these wider measures and measures of treatment harms into informed patient decision aids are an essential step toward reducing apparent treatment resistance
Work with hypertension research community to prevent exclusion of patients with CKD from general hypertension trials and use prespecified analyses with adequate power to describe treatment effects in CKD and resistant hypertension subgroups. Recent trials such as the Systolic Blood Pressure Intervention Trial (SPRINT, 28% eGFR 20–59 mL/min/m²) are a positive step
Clinical trials of hypertension in renal transplant recipients regardless of renal function and patients on dialysis or with eGFR <30 mL/min/m². They remain routinely excluded from all general hypertension trials as well as CKD-specific trials
Perform pragmatic randomized registry-based clinical trials with approved drugs using innovative and flexible designs to permit low running costs. These would answer important clinical questions that are not of commercial interest at a cost that is affordable to public funders.

renin-angiotensin blockade, calcium channel blocker, and a thiazide or loop diuretic. Clinical event outcome data are anticipated. However, the study excluded those with CKD (eGFR <30/mL/min/1.73 m²) perhaps due to the greater risk of treatment-related adverse events. We have summarized unmet needs in outcomes research in resistant hypertension in Table 5.4. Future trials in RH should address these major unmet needs by including those with CKD, indeed the greater event rates, and greater prevalence of RH would be expected to reduce the numbers of participants and time needed to demonstrate clinical effectiveness in this challenging population. Widening the clinical outcomes to incorporate patient-experience measures are also essential to understand and improve drug adherence. In 2008, the American Heart Association Scientific Statement on resistant hypertension made a powerful call to action noting that "the degree to which cardiovascular risk is reduced with treatment of resistant hypertension is unknown" [5]. It is chastening to acknowledge that several years later the question remains largely unanswered. There is an urgent need for clinical trials using pragmatic designs that go beyond traditional measured clinical outcomes to capture the totality of the patient experience [29]. Until then, individualized application of treatment guidelines through shared decision-making with patients will be pursued. Such decision-making should recognize the tradeoff between optimal BP, side effects, cardiovascular risk reduction, and quality of life.

References

1. Judd E, Calhoun DA. Management of hypertension in CKD: beyond the guidelines. Adv Chronic Kidney Dis. 2015;22:116–22.
2. Bangash F, Agarwal R. Masked hypertension and white-coat hypertension in chronic kidney disease: a meta-analysis. Clin J Am Soc Nephrol. 2009;4:656–64.
3. Pogue V, Rahman M, Lipkowitz M, Toto R, Miller E, Faulkner M, et al. Disparate estimates of hypertension control from ambulatory and clinic blood pressure measurements in hypertensive kidney disease. Hypertension. 2009;53:20–7.
4. Modolo R, de Faria AP, Almeida A, Moreno H. Resistant or refractory hypertension: are they different? Curr Hypertens Rep. 2014;16:485.
5. Calhoun DA, Jones D, Textor S, Goff DC, Murphy TP, Toto RD, et al. Resistant hypertension: diagnosis, evaluation, and treatment. A scientific statement from the American Heart Association Professional Education Committee of the Council for High Blood Pressure Research. Hypertension. 2008;51:1403–19.
6. Boswell L, Pascual J, Oliveras A. Resistant hypertension: do all definitions describe the same patients? J Hum Hypertens. 2015;29:530–4.
7. James PA, Oparil S, Carter BL, Cushman WC, Dennison-Himmelfarb C, Handler J, et al. 2014 evidence-based guideline for the management of high blood pressure in adults: report from the panel members appointed to the Eighth Joint National Committee (JNC 8). JAMA. 2014; 311:507–20.
8. Weber MA, Schiffrin EL, White WB, Mann S, Lindholm LH, Kenerson JG, et al. Clinical practice guidelines for the management of hypertension in the community a statement by the American Society of Hypertension and the International Society of Hypertension. J Hypertens. 2014;32:3–15.
9. Tanner RM, Calhoun DA, Bell EK, Bowling CB, Gutiérrez OM, Irvin MR, et al. Prevalence of apparent treatment-resistant hypertension among individuals with CKD. Clin J Am Soc Nephrol. 2013;8:1583–90.
10. Gijón-Conde T, Graciani A, Banegas JR. Resistant hypertension: demography and clinical characteristics in 6292 patients in a primary health care setting. Rev Esp Cardiol. 2014;67: 270–6.
11. Thomas G, Xie D, Chen HY, Anderson AH, Appel LJ, Bodana S, et al. Prevalence and prognostic significance of apparent treatment resistant hypertension in chronic kidney disease: report from the chronic renal insufficiency cohort study. Hypertension. 2016;67:387–96.
12. Daugherty SL, Powers JD, Magid DJ, Tavel HM, Masoudi FA, Margolis KL, et al. Incidence and prognosis of resistant hypertension in hypertensive patients. Circulation. 2012;125: 1635–42.
13. Pierdomenico SD, Lapenna D, Bucci A, Di Tommaso R, Di Mascio R, Manente BM, et al. Cardiovascular outcome in treated hypertensive patients with responder, masked, false resistant, and true resistant hypertension. Am J Hypertens. 2005;18:1422–8.
14. Salles GF, Cardoso CL, Muxfeldt ES. PRognostic influence of office and ambulatory blood pressures in resistant hypertension. Arch Intern Med. 2008;168:2340–6.
15. De Nicola L, Borrelli S, Gabbai FB, Chiodini P, Zamboli P, Iodice C, et al. Burden of resistant hypertension in hypertensive patients with non-dialysis chronic kidney disease. Kidney Blood Press Res. 2011;34:58–67.

16. Salles GF, Cardoso CR, Fiszman R, Muxfeldt ES. Prognostic importance of baseline and serial changes in microalbuminuria in patients with resistant hypertension. Atherosclerosis. 2011; 216:199–204.
17. De Nicola L, Gabbai FB, Agarwal R, Chiodini P, Borrelli S, Bellizzi V, et al. Prevalence and prognostic role of resistant hypertension in chronic kidney disease patients. J Am Coll Cardiol. 2013;61:2461–7.
18. Irvin MR, Booth JN 3rd, Shimbo D, Lackland DT, Oparil S, Howard G, et al. Apparent treatment-resistant hypertension and risk for stroke, coronary heart disease, and all-cause mortality. J Am Soc Hypertens. 2014;8:405–13.
19. Muntner P, Davis BR, Cushman WC, Bangalore S, Calhoun DA, Pressel SL, et al. Treatment-resistant hypertension and the incidence of cardiovascular disease and end-stage renal disease: results from the Antihypertensive and Lipid-Lowering Treatment to Prevent Heart Attack Trial (ALLHAT). Hypertension. 2014;64:1012–21.
20. Sim JJ, Bhandari SK, Shi J, Reynolds K, Calhoun DA, Kalantar-Zadeh K, et al. Comparative risk of renal, cardiovascular, and mortality outcomes in controlled, uncontrolled resistant, and nonresistant hypertension. Kidney Int. 2015;88:622–32.
21. Kaboré J, Metzger M, Helmer C, Berr C, Tzourio C, Massy ZA, et al. Kidney function decline and apparent treatment-resistant hypertension in the elderly. PLoS One. 2016;11:e0146056.
22. Verberk WJ, Kessels AGH, de Leeuw PW. Prevalence, causes, and consequences of masked hypertension: a meta-analysis. Am J Hypertens. 2008;21:969–75.
23. Agarwal R, Pappas MK, Sinha AD. Masked uncontrolled hypertension in CKD. J Am Soc Nephrol. 2016;27:924–32.
24. Bjorklundi K, Lind L, Zethelius B, Andren B, Lithell H. Isolated ambulatory hypertension predicts cardiovascular morbidity in elderly men. Circulation. 2003;107:1297–302.
25. Levey AS, Eckardt KU, Tsukamoto Y, Levin A, Coresh J, Rossert J, et al. Definition and classification of chronic kidney disease: a position statement from Kidney Disease: Improving Global Outcomes (KDIGO). Kidney Int. 2005;67:2089–100.
26. Levey AS, Stevens LA, Schmid CH, Zhang YL, Castro AF 3rd, Feldman HI, et al. A new equation to estimate glomerular filtration rate. Ann Intern Med. 2009;150:604–12.
27. Morisky DE, Green LW, Levine DM. Concurrent and predictive validity of a self-reported measure of medication adherence. Med Care. 1986;24:67–74.
28. Williams B, MacDonald TM, Morant S, Webb DJ, Sever P, McInnes G, et al. Spironolactone versus placebo, bisoprolol, and doxazosin to determine the optimal treatment for drug-resistant hypertension (PATHWAY-2): a randomised, double-blind, crossover trial. Lancet. 2015;386: 2059–68.
29. Carris NW, Smith SM. Quality of life in treatment-resistant hypertension. Curr Hypertens Rep. 2015;17:61.

Chapter 6
Risk Stratification of Resistant Hypertension in Chronic Kidney Disease

Bulent Yardimci and Savas Ozturk

Introduction

Resistant hypertension (RHTN) is an important clinical issue which may arise due to many etiological risk factors and host various comorbidities and is increasing gradually. Due to its negative effect on cardiovascular morbidity and mortality, ultimate care has to be taken as regard to its diagnosis, and it has to be contemplated and treated effectively.

However, sometimes ambiguity may occur in the terminology: According to the American Heart Association (AHA), the definition of treatment-resistant hypertension (TRH) is the arterial blood pressure (BP) values which, pursuant to office measurements, ideally also include diuretic treatment and which are higher than the target value despite three antihypertensive applied at optimal doses or which may be taken (or sometimes may not be taken) under control by means of four or more antihypertensive. In order to be able to make this diagnosis, pseudoresistance (including white coat hypertension) has to be excluded, since while in true resistant hypertension there is a high cardiovascular risk, the risk rate in pseudoresistant hypertension (PRH) is low. Because real distinction cannot be made in the majority of studies, we will use the term "apparent-treatment resistant hypertension (aTRH)". aTRH is defined as arterial blood pressure (ABP) that remains above goal, despite concurrent use of three or more antihypertensive medications from different classes or use of four or more antihypertensive medication classes regardless of ABP level [1, 2] The definitions which maybe classified under RHTN terminology and their potential risks are presented in Table 6.1.

B. Yardimci
Department of Internal Medicine, Nephrology, Istanbul Florence Nightingale Hospital, Istanbul, Turkey

S. Ozturk (✉)
Nephrology Clinic, Haseki Training and Research Hospital, Istanbul, Turkey
e-mail: savasozturkdr@yahoo.com

© Springer International Publishing AG 2017
A. Covic et al. (eds.), *Resistant Hypertension in Chronic Kidney Disease*,
DOI 10.1007/978-3-319-56827-0_6

Table 6.1 Risk factors apart from BP

Type of Hypertension	Definition	Implicated risks
Resistant hypertension (RH)	BP that remains above the target value despite the concurrent use of three antihypertensive agents of different classes [1, 2]. Consequently, patients with a BP that is controlled with four or more drugs should be diagnosed to have RH	The application of ABPM identified a high rate (43% in Nicola's study) of subjects for whom BP control was considered adequate by office measurement but whose conditions were actually suboptimal [3]. ABPM may prevent undertreatment which may be omitted in routine surveillance
Apparent resistant hypertension (aTRH)	Uncontrolled clinic BP (i.e., equal to or greater than 140/90 mmHg) which prevails in spite of the prescription of three or more antihypertensive drugs or which requires the prescription of four or more drugs to be controlled	These patients have higher risks for cardiorenal events. aTRH causes a 1.5 times higher risk (95% CI, 0.8–3.0) of a cardiovascular endpoint in comparison to controlled hypertensives [4]. aTRH also increases the ESRD risk by 2.3 times (95% CI 1.4–3.7) [4]. Following the adjustment of multiple variables: man gender, black race, large waist circumference, diabetes mellitus, history of myocardial infarction or stroke, statin use, and lower eGFR and higher albumin-to-creatinine ratio levels were found to be associated with aTRH among individuals with CKD [5]
True resistant hypertension (TRH)	Uncontrolled clinic BP in spite of being compliant with an antihypertensive regimen which consists of three or more drugs (including a diuretic), each at optimal doses; also uncontrolled BP confirmed by 24-h ABPM	Prevalent in about one-fourth of CKD patients. Very high cardiorenal risk. Presence of mild-to-advanced GFR reduction and/or microalbuminuria amplifies the cardiovascular risk. The combination of ABPM with the diagnosis of RH enables a better risk stratification, especially in CKD patients. TRH may blunt the prognostic value of DM, high proteinuria, or low GFR. TRH is characterized by high sodium sensitivity of BP. Recommended to be surveyed in tertiary care centers and treated aggressively

(continued)

Table 6.1 (continued)

Type of Hypertension	Definition	Implicated risks
Pseudoresistant hypertension	Pseudoresistance refers to poorly controlled hypertension that seems to be treatment resistant but is, in fact, attributable to other factors (e.g., inaccurate measurement of BP, poor adherence to antihypertensive therapy, suboptimal antihypertensive therapy, poor adherence to lifestyle and dietary approaches to lower BP, white coat hypertension)	Pseudoresistant patients are similar to control based on ABPM profiles, target organ damage (prevalence of LVH and severity of renal disease), and long-term prognosis. Pseudoresistant CKD patients should be identified to provide correct prognostic information and, more importantly, to avoid aggressive antihypertensive therapy. A tighter control of BP merely on the basis of the detection of elevated BP in the office might cause patients to be exposed to ischemia-induced worsening of cardiorenal damage [6–8] and eventually convert their prognosis from favorable to unfavorable. In the Spanish ABPM registry, 12% of the 68,045 patients examined were diagnosed as RH; however, after ABPM, as many as 37% of them were identified as pseudoresistant [9]. In clinical practice, lack of adherence is frequently seen. As a matter of fact, about half of the patients with hypertension withdraw from the therapy within the first year following the diagnosis
White coat hypertension	Hypertension in patients with office readings indicating an average of more than 140/90 mmHg and with reliable out-of-office readings indicating an average of less than 140/90 mmHg. Having the BP in the office taken by a nurse or technician, rather than the clinician, may minimize the white coat effect	Cardiovascular risk is not increased or slightly increased compared with normal population. However it poses increased risk for developing persistent HT [7, 8]

Renal and Cardiovascular Risk of RHTN

There is very close correlation between hypertension (HT) and kidney diseases. While HT can lead to kidney disease, it may also become a result of renal disease. Almost all end-stage renal disease (ESRD) patients are hypertensive. In the US, the HT frequency in CKD is around 85% [10]. In Europe, hypertensive nephrosclerosis is one of the most common reasons of ESRD, and its rate in ESRD patients is 17% [11]. On the other hand, the control rate of HT in CKD patients is at quite low levels [12]. There are not enough studies on the TRH frequency in chronic kidney disease (CKD) patients or on its effects on patient survival. According to the US Renal Data

System, the aTRH rate among treated ESRD patients is 24% [13]. In the MASTERPLAN study performed in the Netherlands on 788 CKD patients, the aTRH frequency was demonstrated as 34% according to the office measurements and as 32% according to the ambulatory blood pressure monitoring (ABPM). The study has demonstrated, on a surveillance of an average of 5.3 years, the development of cardiovascular disease (CVD) endpoint in 17% and ESRD in 27% of the aTRH patients [4]. Based on these findings, it may be reported that the kidneys of patients that could not be treated well or that have resistant hypertension are a highly affected end organ. In the Framingham study, the 10-year coronary risk in the aTRH group, which comprises also obesity and CKD, is above 20% [14]. One of the most important studies made on this issue in CKD patients is a study performed by De Nicola et al. [3]. In this study, in which 436 CKD patients from four centers were included, the cardiovascular risk (hazard ratio [95% confidence interval (CI)]) was 1.24 (0.55–2.78) in pseudoresistance, 1.11 (0.67–1.84) in sustained hypertension, and 1.98 (1.14–3.43) in true resistance, compared with control subjects. Corresponding hazards for renal events were 1.18 (0.45–3.13), 2.14 (1.35–3.40), and 2.66 (1.62–4.37), respectively. The authors stated that in CKD, pseudoresistance is not associated with an increased cardiorenal risk, and sustained hypertension predicts only renal outcome and that true resistance is prevalent and identifies patients carrying the highest cardiovascular risk [3]. Moreover, in case of dialysis patients, 45% of the mortality cases result from cardiac events [15]. In the meta-analysis performed by Heerspink et al. [16], the reduction of systolic BP in dialysis patients by 4–5 mmHg and the diastolic BP by 2–3 mmHg significantly reduced mortality. In this regard, the ALLHAT study has been significantly indicative [17]. The patient population of the study was evaluated as a result of an average surveillance time of 4.9 years between the years 1998 and 2002, whereby 33.357 persons were admitted to the study and 14.687 persons concluded it. In the study, aTRH was determined to be in correlation with CVD, coronary heart disease (CHD), peripheral arterial disease, heart failure (HF), and ESRD. In the US National Health and Nutrition Examination Survey, Egan et al. [14] have reported the aTRH rate in hypertensive patients as 11.8%. The problem in the aTRH studies made is that there are quite less findings regarding the real relation between RHTN and CVD as already stated at the beginning. Whereas in the ALLHAT study, these findings were demonstrated clearer. aTRH was found to be in correlation with the study's outcome points, i.e., CHD, stroke, CVD, all-cause mortality, HF, and ESRD. The relationship between aTRH and outcome points are independent from other two important risk factors that are smoking and the estimated filtration rate. Moreover, aTRH also leads to increased risk in the diabetes mellitus (DM) and CHD patients groups.

In some HT studies, true determination of aTRH is quite important as well. In the REACH registry [18], the aTRH systolic/diastolic blood pressure value was taken as ≥140/90 mmHg, whereas in case of DM or chronic renal failure (CKD) as ≥130/80 mmHg. One of the important findings of ALLHAT is that aTRH gives similar results in black and white patients. However, the aTRH rate was found to be higher in black persons in all studies. aTRH was found to be directly associated especially with CVD and renal disease in all studies [17, 18].

Risk Stratification

In the determination of aTRH, it is also important in terms of risk stratification to exclude white coat hypertension in the office measurements. In the study performed by De Nicola et al. [3], ABPM has been made on patients with an office BP of 130/80 mmHg in order to exclude PRH, whereby BP 127/75 mmHg was considered as limit value. As a result of the study, the TRH rate was found to be 23%.

Although the studies focusing prognosis of RHTN in CKD patients are scarce, some new indirect evidence have emerged. In the recently published study, SPRINT study, 28% of the participants were CKD patients; it has been shown that lower systolic BP target ($\leq$120 mmHg) has better cardiovascular outcomes compared with higher systolic blood pressure target ($\leq$140 mmHg) [19]. In this study, renal and composite outcomes were similar between both BP arms, but in non-CKD group, lower BP arm showed significant worse renal outcomes than in the standard-treatment group (defined by a decrease in the eGFR of 30% or more to a value of less than 60 mL/min/1.73 m^2; 1.21% per year vs. 0.35% per year; hazard ratio, 3.49; 95% CI, 2.44–5.10; $P < 0.001$). Although some of resistant HT might be excluded because of the design of the study (patients using too many drugs or with extreme BP were not included), the further analyses of CKD subgroup this study will give invaluable information for both BP goals and the risk management of this CKD group. In their prospective study of 531 RHTN patients, Salles et al. [20] investigated the associations between reduced GFR and endpoints and interaction with microalbuminuria. After a median follow-up of 4.9 years, reduced GFR was an independent predictor of increased cardiovascular morbidity and mortality in these RHTN patients. Moreover, the presence of both reduced eGFR and microalbuminuria significantly increased cardiovascular risk in relation to one or another isolated, with hazard ratios of 3.0 (1.7–5.3), 2.9 (1.5–5.5), and 4.6 (2.2–10.0), respectively, for the composite endpoint, all-cause, and cardiovascular mortality.

In the 2013 ESH/ESC Guidelines for the management of arterial hypertension [21], risk stratification according to BP values was made as shown in Table 6.2. The most remarkable finding here is that in case of CKD prevalence, the patients are included in the high-risk group already from grade 1 hypertension level. The risk factors of this guideline apart from BP were specified as shown in Table 6.3. Here, subjects with an eGFR below 30 ml/min/1.73 m^2 and proteinuria above 300 mg/day, seem to have critical risk. In the JNC-7, published in 2003, cardiovascular risk factors were specified as follows: Major risk factors: target organ damage, hypertension, cigarette smoking, obesity (body mass index $\geq$30 kg/m^2), physical inactivity, dyslipidemia, diabetes mellitus, microalbuminuria or estimated GFR <60 mL/min, age (older than 55 for men, 65 for women), and family history of premature cardiovascular disease (men under age 55 or women under age 65) [22]. On the other hand, in the NKF K/DOQI guidelines [23], it is recommended to adjust antihypertensive treatment doses according to the systolic BP, GFR, and serum potassium follow-up in CKD patients with hypertension, and risk stratification is attempted to be made accordingly (Table 6.4). For CKD patients, ABPM becomes more important

Table 6.2 Stratification of total CV risk in categories of low, moderate, high, and very high risk according to SBP and DBP and prevalence of RFs, asymptomatic OD, diabetes, CKD stage, or symptomatic CVD

Other risk factors, asymptomatic organ damage or disease	High normal SBP 130–139 or DBP 85–89 mmHg	Grade 1 HT SBP 140–159 or DBP 90–99 mmHg	Grade 2 HT SBP 160–179 or DBP 100–109 mmHg	Grade 3 HT SBP ≥180 or DBP ≥110 mmHg
No other RF		Low risk	Moderate risk	High risk
1–2 RF	Low risk	Moderate risk	Moderate to high risk	High risk
≥ 3 RF	Low to moderate risk	Moderate to high risk	High risk	High risk
OD, CKD stage 3 or diabetes	Moderate to high risk	High risk	High risk	High to very high risk
Symptomatic CVD, CKD stage ≥4 or diabetes with OD/RFs	Very high risk	Very high risk	Very high risk	Very high risk

Subjects with a high normal office but a raised out-of-office BP (masked hypertension) have a CV risk in the hypertension range. Subjects with a high office BP but normal out-of-office BP (white-coat hypertension), particularly if there is no diabetes, OD, CVD, or CKD, have lower risk than sustained hypertension for the same office BP

BP blood pressure, *CKD* chronic kidney disease, *CV* cardiovascular, *CVD* cardiovascular disease, *DBP* diastolic blood pressure, *HT* hypertension, *OD* organ damage, *RF* risk factor, *SBP* systolic blood pressure

day by day in terms of risk stratification. The main issue is how to implement this application in practice, because there are also other points to be determined such as TRH. In the ABPM of a group of patients, for whom TRH was not identified and whose office BP was found to be normal, HTN and a CVD increase was determined in them as well. It was demonstrated that masked HTN also constitutes an important risk factor [24]. Hence this circumstance increases the importance of ABPM. One of the important functions of ABPM is that it allows to detect the patients' dipper or non-dipper distinctions. In non-dippers the CVD rate is two times higher [24].

Evaluation of Other Possible Factors

Apart from these, there are many other factors in the development of resistance in CKD. Renal artery stenosis is mostly a result of atherosclerosis, and its rate in CKD is around 5.5%. Since it is mostly asymptomatic, it is hard to know its real rate, and it is a significant RHTN and CVD risk factor. Increased arterial stiffness is a significant risk factor that is frequently seen in CKD patients and that is accompanied by RHTN. In CKD, increased arterial stiffness depends on many pathological

Table 6.3 Definitions and implicated risks related to resistant hypertension

Risk Factors
Male sex
Age (men ≥55 years, women ≥65 years)
Smoking
Dyslipidemia
Total cholesterol >4.9 mmol/L (190 mg/dL)
Low-density lipoprotein cholesterol >3.0 mmol/L (115 mg/dL)
High-density lipoprotein cholesterol: men <1.0 mmol/L (40 mg/dL), women <1.2 mmol/L (46 mg/dL)
Triglycerides >1.7 mmol/L (150 mg/dL)
Fasting plasma glucose 5.6–6.9 mmol/L (102–125 mg/dL)
Abnormal glucose tolerance test
Obesity (BMI ≥30 kg/m²)
Abdominal obesity (waist circumference: men ≥102 cm, women ≥88 cm) (in Caucasians)
Family history of premature CVD (men aged <55 years, women aged <65 years)
Asymptomatic Organ Damage
Pulse pressure (in the elderly) ≥60 mmHg
Electrocardiographic LVH (Sokolow–Lyon index >3.5 mV; RaVL >1.1 mV; Cornell voltage duration product >244 mV.ms)
Echocardiographic LVH (LVM index: men >115 g/m², women >95 g/m² [BSA])[a]
Carotid wall thickening (IMT >0.9 mm) or plaque
Carotid–femoral PWV >10 m/s
Ankle brachial index <0.9
Microalbuminuria (30–300 mg/24 h) or albumin–creatinine ratio (30–300 mg/g, 3.4–34 mg/mmol) (preferentially on morning spot urine)
Diabetes Mellitus
Fasting plasma glucose ≥7.0 mmol/L (126 mg/dL) on two repeated measurements
HbA1c >7% (53 mmol/mol)
Post-load plasma glucose >11.0 mmol/L (198 mg/dL)
Established CV or Renal Disease
Cerebrovascular disease: ischemic stroke, cerebral hemorrhage, transient ischemic attack
CHD: myocardial infarction, angina, myocardial revascularization with PCI or CABG
Heart failure, including heart failure with preserved EF
Symptomatic lower extremities peripheral artery disease
CKD with eGFR <30 mL/min/1.73 m² (BSA); proteinuria (> 300 mg/24 h)
Advanced retinopathy: hemorrhages or exudates, papilloedema

Abbreviations: *BMI* body mass index, *BP* blood pressure, *BSA* body surface area, *CABG* coronary artery bypass graft, *CHD* coronary heart disease, *CKD* chronic kidney disease, *CV* cardiovascular, *CVD* cardiovascular disease, *EF* ejection fraction, *eGFR* estimated glomerular filtration rate, *HbA1c* glycated hemoglobin, *IMT* intima-media thickness, *LVH* left ventricular hypertrophy, *LVM* left ventricular mass, *PCI* percutaneous coronary intervention, *PWV* pulse wave velocity
[a]Risk maximal for concentric LVH: increased LVM index with a wall thickness/radius ratio of 0.42

84 B. Yardimci and S. Ozturk

Table 6.4 Follow-Up evaluation intervals in CKD recommended by NKF K/DOQI Guidelines (23)

Clinical condition	After initiation or increase in dose of antihypertensive therapy	
	4–12 weeks	<4 Weeks
SBP (mmHg)	120–139*	≥140 or <120
GFR (mL/min/1.73 m²)	≥60	<60
Early GFR decline (70)	<15	≥15
Serum potassium (meq/L)	>4,5[a] or ≤4,5[b]	≤4,5[a] or >4,5[b]
	After blood pressure is at goal and dose is stable	
	6–12 months	*1–6 months*
GFR (mL/min/1.73 m²)	≥60	<60
GFR decline (mL/min/1.73 m² per year)	<4 (slow)	≥4 (fast)
Risk factors for faster progression of CKD	No	Yes
Risk factors for acute GFR decline	No	Yes
Comorbid conditions	No	Yes

Clinicians are advised to evaluate each parameter and select the follow-up interval for the parameter that requires the earliest follow-up
[a]For thiazide of loop diuretic therapy
[b]For ACE inhibitor or ARB therapy
*120–129 mmHg to monitor for hypertension;130–139 mmHg to reach blood pressure goal

mechanisms. Vascular calcification, chronic volume loading, inflammation, endothelial dysfunction, oxidative stress, and activation of the renin angiotensin aldosterone system are the known mechanisms. Obesity and obstructive sleep apnea (OSA) are other risk factors. The relation between RHTN and OSA is known and has also been shown in the studies made with dialysis patients [25].

The inaccuracy and insufficiencies in the use of antihypertensive medicine or the uncontrolled use of other drugs effecting BP are significant reasons of RHTN. Nonsteroidal anti-inflammatory drugs and cyclooxygenase-2 inhibitors are drugs that are used very commonly and affect BP control easily. Sympathomimetic agents (including decongestants, diet pills, and cocaine), glucocorticoids, and corticosteroids are further significant drug groups that lead to RHTN. Other agents include oral contraceptives, erythropoietin, cyclosporine, herbal compounds, and natural licorice [26]. Obesity (BMI ≥30), age above 55 for men and 65 for women, and smoking (especially 20 cigarettes/day and above), and alcohol consumption of more than three portions a day may be stated as the other risk factors [21, 26].

A subject that should not be disregarded in CKD patients is the resistance caused by secondary diseases. There are prospective and retrospective studies which demonstrate that primary hyperaldosteronism is prevalent in 11–20% of resistant hypertension patients [27, 28]. Endocrinological diseases such as pheochromocytoma, Cushing syndrome, and hyperparathyroidism are further secondary reasons for resistance [27, 28].

Apart from all these, in about 10% of the RTHN patients, there cannot be identified any risk factor, considering them to be associated with genetic and environmental factors [29].

It should not be disregarded that in CKD patients, DM is an important risk factor and that it shall cause the disease to progress rapidly particularly when combined with uncontrolled hypertension [30]. Likewise dyslipidemia, which is often accompanying hypertension, is a frequently seen cardiac risk factor in CKD patients [30, 26].

Along with all these risk factors, the extension of resistant hypertension duration in CKD patients increases CVD and mortality significantly [5, 31, 32]. Particularly, in patients with a low glomerular filtration rate and high urinary albumin creatinine ratio, RHTN is higher. The use of these laboratory findings in risk assessment shall be useful for the treatment approach [32, 33].

An algorithmic approach to the RHTN for stratification of the renal and cardiovascular risk was presented in Fig. 6.1.

Conclusions

RHTN is a significant reason for morbidity and mortality in CKD patients. A major part of the patients die due to cardiac reasons. First of all, it should be identified whether these patients are true RTHN, and risk stratification should be determined well by taking into consideration all risks explained. Every successful treatment approach to be made towards risk factors shall reduce morbidity and mortality significantly.

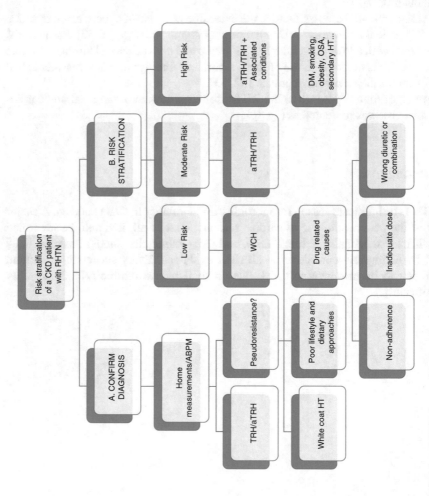

Fig. 6.1 Algorithmic approach to RHTN for renal and cardiovascular risk stratification

References

1. Kumar N, Calhoun DA, Dudenbostel T, et al. Management of patients with resistant hypertension: current treatment options. Integr Blood Press Control. 2013;6:139–51. doi:10.2147/IBPC.S33984.
2. Borrelli S, De Nicola L, Stanzione G, et al. Resistant hypertension in nondialysis chronic kidney disease. Int J Hypertens. 2013;2013:929183. doi:10.1155/2013/929183.
3. De Nicola L, Gabbai FB, Agarwal R, Chiodini P, Borrelli S, Bellizzi V, et al. Prevalence and prognostic role of resistant hypertension in chronic kidney disease patients. J Am Coll Cardiol. 2013;61(24):2461–7.
4. de Beus E, Bots ML, van Zuilen AD, et al.; on behalf of the MASTERPLAN Study Group. Prevalence of apparent therapy-resistant hypertension and its effect on outcome in patients with chronic kidney disease. Hypertension. 2015;66:998–1005.
5. Tanner RM, Calhoun DA, Bell EK, Bowling CB, Gutiérrez OM, Irvin MR, et al. Prevalence of apparent treatment-resistant hypertension among individuals with CKD. Clin J Am Soc Nephrol. 2013;8(9):1583–90.
6. Lewis JB. Blood pressure control in chronic kidney disease: is less really more? J Am Soc Nephrol. 2010;21(7):1086–92.
7. Mancia G, Bombelli M, Brambilla G, Facchetti R, Sega R, Toso E, Grassi G. Long-term prognostic value of white coat hypertension: an insight from diagnostic use of both ambulatory and home blood pressure measurements. Hypertension. 2013;62(1):168–74.
8. Pierdomenico SD, Cuccurullo F. Prognostic value of white-coat and masked hypertension diagnosed by ambulatory monitoring in initially untreated subjects: an updated meta analysis. Am J Hypertens. 2011;24(1):52–8.
9. De La Sierra A, Segura J, Banegas JR, Gorostidi M, de la Cruz JJ, Armario P, et al. Clinical features of 8295 patients with resistant hypertension classified on the basis of ambulatory blood pressure monitoring. Hypertension. 2011;57(5):898–902.
10. Whaley-Connell AT, Sowers JR, Stevens LA, Norris KC, Chen SC, Li S, et al.; Kidney Early Evaluation Program Investigators. CKD in the United States: Kidney Early Evaluation Program (KEEP) and National Health and Nutrition Examination Survey (NHANES) 1999–2004. Am J Kidney Dis. 2008;51(4 Suppl 2):S13–20.
11. ERA-EDTA Registry. ERA-EDTA registry 2003 annual report. Amsterdam: Academic Medical Centre; 2005.
12. Süleymanlar G, Utaş C, Arinsoy T, Ateş K, Altun B, Altiparmak MR, et al. A population-based survey of chronic renal disease in Turkey—the CREDIT study. Nephrol Dial Transplant. 2011;26(6):1862–71.
13. US Renal Data System. USRDS 2004 annual data report: atlas of end-stage renal disease in the United States. Bethesda: National Institutes of Health, National Institute of Diabetes and Digestive and Kidney Diseases.
14. Egan BM, Zhao Y, Axon RN, Brzezinski WA, Ferdinand KC. Uncontrolled and apparent treatment resistant hypertension in the United States, 1988 to 2008. Circulation. 2011;124(9):1046–58.
15. Collins AJ, Foley R, Herzog C, Chavers B, Gilbertson D, Ishani A, et al. Excerpts from the United States Renal Data System 2007 annual data report. Am J Kidney Dis. 2008;51(1 Suppl 1):S1–320.
16. Heerspink HJ, Ninomiya T, Zoungas S, de Zeeuw D, Grobbee DE, Jardine MJ, et al. Effect of lowering blood pressure on cardiovascular events and mortality in patients on dialysis: a systematic review and meta-analysis of randomised controlled trials. Lancet. 2009;373(9668):1009–15.
17. Muntner P, Davis BR, Cushman WC, Bangalore S, Calhoun DA, Pressel SL, et al.; for the ALLHAT Collaborative Research Group. Treatment-resistant hypertension and the incidence of cardiovascular disease and end-stage renal disease results from the Antihypertensive and

Lipid-Lowering Treatment to Prevent Heart Attack Trial (ALLHAT). Hypertension. 2014;64(5):1012–21. doi: 10.1161/HYPERTENSIONAHA.114.03850.
18. Kumbhani DJ, Steg PG, Cannon CP, Eagle KA, Smith SC Jr, Crowley K, et al.; REACH Registry Investigators. Resistant hypertension: a frequent and ominous finding among hypertensive patients with atherothrombosis. Eur Heart J. 2013;34(16):1204–14.
19. SPRINT Research Group, Wright JT Jr, Williamson JD, Whelton PK, et al. A randomized trial of intensive versus standard blood-pressure control. N Engl J. 2015;373(22):2103–16.
20. Salles GF, Cardoso CR, Pereira VS, Fiszman R, Muxfeldt ES. Prognostic significance of a reduced glomerular filtration rate and interaction with microalbuminuria in resistant hypertension: a cohort study. J Hypertens. 2011;29(10):2014–23.
21. Task Force for the management of arterial hypertension of the European Society of Hypertension, Task Force for the management of arterial hypertension of the European Society of Cardiology. 2013 ESH/ESC guidelines for the management of arterial hypertension. Blood Press. 2013;22(4):193–278.
22. Chobanian AV, Bakris GL, Black HR, et al.; National Heart, Lung and Blood Institute Joint National Committee on Prevention, Detection, Evaluation and Treatment of High Blood Pressure; National High Blood Pressure Education Program Coordinating Committee. The seventh report of the Joint National Committee on Prevention, Detection, Evaluation and Treatment of High Blood Pressure: the JNC 7 report. JAMA. 2003;289(19):2560–72. Erratum in: JAMA. 2003 Jul 9;290(2):197.
23. Kidney Disease Outcomes Quality Initiative (K/DOQI). K/DOQI chronic kidney disease. Am J Kidney Dis. 2004;43(5 Suppl 1):S1–290.
24. Pierdomenico SD, Lapenna D, Bucci A, Di Tommaso R, Di Mascio R, Manente BM, et al. Cardiovascular outcome in treated hypertensive patients with responder, masked, false resistant and true resistant hypertension. Am J Hypertens. 2005;18(11):1422–8.
25. Drexler YR, Bomback AS. Definition, identification and treatment of resistant hypertension in chronic kidney disease patients. Nephrol Dial Transplant. 2014;29(7):1327–35.
26. Vega J, Bisognano JD. The prevalence, incidence, prognosis and associated conditions of resistant hypertension. Semin Nephrol. 2014;34(3):247–56.
27. Calhoun DA, Nishizaka MK, Zaman MA, Thakkar RB, Weissmann P. Hyperaldosteronism among black and white subjects with resistant hypertension. Hypertension. 2002;40:892–6.
28. Douma S, Petidis K, Doumas M, Papaefthimiou P, Triantafyllou A, Kartali N, et al. Prevalence of primary hyperaldosteronism in resistant hypertension: a retrospective observational study. Lancet. 2008;371(9628):1921–6.
29. Calhoun DA, Jones D, Textor S, Goff DC, Murphy TP, Toto RD, et al. Resistant hypertension: diagnosis, evaluation and treatment. A scientific statement from the American Heart Association Professional Education Committee of the Council for High Blood Pressure Research. Hypertension. 2008;51(6):1403–19.
30. Garg JP, Elliott WJ, Folker A, Izhar M, Black HR; RUSH University Hypertension Service. Resistant hypertension revisited: a comparison of two university-based cohorts. Am J Hypertens. 2005;18(5 Pt 1):619–26.
31. Bakris G, Vassalotti J, Ritz E, et al.; for the CKD Consensus Working Group. National Kidney Foundation consensus conference on cardiovascular and kidney diseases and diabetes risk: an integrated therapeutic approach to reduce events. Kidney Int. 2010;78(8):726–36.
32. Borrelli S, De Nicola L, Stanzione G, Conte G, Minutolo R. Resistant hypertension in nondialysis chronic kidney disease. Int J Hypertens. 2013;2013:929183.
33. Palmer BF. Renal dysfunction complicating the treatment of hypertension. N Engl J Med. 2002;347(16):1256–61.

Chapter 7
Pathophysiological Insights in Resistant Hypertension

Alexandru Burlacu and Adrian Covic

Introduction

Background: Exploring Paradigms and Controversies

Resistant hypertension (RH) is an entity still incompletely explained and studied from the perspective of the physiopathological mechanisms, no more than it is its "mother" condition, essential hypertension.

Therefore, our endeavor in the pathophysiologic characterization of RH must start with an "essential" question: is RH really a distinct entity or is it just:

(a) The same disease as essential hypertension, with the same pathways, but in an advanced stage?

Corollary 1. Is there a borderline from which a "regular" essential hypertension becomes true resistant (e.g., contexts like obesity, sleep apnea, diabetes mellitus, in which hypertension can be managed at first but later becomes permanent and irreversible)?

(b) The same disease which implies/recruits more neurohumoral and molecular mechanisms than "regular" hypertension?

Corollary 2. Are there specific mechanisms involved from the very beginning (genetic mutations – Na+ absorption, bone marrow and neuroinflammation, hyporeninemic hypertension in Afro-Americans), or are we talking about the progressive

A. Burlacu (✉)
Department of Interventional Cardiology,
Cardiovascular Diseases Institute – Iaşi, Iaşi, Romania
e-mail: alburlacu@yahoo.com

A. Covic
Professor Internal Medicine & Nephrology, Grigore T. Popa University of Medicine,
Iaşi, Romania

© Springer International Publishing AG 2017
A. Covic et al. (eds.), *Resistant Hypertension in Chronic Kidney Disease*,
DOI 10.1007/978-3-319-56827-0_7

involvement of different mechanisms through the expansion of organ damage (excessive proinflammatory factors, endothelin, adiponectin)?

(c) The same disease, with the same mechanisms, but the arbitrary cutoffs used for definition are imperfect (old age, morbid obesity)?

The polemics start from the fact that RH is an entity identified retrospectively, following a dead-end reached in the treatment of firstly presumed essential hypertension, and based on two fundamental suppositions: (1) we presume the hypertension is essential, and (2) we must exclude secondary hypertension, the causes for noncompliance to treatment, and pseudo-resistant hypertension. Hence, if we are to be completely honest, in approaching and characterizing a true RH, we do not know with absolute certitude if it is secondary hypertension, if there are certain underlying causes for a pseudo-resistance, or if it is, indeed, a true RH.

The treatment entails rules applicable to a majority of patients, who would respond out of "common sense" to the current treatment schemes. Thus, the criteria for "resistance" to treatment also represent the criteria in the diagnosis of RH. Concurrently, this provides us with the possibility (at least in theory) that the definition of RH could (and would) be modified with the identification of a new class of drugs or the adjustment of the therapeutic strategy.

Within this context, we believe that, despite the ESC classification, the reversible forms of RH triggered by various extrinsic factors such as excessive alcohol consumption, high sodium intake, and vasopressor drugs should be excluded from the definition of true resistant hypertension, as removal of the external causes leads to the reversibility of the condition.

Furthermore, we can place at the border between essential and secondary hypertension the particular form of RH associated with various comorbidities/cardiovascular risk factors (diabetes mellitus, obesity, chronic kidney disease, sleep apnea). We can argue that the interaction between the induced neuro-metabolic and vascular alterations due to comorbidities and the specific mechanisms involved in essential hypertension has an augmenting effect, which generates a form of RH with partial reversibility and treatment resistance. Conversely, since the evolution of RH cannot be predicted through the strict management of these conditions, they fall within the category of borderline true RH which we will discuss further in this chapter.

As we begin our exploration of the physiopathological mechanism underlying this ambiguous and dynamic condition, there still remain several uncharted territories. Two issues that still remain under debate are as follows: (1) Is there a genetic or molecular determinism to be investigated in resistant hypertension? (2) To what extent do common cardiovascular risk factors bear an influence upon the response of any form of essential, borderline, or resistant hypertension to treatment?

We believe that searching and/or identifying completely the core mechanism of this entity would allow (1) the identification of novel therapeutic pathways and (2) the upgrade of the inclusion criteria of clinical trials (e.g., renal denervation), which would lead to more veridical and useful results (free from intervention of subjective factors such as adherence to treatment).

We underline the fact that, even if the pathophysiological mechanism lying behind RH is a complex multifactorial edifice founded on the sensible imbalance between various elements in several key locations in the body, for theoretical purposes we will discuss each of these elements separately, in an attempt to highlight their individual contribution. Moreover, each pathway influences to a greater extent the other described mechanisms.

Neurogenic Pathways

The neurogenic pathways involved in RH are based on the over-activation of already known pathogenic pathways of essential hypertension. Thus we can identify a central and a peripheral neurogenic dysfunction, which are discussed individually.

Central Neurogenic Dysfunction

Sympathetic Over-Activation

Hyperactivity of the central autonomic nervous system triggers neurogenic resistant hypertension, and it is associated with abnormal homeostatic reflex control. Over-activation of the sympathetic nervous system (SNS) is characteristic for young individuals (<45 years old) with effects on skeletal muscle vasculature, kidneys, and heart, resulting in insulin resistance and hyperinsulinemia (through the effects on glucose delivery), as well as left ventricular hypertrophy [1, 2]. The *sympathetic pathway plays an essential role in the development and evolution of RH*, from triggering to resistance and progression [3]. Recent researches recorded two to three times higher rate of sympathetic nerve firing in patients with true resistant hypertension, regardless of the design of the multidrug therapy [4].

In the activation of the sympathetic pathway, there are involved both specific autonomic territories and peripheral reflex mechanisms comprising arterial baroreceptors, arterial chemoreceptors, and cardiopulmonary mechanoreceptors.

The possible origin of the sympathetic pathway is in the neurons from the *ventrolateral periaqueductal gray*, which send projections to the rostral ventrolateral medulla in the brain stem. This integrative structure that also incorporates similar projections from several locations plays an essential role in the control of tonic sympathetic activation and tonic arterial pressure, as it has a direct connection with the superior segment of the medulla through the upper centers of modulation for the vasomotor sympathetic nerve discharge and blood pressure [5].

The SNS pathway is a subunit of the arterial baroreflex system which connects the autonomic nervous system with the cardiovascular system, and therefore its response is determined by the input received from the mechanoreceptors in the carotid artery [6]. Thus, the afferent signals of the baroreceptors in the peripheral system trigger the release of a signal from the *nucleus tractus solitarius* in the medulla with twofold destination: decrease of the heart rate through parasympathetic vagal stimulation and lowering of blood pressure through tonic inhibition of neurons in the rostral ventrolateral medulla, with the intervention of non-catecholaminergic depressor neurons in caudal ventrolateral medulla. It is currently believed that the sympathetic over-activation in RH is generated by a *disproportion* between the catecholaminergic neurons in the brain stem and decrease or even loss of the inhibitory function of the non-catecholaminergic neurons in the *rostral and caudal ventrolateral medulla*; however, this hypothesis has not been directly investigated [7].

Another involvement of rostral ventrolateral medulla in RH genesis is *neurovascular compression* induced by the posterior inferior cerebellar artery and vertebral artery. This process causes loss of the same inhibitory effect on blood pressure, mainly transmitted via vagus and glossopharyngeal nerves. Thus, sympathetic nerve activity, arterial pressure, heart rate, and plasma levels of epinephrine and norepinephrine were increased by pulsatile compression of these neurons [8].

Furthermore, the "adrenaline hypothesis" currently still under debate takes into account the role of neurotransmitter in the self-maintenance of essential hypertension, through a positive feedback loop developed at the level of the presynaptic beta-adrenoceptors [9].

Vagal Modulation

Since hypertension is characterized by an increased sympathetic tone, the evaluation of the sympathovagal balance could ascertain more accurately the possibility that *vagal tone* could also be involved in RH pathogenesis. Rhythmic components of heart rate variability (HRV, evaluated by RR interval recordings) permit to evaluate autonomic activity at baseline conditions and to separate the different components of variability which seem to reflect specific regulatory mechanisms. The high-frequency (HF) component is a marker of vagal activity, while the low-frequency (LF) component is a marker of sympathetic and vagal activity. The LF/HF ratio is considered as a marker of sympathovagal balance [10, 11].

It is a known fact that vagal nerves influence blood pressure variability more than the sympathetic system [12]. Moreover, blood pressure variability is related to variability of heart rate which is largely influenced by vagal tone [13].

Therapeutic correlation Modulating parasympathetic system by direct vagal nerve stimulation is an emerging interventional therapy [14]. A recent study using a new technique of tripolar stimulation decreased blood pressure in rats without inadvertent stimulation of non-baroreceptive fibers (reducing the side effects like bradycardia and bradypnea) [15].

Peripheric Dysfunction

Carotid Baroreflex

The peripheral unit of the *arterial baroreflex system* consists of the baroreceptors in the cardiovascular unit located in the arterial, venous, and ventricular walls, of which the most investigated are those in the aorta and carotid sinuses. Their activation is prompted by the distension of the vessel wall, as a consequence of the transmural pressure [14]. These mechanoreceptors are activated by the stretch, sending signals that join the glossopharyngeal nerves to the nucleus tractus solitarius and nucleus ambiguus before eventually being modified in the hypothalamus. The hypothalamus is then responsible for the increased parasympathetic efferent activities slowing HR and decreasing blood pressure [6].

Thus, an *impaired activation of the baroreceptors* elicits an increased response from the central nervous system, with a subsequent increase in vascular tonus and decrease in renal excretory function, generating RH [16].

Therapeutic correlation   Recent studies on electrical carotid sinus stimulation with positive results in the management of hypertension have ascertained the important role of the carotid structures in the efficient regulation of blood pressure. The idea behind electrical stimulation of baroreceptors or baroreflex afferent nerves is that the stimulus is perceived as high blood pressure, and then, baroreflex efferent structures are involved to counteract the perceived blood pressure increase [17]. FDA approved a phase II clinical trial for baroreflex activation therapy (Rheos Feasibility Trial) to study the efficacy of the technique and investigate the safety of results [18].

Chemoreceptors

The function of chemoreceptors situated in the carotid body [19] consists in detecting alterations in arterial PO_2, PCO_2, and pH, consequently generating respiratory, autonomic, and cardiovascular corrections such as minute ventilation and arterial pressure increase, in order to prevent oxygen impairment of the brain. Their input is integrated by the *pre-sympathetic neurons* in the medulla and hypothalamus [20]. There is recent evidence that the sympatho-excitatory reflex response is increased in RH, which has led to the introduction of the *carotid body tone concept*. It appears that carotid body tonicity drives sympathetic vasomotor tone, while it does not involve cardiac autonomic activity or ventilation [21].

Therapeutic correlation   Currently, ablation of one of the carotid bodies is investigated as a relatively safe treatment option, and it requires previous determination of abnormal carotid body tone. However effective, this procedure still represents an organ-specific approach, and it must be corroborated with other procedures or therapeutic schemes for the customized management of each individual case [22].

Neural Regulation of the Kidney

The renorenal reflexes have an inhibitory action on excitatory reflexes. Renal mechanosensory nerves lower efferent renal sympathetic nerve activity (ERSNA) and increase urinary sodium excretion, an *inhibitory renorenal reflex*. There is an interaction between efferent and afferent renal nerves, whereby increases in ERSNA increase afferent renal nerve activity (ARNA), leading to decreases in ERSNA by activation of the renorenal reflexes to maintain low ERSNA to minimize sodium retention [23].

Sympathetic neural regulation of renin release and fluid reabsorption may influence fluid balance and, in the longer term, the level at which blood pressure is set. The imbalance in the sympathetic neural innervation of these mechanisms is involved in *resistance to antihypertensive medication* [24].

Therapeutic correlation Recently, bilateral selective renal sympathetic denervation has been performed for patients with resistant hypertension, yielding several benefits in decrease of renal norepinephrine spillover and renin activity, with increase in renal plasma flow and overall prolonged reduction of blood pressure. The procedure consists in ablation through radio frequency of the afferent and efferent innervation of the kidney, with consequent *isolation of renal parenchymal and juxtaglomerular structures from abnormal stimulation* of the efferent adrenergic system, thus severing the link between the over-activated efferent adrenergic system and the renal structures involved in regulation of blood pressure [25, 26].

The kidney is also involved in the development of *salt-sensitive hypertension*, common in the elderly, diabetics, African-Americans, and obese patients, which increases the risk for glomerulosclerosis and renal failure, as a result of augmented glomerular capillary pressures. An important component of the fine autoregulation mechanism of renal blood flow, the *myogenic response*, consists of the constriction of the afferent arteriole triggered by increases in perfusion pressure, which, due to its very short activation delay, can be used in the isolation of glomerular capillaries from the variations in renal perfusion pressure. The myogenic response is mediated by the action of extracellular ATP on *P2X receptors*, their activation being mediated by 20-hydroxyeicosatetraenoic acid (20-HETE) [27]. There are several researches that investigate the involvement of 20-HETE in the control of arterial pressure, regulation of vascular tone and of renal function, as well as protection of glomerular permeability barrier [28]. The *impaired ability of the kidney to synthesize 20-HETE* leads to an increased Na+ transport in the proximal tubule and thick ascending loop of Henle, which consequently generates sodium retention, generating salt-sensitive forms of hypertension.

Therapeutic correlation Given the significant evidence that substantiates the role of 20-HETE in hypertension, new therapies have been established based on antihypertensive agents that function as inhibitors of synthesis of 20-HETE and 20-HETE agonists and antagonists (such as 20-hydroxyeicosa-5(Z),14(Z)-dienoic acid (5-,14-,20-HEDE), *N*-[20-hydroxyeicosa-5(Z),14(Z)-dienoyl]glycine (5-,14-,20-HEDGE) and are associated with PPAR-α (fibrates) or gene therapy, which upregulate 20-HETE synthesis. Another outcome of this therapy could possibly be obtained in hindering the progression of glomerular fibrosis and renal fibrosis [27].

New Theories

Gαi2-Protein-Gated Pathways

A new hypothesis introduced in the attempt to decipher the complex framework of salt-resistant hypertension advances the involvement of paraventricular nucleus *Gαi2-protein-gated signal transduction pathways* in the sympathetically mediated process of renal sodium retention. Experimental investigations on naive Brown Norway, Dahl salt-resistant, and scrambled oligodeoxynucleotide-infused Dahl salt-resistant but not DSS rats have demonstrated that this central molecular pathway plays an important role in the mediation of sympathoinhibitory renal nerve-dependent responses triggered in the mechanism of sodium homeostasis and of a salt-resistant phenotype [29].

Microglia

Currently, the possibility to take into account microglia as a new target for treatment of RH is being investigated, as the activation of these cells in autonomic brain regions is characteristic for the neuroinflammation in neurogenic hypertension [30]. Apparently, the microglia are the main cellular factors in the mediation of neuroinflammation and the modulation of neuronal excitation, mechanisms involved in elevated blood pressure. The hallmarks of *microglial activation are microgliosis and proinflammatory cytokine upregulation.* Moreover, research has ascertained that angiotensin II-induced hypertension is correlated with activation of microglia and increases in proinflammatory cytokines [31] in the paraventricular nucleus.

Therapeutic correlation Studies performed on rats have proved that the targeted depletion of microglia has decreased neuroinflammation, glutamate receptor expression in the paraventricular nucleus, plasma vasopressin level, kidney norepinephrine concentration, and blood pressure [32]. Moreover, the transfer of preactivated cells into the brains of normotensive mice determined a considerably prolonged pressor response to intracerebroventricular injection of angiotensin II, while the inactivation of microglia leads to the disappearance of these effects [33].

Bone Marrow

Bone marrow contribution to the mechanisms of hypertension resides in the increase of peripheral inflammatory cells and their extravasation into the brain (BM – brain interaction) [30]. Moreover, the hypothesis advancing the involvement of

BM-derived cells in neuroinflammation is currently being investigated. Experimental evidence indicates that *minocycline*, an inhibitor of microglial activation, could represent an effective therapy due to its ability to alter neurogenic components of hypertension.

Renalase

Several researches unveiled a new mechanism involved in regulation of cardiac function and blood pressure: *the renalase pathway*. Renalase is an amine oxidase synthetized in the kidney, inactive at baseline, which metabolizes *circulating catecholamines*. Its activation is very swift, and it is triggered by any small variation in blood pressure and plasma catecholamines, leading to an important decrease in blood pressure [34]. Damages in synthesis of renalase are connected with elevated blood pressure and increases in circulating catecholamines. Currently, the mechanisms responsible for the involvement of renalase deficiency in hypertension, as well as the possible contribution of renalase to the regulation of renal dopamine system, are not well described [35].

Gut Microbiota

Recent research on Dahl rats have proven the correlation between gut microbial content and *blood pressure regulation*, with further perspectives opened for investigation regarding the possible association between the host genome and microbiome within the context of blood pressure regulation [36].

GABAA Receptors

Studies on BPH/2J mice demonstrated the cardiovascular effects of chronic activation of GABAA receptors. It seems that their impairment may play a role in the mechanism of neurogenic hypertension by the *failure to suppress arousal-induced sympathetic activation* within the amygdala and hypothalamic nuclei [37].

RAAS Mechanisms

Angiotensin-Aldosterone Escape Pathway

The mechanisms underlying the renin-angiotensin-aldosterone system (RAAS) have been extensively investigated and described. However, recent research has ascertained that the processes are much more complex than a straightforward cascade renin-angiotensinogen-angiotensin I-angiotensin II-aldosterone. The mere understanding of these molecules of the location for their initial (and prevalent) synthesis and knowledge of currently used drug classes (recommended by guidelines) in the therapeutic targeting of the RAAS does not provide any more a complete grasp on the multifaceted aspects of its deficient functioning in RH.

Thus, studies have shown that, once treatment with one of RAAS modulators is initiated, various escape mechanisms are triggered, which are far less known and investigated and which will represent the center of our discussion onward.

Firstly, pathological changes involving aldosterone extend far beyond dysregulations in the sodium and potassium balance, inflammation, cardiovascular remodeling, and renal injury [38]. Vascular smooth muscle cell hypertrophy and hyperplasia, vascular matrix impairment, endothelial dysfunction, decreased vascular compliance, increased peripheral vascular resistance, impaired autonomic vascular control, myocardial norepinephrine release, and decreased serum high-density lipoprotein cholesterol represent all consequences of aldosterone-impaired function [39]. These actions occur through both mineralocorticoid-dependent and mineralocorticoid-independent pathways, and they are either delayed (genomic) mechanisms or rapid (nongenomic) [40]. While some of these effects may be compensated by chronic treatment with angiotensin-converting enzyme inhibitors (ACE-I) and angiotensin receptor blockers (ARB), research has shown that there exists an escape mechanism which brings aldosterone concentrations back to baseline value, possibly reversing the beneficial effects of the treatment on left ventricular hypertrophy [41] and increasing renal damage for patients with type 2 diabetes mellitus [42].

There appears to be a secondary synthesis site besides the adrenal cortex at the vascular level.

Studies have recorded the angiotensin II reactivation and aldosterone escape during treatment with ACE-I or ARB [42], possibly due to accumulation of renin and angiotensin I and to the recently discovered renin-dependent but ACE-independent pathways, which account for 30 to 40% of angiotensin II formation in the normal status. However, experimental studies have shown that the direct renin-prorenin interaction has no direct contribution to the increasing aldosterone levels, which indicates that there exists also and angiotensin II escape pathway involved [43].

Furthermore, it appears that ACE gene polymorphisms [44] intervene in the adequate regulation of the neurohormonal response to long-term treatment, involving the angiotensin II type 2 receptor (AT2R) [45], which, although its functional effects are still unclear, influences hemodynamic function and circulating RAS mediators. Moreover, for chronic heart failure patients, a higher prevalence of the DD phenotype for ACE has been described [46].

The same receptor is the main character in the escape pathway for ARB treatment, which is related to an AT2R-dependent mechanism correlated with target-organ damage in animal models. Recent studies investigate the involvement of proteins expressed by the extracellular matrix in the adrenal cortex, such as bone morphogenetic protein (BMP) [47] and endothelin-1 (ET-1) in the design and function of the aldosterone escape pathway.

Hence, the presence of the BMP system, which has been shown to stimulate angiotensin II-induced aldosterone production, appears to be an event pertaining to the aldosterone cellular escape pathway, triggered under the influence of long-term ARB treatment [48]. Additionally, the role of the endothelin system is being investigated within the framework of chronic heart failure. It has been shown that endothelin-1 (ET-1) system functions as a stimulating factor for aldosterone secretion via both A and B receptors, while the ET peptide ET-1(1–31) seems to be a contributor to adrenocortical growth [49].

Therapeutic correlation   Given the important role played by the ET-1 system in the aldosterone escape pathway and the connection with secondary organ damages associated with RH, the potential use of endothelin antagonists in the prevention of cardiovascular disease is being discussed [50].

The main initiator of the escape process appears to be an important decrease in the levels of thiazide-sensitive NaCl cotransporter (NCC) in the distal convoluted tube, while concurrently increasing in the apical Na/H exchanger of the proximal tubule (NHE3), events which have shown to be nitric oxide dependent [51].

Also related to the aldosterone homeostasis is the expression of human prostasin transgene, which regulates the RAAS and kallikrein-kinin systems, and the circulatory levels of the atrial natriuretic peptide [52], although further research is necessary in order to enable their possible therapeutic targeting [53].

Finally, oxidative stress is a contributing factor which mediates the pathogenesis of chronic cardiovascular and renal damage associated to the malfunctions in the RAAS system and aldosterone homeostasis such as activation of the nuclear transcription factor kappaB and stimulation of pathways and genes that promote vasoconstriction, endothelial dysfunction, cell hypertrophy, fibroblast proliferation, inflammation, excess extracellular matrix deposition, atherosclerosis, and thrombosis [54].

Aldosterone/Renin Ratio

With respect to mineralocorticoid receptors, specialists differentiate two subtypes of RH, associated with high and with normal plasma levels of aldosterone. The first subtype is characterized by primary aldosteronism, obstructive sleep apnea, aldosterone escape mechanism previously described, and increased aldosterone/renin ratio [55], with increased plasma aldosterone levels, but without primary aldosteronism features. The second subtype of hypertension is described by obesity, diabetes mellitus, chronic kidney disease, and polycystic ovary syndrome, and it is mediated by mineralocorticoid receptor activation through individual MR pathways.

Primary aldosteronism holds a special position in the physiopathology of resistant hypertension since it seems to be particularly characteristic for this subgroup of patients, therefore providing potential grounds for designing a screening protocol. Moreover, as advances in identifying confirmatory testing, subtype differentiation and assay methodology are accumulating, and new treatment approaches are also elaborated [56].

Therapeutic correlation Increased plasma aldosterone levels and primary aldosteronism are associated with the absence of aldosterone escape phenomenon in the context of long-term treatment with ACE-I or ARB, which provides the opportunity to use a first-line therapy with mineralocorticoid receptor antagonists [57]. Conversely, for resistant hypertension associated with normal plasma aldosterone levels, ARB or ACE-I may be used as first-line therapy with the introduction of an MR antagonist as an add-on agent [58].

Furthermore, it has been proved that decreased expression of regulators of G protein signaling 2 (RGS2) contributes, together with increased plasma aldosterone levels and high aldosterone/renin ratio, to the development of resistant hypertension [59]. It has also been suggested that increased levels of corticotropin could determine the increase in aldosterone, as well as in brain and atrial natriuretic peptide levels [60].

Therapeutic correlation Experimental studies have shown that the subacute modifications in RAAS activity during ACE-I treatment, reflected in increases in the urinary aldosterone/creatinine ratio, indicate an incomplete blockade of the system and the presence of escape mechanisms, which could prove useful in evaluation of effectiveness of therapy and a better management of the disease [61].

Renin and Prorenin

Within the current trend of optimization of RAAS blockade in RH, a special interest is dedicated to the prorenin receptor (PRR). This component of the RAAS system is located in the kidneys, within mesangial cells, renal arterioles, and distal nephron segments, and has four distinct functions: (1) To bind renin and prorenin in the production of angiotensin I, increasing renin catalytic activity and activating prorenin. (2) To activate intracellular signals when a ligand binds to PRR, upregulating the expression of profibrotic genes. (3) To contribute to the functions of vacuolar proton ATPase. (4) To take part in the Wnt signaling pathways [62], which play a critical role in adult and embryonic stem cell biology, embryonic development, and various diseases such as cancer [63].

Additionally, given that the stimulatory effects of prorenin on microglial activation and production of proinflammatory cytokines have been ascertained, the PRR could also be involved in the development of RAAS-induced neurogenic hypertension [64].

While results of animal studies did not clearly ascertain the significance of PRR in hypertension or in organ damage, human studies indicated that there exists a correlation between a polymorphism of the PRR gene and blood pressure [65]. Moreover, while the mechanisms involved in regulation of renin in the collecting duct are not elucidated yet [66], it appears that increase in renin synthesis and activity independent of blood pressure at this location may contribute to the additional production of intrarenal and intratubular angiotensin II, while renin-PRR interactions could be involved in the development of hypertension and kidney disease [67]. Several researches have shown a stimulating effect of the intrarenal angiotensin II on PRR expression [68] through a succession of processes which involves the cyclooxygenase-2-prostaglandin E2 pathway with vasoconstrictor effects [69] and the prostaglandin E-prostanoid 4 receptor [70], therefore leading to the development of angiotensin II-dependent hypertension [71].

Therapeutic correlation   Even though experimental research has not been yet able to fully understand the involvement of PRR in each cell and disease context, the usage of PRR as potential target in RH prevention and treatment is currently being considered, as it has been shown that neuron-specific PRR knockout hinders the development of salt-sensitive hypertension [72]. Therefore, the addition of a renin inhibitor in the treatment of RH and associated organ damage could increase the efficiency of RAAS blockade in tissues [73].

Angiotensin Receptors

The role and interaction of angiotensin receptors have also been investigated within the context of RH. While the physiological functions of angiotensin type 1 receptor (AT1R) are well ascertained and described, the involvement of type 2 receptor (AT2R) is far less investigated. The location of AT2 expression largely in vascular endothelial cells and muscular media in resistant arteries and in the perivascular nerve fibers as well indicates its involvement in systemic and neuronal blood pressure regulation [74]. Also, experimental studies on insulin-resistant hypertensive rats have shown that one function of AT2R is to counterbalance the effects of AT1R on blood pressure and glucose metabolism [75], while the actions of both receptors are dissociated from their involvement in glucose metabolism. With respect to AT1R, studies have shown that various factors are involved in its regulation in salt-sensitive HT such as the renin-angiotensin system [76] and estrogenic hormones [77]. Furthermore, it has been reported that polymorphism of AT1 A-C1166 gene could be involved in the defective regulation of blood pressure of RH patients [78]. Activation of AT1R in cardiac hypertrophy appears to be mediated by autocrine and paracrine effects of locally produced angiotensin II, although there are studies which indicate an angiotensin-independent activator effect for mechanical stress [79]. Further studies are required in order to complete the description of the pathophysiological functions for this receptor.

Chymase

As part of the effort to optimize the effects of RAAS blockade, investigations regarding production pathways for angiotensin II have introduced chymase as an essential enzyme involved in this process [80]. Chymase is synthesized in mast cells and endothelial cells in the human heart [81], as well as in cardiac interstitium [82]. Its activity results in continuing conversion of angiotensin I to angiotensin II despite effective ACE-I treatment, with apparently higher specificity for angiotensin than ACE. Chymase-dependent mechanisms may be involved in progression of chronic kidney disease [83] as well as adverse atrial and ventricular remodeling.

On the other hand, the involvement of neutral endopeptidase 24.11 in cleavage of atrial natriuretic peptide and angiotensin II has been investigated, establishing that inhibition of the enzyme modulates circulating levels of angiotensin II when basal levels are above normal [84].

Therapeutic correlation Therapeutic targeting of RAAS system is currently being redesigned by the inclusion of the alternate pathways for the generation of angiotensin peptides. Additionally, to renin inhibitors, dual inhibitors of ACE and endopeptidase 24.11 are being considered, as well as gene therapy or antibody treatment.

Intracellular RAAS

The recent discovery of locally generated angiotensin products (angiotensin II, III, and IV and Ang 1–7) in several tissue and organs such as the brain, bone marrow, adipose tissue, epididymis, carotid body, liver, and pancreas [85], together with new evidence that the prorenin/renin molecule is an intracrine enzyme, has led to the introduction of the concept of intracellular RAAS [86], which describes independent intracrine/autocrine/paracrine subsystems located in tissues throughout the entire organism, opposing the endocrine system paradigm [87]. Thus, RAAS system is proving out to be a continuous process involving both large and small structures, with independent control at several levels. Recent evidence establishes that in its structure enter four main axes: (1) the classical renin-ACE-angiotensin II; (2) the prorenin-PRR-MAP kinase; (3) the ACE2-Ang 1–7/Mas receptor, with seemingly antagonistic effect; and (4) the angiotensin IV-insulin-regulated aminopeptidase [88]. The locally generated angiotensin peptides apparently have multiple and new functions such as cell growth, antiproliferation, apoptosis, reactive oxygen species generation, hormonal secretion, promotion of inflammation and fibrosis, and vasoconstriction and vasodilation.

Although the pathophysiological functions of these systems have yet to be described in detail, evidence indicates the involvement of tissue intracrine systems in etiopathogeny of cardiovascular disease and in cardiovascular structural remodeling [89]. There appears to be also an angiotensin-regulated synthesis of aldosterone in the cardiac tissue, which indicates the possible existence of an RAAS local cardiovascular system [90]. Experimental studies show that in diabetic conditions, the cardiac intracellular RAAS is activated, increasing oxidative stress and cardiac fibrosis [91]. Moreover, local RAAS seems to be involved in control of cell communication and inward Ca(2+) current [92].

Recent studies have shown the involvement of kidney local angiotensin II production in regulation of blood pressure and proximal tubular reabsorption [93] on rats and mice [94]. Moreover, as internalization of angiotensin II has been demonstrated, it is still uncertain if this process is involved in intracrine and signaling pathways [95].

Similarly, the RAAS in the hematopoietic bone marrow is involved in mediation of pathobiological dysregulations of hematopoiesis, while the presence of ACE has been ascertained in human primitive lymphohematopoietic cells, as well as in embryonic, fetal, and adult hematopoietic tissues [96]. It appears that angiotensin II triggers the proliferation and differentiation of CD34+ stem cells through binding with angiotensin II type 1a membrane receptors. Moreover, the human umbilical cord blood seems to comprise a local RAAS, and expression of renin, angiotensinogen, and ACE mRNAs has been demonstrated, with possible involvement in cellular growth in several tissues [97].

Existence of local RAAS in the brain has been demonstrated in dendritic processes of neurons in the medial nucleus tractus solitarii and area postrema [98], areas involved in central cardiovascular effects triggered by angiotensin II, through identification of intracellular and plasmalemmal AT1 receptors and of intraneuronal production of angiotensin II [99].

In the pancreas, the local RAAS has been identified in pancreatic acinar, isled, duct, endothelial, and stellate cells, while its expression is modulated in accordance with various stimuli such as hypoxia, pancreatitis, islet transplantation, hyperglycemia, and diabetes mellitus [100].

The presence of local intracrine RAAS has been ascertained in the liver as well, where it has been reported to act in concert with or independently of the endocrine renin system [101].

Tissue Kallikrein-Kinin

Within the framework of these new concepts introduced in the description of RAAS, it seems that hypertension could be in fact the consequence of an imbalance between the vasodepressor and vasopressor hormonal systems. Moreover, local hormonal systems could be put together by vasodepressor hormones such as kinins, prostaglandins, and endothelium-derived relaxing factor. The tissue kallikrein-kinin system could be involved in local regulation of circulation, renal function, as well as in the acute antihypertensive effect of ACE-I [102].

Involved in several intracellular signaling pathways, angiotensin II contributes significantly to the organ damage associated with RH. While the upregulation of its intracellular signaling increases the risk for kidney damage in hypertension [103], its inhibitory influence on several receptors and regulatory proteins in the insulin signaling pathways leads to a higher insulin sensitivity, thus decreasing the risk for type 2 diabetes mellitus [104]. The pathological changes in the heart and blood vessels generated by the abnormal activity of fibroblasts involve multiple intracellular pathways, which, although still incompletely elucidated, implicate angiotensin II as activating factor for an extracellular signal-regulated kinase (ERK1/2) [105]. On the other hand, excessive angiotensin II signaling leads to high levels of intracellular calcium recruitment in fibroblasts, though recent research has shown that this event is diminished by insulin in insulin-sensitive individuals [106]. Hence, since the insulin resistance appears to be related to a subnormal Galpha(i2)-mediated signal transduction, it could provide a pathway for regulation of angiotensin II signaling pathway.

Protective Pathways

Several studies have reported protective roles for some of the elements described above. Thus, the AT1R is one of the main characters of the ACE-angiotensin II-AT1R pathway, which functions as a counter-regulatory axis for RAAS. It has been suggested that AT1R functions as stimulatory factor on sodium reabsorption as they are related to the increased expression of specific tubular sodium transporters [107], while AT2R has the reverse action, increasing natriuresis and lowering blood pressure through an autocrine cascade including bradykinin, nitric oxide, and cyclic GMP and controlling vasodilator prostaglandins [108]. It seems that the interaction between these renal pathways bears significance for the increase of long-term effective management of blood pressure, with AT2R having an opposite protective role to that of AT1R. Moreover, experimental studies have shown that AT2R stimulation mediates vasodilatory and natriuretic effects, increasing renal function especially in women, which indicates a potential therapeutic target for cardiovascular disease [109].

Several studies have attributed a protective role for plasma angiotensin 1–7 in the vascular smooth muscle, through reversal of vascular proliferation [110], as well as a role in regulation of metabolic pathways related to cell death and survival in human endothelial cells [111]. Furthermore, it seems that the protective signaling of angiotensin 1–7 against diastolic dysfunction is independent of blood pressure regulation [112] and is mediated through activated pathways contributing to Ca2+ handling, hypertrophy, and survival. Moreover, another counter-regulatory axis for RAAS, the ACE-angiotensin 1–7-Mas receptor pathway, plays a significant role in cardiovascular repair [113], with antihypertrophic and antifibrotic actions [114], through stimulation of CD34+ stem/progenitor cells, which are cardiovascular protective [115]. Although the renal protective action of this peptide hormone is reported, especially against endothelial dysfunction or angiotensin II-stimulated tubular damage, its involvement in glomerular function is not yet fully elucidated [116]. Conversely, it appears that the involvement of angiotensin 1–7 in blood pressure regulation is mostly indirect, through interaction of bradykinin and nitric oxide signaling [114], while there are studies which suggest it could act as an endogenous ACE inhibitor [117], given increased levels of angiotensin 1–7 during ACE-I administration [118].

Among other protective agents in the pathophysiological dynamics of RH, studies report that vitamin D could ameliorate HT and renal damage, through genomic and extra-genomic pathways [119], while vitamin D receptor-modulated expression of heat-shock protein 70 has a protective intervention against angiotensin II-induced HT and renal damage [120]. Estrogens have proven to be intervening in reduction of vascular damage, mainly through the nuclear estrogen receptor alpha, and protecting against angiotensin II-induced hypertension [121]. Additionally, overexpression of Smad7 protein has a protective role in angiotensin II-mediated hypertensive cardiac remodeling as well [122]. Downregulation of p22hox, an important component of NADPH oxidase complex, plays a protective anti-inflammatory effect in angiotensin II-induced oxidative stress, through suppression of MAPK and NF-kB signaling pathways [123]. Melatonin hormone is involved in protection against hypertension, as melatonin receptors are involved in regulation of the RAAS system [124]. Finally, local kallikrein-kinin system (KKS) pathways are significantly implicated in endogenous cardiovascular protective mechanisms [125], while studies substantiate the finding that kinins are mediators of these mechanisms, their role in the cardiovascular system, as well as the interaction between KKS and RAAS being still insufficiently investigated [125].

Sodium Involvement in Resistant Hypertension

Dopamine

The complex network of mechanisms involved in regulation of sodium balance in physiological and pathological circumstances is extensively investigated in relation with the events describing the genesis of RH. The processes surrounding sodium excretion and reabsorption involve the interactive relationship between the renin-angiotensin-aldosterone system (previously described in "RAAS Mechanisms" section.) and the renal dopaminergic system, centered on the synthesis and activity of intrarenal dopamine [126].

Increased levels of dopamine and the consequent over-activation of dopaminergic receptors are triggered by high NaCl intake and result in decreased epithelial sodium transport and increased sodium excretion, with additional stimulation of antioxidant and anti-inflammatory pathways. Therefore, alterations in the essential processes featuring dopamine such as biosynthesis, receptor expression, and signal transduction are consistent with the imbalance in renal sodium excretion characteristic for hypertension [127].

Therapeutic correlation   Due to its essential role in sodium processing and regulation of renal blood flow, current research brings about the possibility to use dopamine as a nephroprotective agent in order to prevent renal failure. Further investigation will have to show if this strategy is a viable option for critically ill patients.

The activating factors of these deficiencies are still not identified [126], although recent research seems to indicate high sodium intake and elements that favor the insulin resistance state such as diets high in carbohydrates and fat. There are also surging issues regarding the altered abilities of intrarenal sodium sensors, given the sensitization effects of high sodium intake and volume expansion on the renal dopaminergic system. Experimental studies have ascertained the correlation between impaired renal dopamine production and failure to eliminate acute increase in sodium load on genetically altered rat populations [127].

There are two types of receptors associated with the physiology of dopamine, namely, D1-like receptors (D1 and D5) and D2-like receptors (D2, D3, and D4) [128]. In normal status, dopamine synthesized at the renal level behaves as an autocrine/paracrine/natriuretic hormone and initiates the inhibition of apical and basolateral ion transports and exchanges resulting in decreased tubular sodium reabsorption [129]. The binding of stimulatory guanine nucleotide-binding proteins (G proteins, such as Gαs and Golf) on D1-like receptors leads to the activation of multiple cellular signaling systems such as adenylyl cyclase and phospholipase C (PLC) [130]. Therefore, it seems that a defective coupling of the D1-like receptors to their G protein complex could be responsible for the disturbances in the sodium processing systems which are recorded in hypertension [131]. Current research suggests that in rats as well as in humans the uncoupling of D1-like receptors from the G protein/effector complex could be caused by their ligand-independent hyperphosphorylation and desensitization [132]. These processes may be determined by the inability of D1-like agonists to increase the activity of a specific enzyme, protein phosphatase 2A [133], which plays an essential role in the regulation of the G protein-coupled receptor function.

Therapeutic correlation Recent studies show that direct interstitial stimulation of D1-like receptors with fenoldopam, a selective receptor agonist, triggers natriuresis via an angiotensin type 2 receptor mechanism, with possible further implications in the therapeutic management of hypertension [134].

On the other hand, experimental research identified the genetically determined defective coupling of D1 receptors to the G protein/adenylyl cyclase complex as the possible culprit in the impairment of the renal dopaminergic system [132]. The defect is identifiable prior to the initiation of hypertension and is consistent with the hypertensive phenotype while not being relayed to other humoral agents. It appears to be a "mistargeting" mechanism which is not caused by a mutation in the primary sequence and is yet to be identified [135]. Moreover, the defect could not be recorded in other renal locations outside the proximal tubules. This receptor impairment results in the failure of D1 agonists to inhibit Na+/H+ exchange activity. Furthermore, apparently, the decreased renal sodium excretion after dopamine administration is related to decreased cyclic AMP synthesis and to the impaired ability of dopamine to inhibit Na+,K + −ATPase activity. Besides dopamine, experimental studies on rats show that toxin-sensitive G proteins (pertussis and cholera toxin) are directly involved as well in the regulation of proximal tubule Na+, K+-ATPase activity, their activity being abnormal in hypertensive rat populations, resulting in enhanced salt reabsorption in the kidney [136].

In normal status, D1-like and D2-like receptors are the initiators of several signaling pathways which result in activation of adenylyl cyclase, increased cyclic adenosine 3′,5′-monophosphate (cAMP) levels, protein kinase activation, stimulation of phospholipase Cβ1 in renal tubules, suppression of protein kinase B signaling pathway, and activation of mitogen-activated protein kinase while concurrently interacting with one another and creating new signaling pathways, which in turn increase phospholipase C (PLC) stimulation in renal cortical cells [129].

Deficiencies in these signaling pathways lead to inhibition of Na+, K+-ATPase determined by an impaired activation of phospholipase C and protein kinase C. Recent experimental investigations bring supplementary evidence as to the signification of the decrease in levels of the specific antipeptide Gq/11 alpha and impaired metabolism of arachidonic acid, a product of phospholipase A2, which, together with the decreased activation of G proteins, contribute to the decreased dopaminergic inhibition of sodium pump activity [137]. Additionally, it has been suggested that the dopamine D1 receptor-mediated stimulation of PLC is a consequence of protein kinase A activation, which increases PLC-gamma in cytosol and cell membrane with the contribution of protein kinase C activation [138].

Therapeutic correlation   Studies on black normotensive and hypertensive salt-sensitive versus salt-resistant subjects have shown a deficiency in the renal dopaminergic system that triggers the natriuretic response to high sodium intake only in salt-resistant subjects and only under low-sodium diets. It seems that this deficiency is associated with a decreased decarboxylation of dopa into dopamine [139].

Epithelial Na+ Channel Proteins

The traditional approach of epithelial Na+ channel (ENaC) proteins discusses them from the point of view of their involvement in the salt and water processes involved in blood pressure regulation from the aldosterone-sensitive renal cortical-collecting duct, as the closing effector element of the renin-angiotensin-aldosterone system (RAAS) [140].

Nevertheless, recent studies have brought evidence in support of three essential nontubular roles of these proteins [141]. The first role is related to their activity in the central nervous system. Thus, ENaC from the choroid plexus and cardiovascular-regulatory brain stem nuclei act as sensors of the cerebral spinal fluid for variations in sodium balance and participate in sodium regulation mechanism by eliciting an increased sympathetic activity as response to high sodium levels in order to induce vasoconstriction and proximal tubule natriuresis. Moreover, a recent study reports that enhanced expression of ENaC generates salt-induced pressor activity [142].

The second location for ENaC intervention is at the vascular level, where one of their roles is the intervention in endothelial cell function, where they mediate shear stress and endothelial membrane stiffness, in a newly discovered, but still incompletely investigated, pathway for regulation of vascular tone, while the second role is as mechanosensors that initiate the vascular smooth muscle cell-mediated myogenic constriction, independent of neural influences. Their role as mediators in the mechanism of renal blood flow autoregulation and protection from increased systemic pressure has been supported by experimental studies as well, which have correlated high blood pressure with increased level of ENaC proteins.

Ultrastructurally, the ENaC proteins consist of four homologous subunits (α, β, γ, and δ) encoded by genes SCNN1A, SCNN1B, SCNN1G, and SCNN1D, which belong to the ENaC/degenerin superfamily, together with other related proteins such as degenerin, described in nematodes, and acid-sensing ion channel (ASIC) family, recorded in mammals. Their protein structure reflects the function of extracellular proton and/or mechanosensors for either extracellular Na+, shear stress, or strain [143].

Through their extracellular domain which interacts with the extracellular environment, the ENaC proteins function as fine-tuning mechanisms on the long-term regulation of renal Na+ and water balance and hence of blood pressure. Thus, ENaC functions as convergence point of these signaling pathways as activation in central ENaC leads to increased renal vascular resistance and increased Na+ renal reabsorption, while concurrently stimulating the RAAS system, which brings about supplementary consequences in renal hemodynamics and salt/water transport. Simultaneously, the functions of ENaC at the vascular level resulting in vasodilation and myogenic-mediated vasoconstriction lead to increased renal tubular Na+/water transport due to alterations in peritubular capillary pressure. Long-term loss of myogenic constriction results in renal injury associated with hypertension.

Therapeutic correlation Given their essential role in regulation of body salt and water homeostasis, ENaC and ASIC proteins represent viable therapeutic targets for a possible long-term control of resistant hypertension [144]. Studies report that H2S prevents advanced glycation end products (AGEs)-induced ENaC activation in A6 cells, which could have an important significance in the management of diabetic hypertension [145].

Furthermore, the inhibitory regulation of ENaC has been attributed to the intervention of an intrinsic purinergic signaling system, which involves the metabotropic P2Y2 purinergic receptor in the relay of paracrine ATP signaling. It has been shown that mutations involving ENaC activity and defective regulation of this channel, such as loss of purinergic inhibition or stimulation of P2Y2, result in abnormal variations in blood pressure and Na excretion, which support the possible causative role of purinergic signaling pathway of the distal nephron for specific form of hypertension [140]. As to the stimulatory regulation of ENaC, experimental research has shown the contribution of norepinephrine [146], by observing the presence of noradrenergic nerve fibers in close proximity to ENaC-expressing cells, and of ethanol, which probably increases intracellular oxidative stress through acetaldehyde [147].

These findings support the hypothesis that RH associated with alcohol consumption does not fall within the category of true RH, and could be of a transient nature, even if there are no studies investigating the degree of its reversibility in the circumstances of complete alcohol abstinence. Moreover, effects of ethanol exposure involved both ENaC gating, by increasing open state probability and also surface abundance, increasing ENaC availability at the apical membrane, which proves that the mechanism in which ethanol interferes with salt and water transport is extremely complex. Further research is required in order to ascertain the relevance of ethanol concentration and chronic consumption in the etiology and dynamics of RH, and, given that oxidative stress is the main culprit for the variations in ENaC activity after ethanol administration, it is essential to understand the reasons for which it enhances ENaC activity under the influence of certain factors (such as ethanol) [148].

Genetic mutations through targeted substitution of the tryptophan residues in the transmembrane domain lead to an increased steady state at hyperpolarizing voltage potentials associated with transient activation times [149], while through site-directed mutagenesis the inhibitory effect of external sodium concentrations can be altered, an acidic cleft being the main ligand-binding locus for ENaC and possibly for other members of the ENaC/ASIC superfamily [150].

Other Molecules

The sodium pump ligand, ouabain, is currently investigated as a possible main character in the etiopathogeny of salt-dependent hypertension, as high levels of ouabain appear to be involved in the sustained increased of sympathetic nerve activity elicited by high sodium intake, participating in a hypothalamic signaling pathway together with aldosterone, ENaC, and angiotensin II, while at the periphery ouabain synthesized by the adrenal cortex increases vasoconstriction through specific signaling pathways [151].

At the cardiovascular level, ouabain, through its function as a growth factor, may be involved in the vascular remodeling associated with RH, and it has been associated both to left ventricular dysfunction and hypertrophy.

Ouabain seems to be a component of a new CNS-humoral axis, which interconnects the central nervous system with RAAS and sodium regulation system, contributing to the chronic pressor effect of brain angiotensin II [152]. Within the same framework, ouabain seems to stimulate through specific pathways, activated also by sympathetic activity, the endogenous ligand of alpha(1) sodium pump, adrenocortical marinobufagenin, which inhibits renal Na-K-ATPase and increases blood pressure [153, 154]. Moreover, a genetic pathway has been described, associated with both acute and chronic salt variations, that involves the uromodulin gene [155], which modulates tubular sodium excretion, while the lanosterol synthase gene, related to the synthesis of endogenous ouabain, influences vasoconstrictor activity which modulates circulating ouabain levels.

Therapeutic correlation The complex physiopathologic relationship between salt intake, genetic control of renal sodium processing, and endogenous ouabain effect is still incompletely deciphered. However, new antihypertensive agents [156] are being currently tested that selectively antagonize the effects of ouabain and another associated protein, adducin, in enhancing the Na-K function and increasing sodium reabsorption and blood pressure.

Among the mechanisms involved in RH pathogeny, experimental studies have described the involvement of the α2-Na+ pump, whose pathologic upregulation leads to excessive Ca(2+) entry and signaling, contributing significantly to blood pressure elevation [157]. Moreover, several trials have attributed the molecular identity of the H(+) transport pathway to the voltage-gated proton channel, HV1, which promotes superoxide production in medullary thick ascending limb nephron segments in the presence of decreased levels of intracellular sodium, thus contributing to the development of hypertension and renal disease [158].

Oxidative Damage and Inflammation

In recent years, there has been increasing evidence related to the involvement of the *immune system* in the pathogenic mechanism of hypertension. A *neuroimmune axis* [159] has been proposed which connects the sympathetic nervous system, immune cells, the production of cytokines, and vascular and renal dysfunction, orchestrated in a complex interaction that brings about severe and resistant hypertension. As our discussion on the implication of the immune system will unfold, we will attempt to present the latest data that seem to substantiate the theory that one of the multiple facets of RH could be that of *autoimmune disease* [160].

Thus, studies have reported the accumulation of macrophages and long-lived memory T cells [161] in the kidneys and blood vessels of humans and experimental animals with RH, and the impaired blood pressure response of lymphocyte-deficient mice to several stimuli (such as angiotensin II, increased salt levels, and norepinephrine) can be restored by the adoptive transfer of T cells. Immune cell activation in hypertension is apparently regulated via the central nervous system, since experimental data has shown that damage to the anteroventral third ventricle impedes T-cell activation triggered by angiotensin II.

It is therefore likely that the initial increase in blood pressure termed as "prehypertension" [162], caused by over-activation of the sympathetic pathway in response to common mild hypertensive stimuli, *generates neoantigens* by modifications in protein structure caused by oxidative stress [163]. It is reported that proteins modified through oxidation by highly reactive γ-ketoaldehydes (*isoketals*) are synthesized by dendritic cells due to hypertensive stimuli administrated to animal models [164]. Accumulation of isoketals leads to the activation of the antigen-presenting function of these cells and represents the *source of self-antigens*. The immune cascade is consequently initiated, the dendritic cell playing an essential role through its function in processing and presenting the neoantigens and neopeptides resulted. Activation of dendritic cells results in increased production of IFN-γ and IL-17A and increased proliferation of T cells, mainly CD8+. Furthermore, experimental studies show that an important contribution in the consequent activation of CD8+ T lymphocytes may be played by the co-stimulatory molecules CD70, CD80, and

CD86 expressed by dendritic cells, as well as IL-15, a cytokine synthesized by renal epithelium as a result of inflammation [165].

The subsequent migration of activated T cells and macrophages in the kidney and blood vessels contributes to the renal and vascular impairment through synthesis of inflammatory cytokines (IL-6, interferon-γ, and IL-17) [162]. At the *vascular level*, the inflammatory cytokines synthesized by activated T cells lead to increased arterial stiffness, as studies report detectable levels of IL-1β in patients with resistant hypertension, while apparently TNF-α is likely to intervene in the mediation of vascular damage as well [166, 167]. Other inflammatory biomarkers involved in the vascular dysfunction associated with resistant hypertension are E-selectin, P-selectin, and MCP1, high levels there of being recorded in the serum of patients with hypertension [168].

Therapeutic correlation Due to the involvement of memory T cells in cytokine synthesis, which leads to angiotensinogen production and Na+ retention, prevention of end-organ damage and hypertension could be achieved through interventions which would target the formation or accumulation of specific subsets of memory T cells in the kidney [169]. On the other hand, there are also recent discussions about the design of a vaccine for hypertension [170] which would target the specific peptides involved in the pathogenic mechanism. Furthermore, given that isoketal scavengers prevent the development of the immune cascade associated with hypertension, these modified proteins represent a potential target for new treatment strategy in resistant hypertension [164].

In addition to the dynamics of the cellular processes involved in the immune aspect of RH, studies also assign an important contribution to *oxidative stress* in the increase of hypertension, although the etiopathogenic signification has not been proven yet in humans. Nevertheless, it has been ascertained that RH patients display *higher oxidative stress levels*, reflected in the endothelial dysfunction and cardiovascular modifications specific for hypertension [171].

Oxidative stress (involving reactive oxygen species – ROS) is generated by the family of nicotinamide adenine dinucleotide phosphate (NADPH) oxidase family (Nox1, Nox2, Nox4, and Nox5), mitochondrial enzymes, xanthine oxidase, and uncoupled *NO synthase* (NOS), through a complex molecular mechanism which results from the interaction between the increased expression of adhesion molecules, synthesis of proinflammatory and pro-thrombotic factors, and increased endothelin-1 secretion [172]. Consequently, in the dynamics of the molecular processes, increased levels of oxidative stress also lead to decrease of *nitric oxide levels* [15, 173], with the involvement of COX-2 enzyme of the cyclooxygenase family, whose increased levels were recorded in essential hypertensive patients, and also to the impaired antioxidant ability of the cardiovascular, renal, and nervous systems [174].

There is also a subtle interaction between these processes at the level of the central nervous system, as research has shown that the genetic manipulation of oxidative stress in the subfornical organ on the dorsal part of the third ventricle influences hypertension as well as T lymphocyte activation [162]. As we have already discussed in section the section on Neurogenic Pathways, bone marrow is involved as well in neuroinflammation, since it is the source for the proliferation of peripheral inflammatory cells and their transport into the brain [30].

Therapeutic correlation Clinical trials have investigated the effects of antioxidants in hypertensive patients, and although they have not proven to be an operational treatment, current research advances the idea of targeting Noxs in an isoform-specific manner in the attempt to balance the levels of oxidative stress.

The hypothesis of RH as autoimmune disease is completed by the involvement of *complement system* and standard and *high-sensitive C reactive protein* [175], their increased levels being reflected in the endothelial damage and arterial stiffness [176, 177]. Currently, the role of matrix metalloproteinases/tissue inhibitors of metalloproteinases (MMPs/TIMPs) system in the pathogeny of hypertension is being investigated, indicating a possible contribution to the determination of arterial function [178].

Therapeutic correlation Aside from providing partial control of resistant hypertension, *renal denervation* brings supplementary evidence as to the sympathetic control of chronic vascular inflammation [179, 180], since the procedure has beneficial outcomes in the decrease of inflammation biomarkers and reduced T-cell activation as well [181].

Genetic Perspectives on Resistant Hypertension

Each previous section on physiopathological mechanisms of RH (neural, RAAS, Na, inflammation) includes gene involvement and influence on the various sites, such as receptor, ligand, enzyme, or intracellular mechanism. Mutations in the gene that codes the respective receptor/enzyme/ligand lead to dysregulation of the entire mechanisms and, consequently, to an exaggerated pressor response or insufficient inhibition.

An excellent summarization of the research on gene variants involvement in RH was recently published by El Rouby and Cooper-DeHoff [182].

We identified three main directions in the approach of RH gene framework:

- Understanding of the mechanisms behind the inadequate/exaggerated pressor response
- Understanding the reasons for the absence of response to usual antihypertensive medication
- Elaboration of new treatment approaches

Mainly, the pharmacogenomics of RH envisages the identification of genetic markers for the prediction of the response to antihypertensive medication, therefore optimizing the treatment scheme and possibly decreasing prevalence of RH [183]. Response or lack thereof to treatment is associated with several gene polymorphisms (e.g., ADRB1, CACNB2, NEDD4L) [184].

Genetic profiling will probably lead to the redefinition of the RH paradigm and introduce different diagnosis criteria, identifying an entity by the gene/cluster involved and not by number of antihypertensive drugs, which will consequently determine adequate tailoring of treatment or even the design of new therapeutic solutions (e.g., vaccine).

To date, we cannot attempt an exhaustive description of gene mechanisms involved, not for RH population subgroup and even more not for the entire essential hypertension population, as we are in the midst of a hunting for genes direction. The Millennium Genome Project (MGP) for Hypertension launched at the beginning of 2000 is a complex endeavor, aiming to identify genetic variants conferring susceptibility to hypertension, in the attempt of enriching knowledge and understanding of HT etiopathogenesis and designing genome-based personalized medical care. The investigation approach is based on two different multilateral directions: (1) genome-wide association analysis (GWAS) using single nucleotide polymorphisms (SNPs) and microsatellite markers and (2) systematic candidate gene analysis, based on the hypothesis that common variants play a significant role in the etiopathogeny of common diseases. These approaches singled out ATP2B1 as gene responsible for hypertension in Japanese and Caucasian populations. The increased risk for high blood pressure granted by specific alleles of ATP2B1 has been widely replicated in several populations [185].

However, the simple identification of genetic variants may not fully explain the complexity of RH etiopathogenic mechanisms, since their effects may be influenced by gene-gene or gene-environment interactions. A suggestive example is a recent study which assessed the interaction between gene polymorphisms for ACE (rs1799752), angiotensinogen (M235 T, rs 699), and nitric oxide endothelial synthase (Glu 298Asp, rs 1,799,983) and environmental factors (age, gender, biologic parameters), reporting that the AGT 235 allele represents an independent risk factor for RH, especially associated with over 50 years of age [186].

Both in essential and resistant hypertension, gene analysis reveals the involvement of several genes and interactions between genes and nongenetic factors, as opposed to monogenic conditions where genetic analysis can be complete and clear. Currently, the gathering of extensive collections of SNPs which can be used as markers in GWA studies with the aim to identify hypertension susceptibility loci. Therefore, it is expected that markers interrogating SNPs involved in inheritance of disease susceptibility will emerge through their association with this trait in the afflicted population [187].

There are large studies comprising genetic subinvestigations which have examined antihypertensive treatment in essential HT and considered the reasons for the lack of response to various medication classes (NORDIL, GITS, INSIGHT – calcium –antagonists, GENRES, and MILAN, diuretics). Furthermore, the analysis of response to diuretic (hydrochlorothiazide) is based on SNPs (in PEAR and GERA studies), while in pharmacogenomics studies it is investigated response to beta blockers and diuretics [188, 189].

There are few data on genetic variants associated with RH. One study aimed to identify SNPs associated with RH in hypertensive participants with coronary artery disease (CAD) from INVEST-GENES (the International VErapamil-SR Trandolapril STudy-GENEtic Substudy). They concluded that ATP2B1 rs12817819 A allele is associated with increased risk for RH in hypertensive participants with documented CAD or suspected ischemic heart disease [190].

A recent analysis from the Genetics of Hypertension Associated Treatment Study assessed the association of 78 candidate gene polymorphisms with RH and concluded that The Met allele of rs699 and the G allele of rs5051 were positively associated with RH [191]. Recent GWA studies have revealed that the ATP2B1 gene is associated with HT not only in people of European origin but also in Japanese, Chinese, and Koreans, while recently investigations have suggested that the ATP2B1 gene may be involved in mechanisms responsible for calcium homeostasis [192].

Ethnic Differences in Genetic Predisposition to Hypertension

Transethnic meta-analyses of GWA studies have identified eight blood pressure-associated loci which seem to be shared by three ethnic groups – Europeans and East and South Asians. The possible sources of heterogeneity have been outlined by four genetic mechanisms, from incidence of allelic heterogeneity to variations in linkage disequilibrium structure, to gene-gene and gene-environment interactions, and, finally, to deficiencies of target variants in other ethnic groups. These mechanisms appear to be the foundation for the considerable ethnic differences reported in clinical presentation of HT, response to treatment, salt sensitivity, and impact of obesity. It is currently believed that the transethnic meta-analyses are the most useful investigation approach which could prove of use in identifying new susceptibility loci and pathophysiological pathways and in enabling fine mapping of common variants [193].

One GWA study reported results of the Korean Association REsource (KARE, 8842 subjects) and recorded ten SNPs that showed significant association with hypertension. Of these ten SNPs, three were replicated in the Health2 project (7861 subjects) with the aim to identify an association with systolic or diastolic blood pressure. The three significant SNPs were located on four distinct genes: the previously reported ATP2B1 (rs17249754), the c-src tyrosine kinase gene (rs1378942), and the arylsulfatase G gene (rs12945290). Another SNP was associated with the increased risk of hypertension, namely, rs995322, located in the CUB and Sushi multiple domains 1 (CSMD1) [194].

Future research in this area will be facilitated by enhancing collaboration between research groups through consortia such as the International Consortium for Antihypertensive Pharmacogenomics Studies, with the goal of translating replicated findings into clinical implementation [195] and into the design and implementation of the concept of genetic risk score.

Physiopathological Mechanisms of RH in Obesity/Metabolic Syndrome

While studies report that 30–40% of RH are obese [196–198], the ESC Arterial Hypertension Guidelines [199] suggest that weight loss leads to control of hypertension with less medication [200, 201]. Therefore, it is possible that obesity-associated hypertension may fall out of criteria for true RH and become essential hypertension, since it can be controlled with less than three drugs.

Moreover, the reversibility of RH through weight loss could signify that the obesity-associated hypertension is *transiently resistant* and does not involve exactly the same mechanisms as "true" *RH*. Hence, one can describe different entities which only in specific contexts manifests a resistance (transient or sustained) to treatment. A solid argument that supports this hypothesis is the lack of response to renal denervation in obesity-associated RH [202].

However, weight loss reverses some of the physiopathological mechanisms, decreasing sympathetic activation, plasma renin activity, and circulating leptin and insulin levels, while determining an improvement in blood pressure and in vasodilatory effect of adiponectin and diminishing other risk factors for atherosclerosis [203]. Nevertheless, recent research shows that blood pressure decrease reported in weight loss studies may not be sustained, regardless of weight status, which raises the need for long-term studies.

The phenotype of RH in obesity comprises insulin resistance and obesity/proinflammatory molecules, together with the correlation between demographics, lifestyle, genetic factors, and environmental fetal programming [204]. Within this framework, insulin resistance holds an important place due to its involvement in activation of sympathoadrenal system, which, converging with increased glomerular filtration of glucose doubled by its reabsorption accompanied by sodium, leads to hypervolemia and increased levels of sodium and calcium in vascular walls [205]. Thus, the spasm generated determines the increase of peripheral vascular tension, while narrowing of the vessels due to insulin-stimulated fibroblast and vascular smooth muscle cell proliferation leads to activation of RAAS and, finally, hypertension [206].

Another factor contributing to the pathogenesis of obesity-associated RH is represented by abnormal production of adipocytokines [207] such as leptin, resistin, perivascular relaxation factors, and adiponectin triggered by excessive fat mass [208], which results in imbalances in blood pressure control and, due to their functions as inflammatory, immune, or hormonal signalers, has an impact on insulin resistance and cardiovascular risk [209]. Moreover, they are correlated with hyperactivity of sympathetic and RAAS and contribute to the target-organ damage associated with HT, being involved in the development of arterial stiffness [210]. Research advances the hypothesis that *adipokines* are the missing link between insulin resistance and obesity, as they are the *pivotal element* that links the external factors involved in obesity pathogenesis with the molecular elements generating the cluster of conditions associated with obesity such as metabolic syndrome, inflammatory and/or autoimmune diseases, and rheumatic diseases [211, 212].

Adiponectin, either systemically derived or from perivascular fat, promotes endothelial-dependent vasodilation [213]. These effects are diminished with obesity in which low levels of plasmatic adiponectin generate higher NO inactivation and decreased NO production [214].

Therapeutic correlation An optimized treatment for RH associated with obesity will have to take into account the design of strategies for the regulation of adipokine synthesis and release.

On the other hand, studies report the interaction between adipokines and the *immune system*, since decreased leptin levels reduce T-cell responses [215], while several inflammatory conditions have been associated with modified adipokine levels. Additionally, interleukin-6 and TNF-α secreted by adipocytes trigger the induction of CRP production and lead to installation of inflammatory state [216]. High levels of adipose stem cell proliferation, resulting in increased synthesis of inflammatory cytokines, have been correlated with impaired blood pressure control in obese subjects [213]. However, the mechanisms by which adipokines intervene in the etiopathogenic process of hypertension have not been completely elucidated [217].

The central control mechanism of hypertension is also impaired by obesity, as experimental studies report that the sympathoinhibitory reflexes such as the baroreflex arc and the reflex induced by the gastrointestinal hormone cholecystokinin are significantly diminished by abnormal weight, resulting from aberrant central signaling triggering decreased responses of rostroventrolateral medulla neurons [218].

Finally, experimental studies reported that the insulin receptor substrate 2 (IRS2) intervenes in the effect elicited by the action of insulin on proximal tubule transport, through the insulin/PI3-K pathway, with specific regulatory mechanisms [219]. It is therefore possible that preserved stimulation of this mechanism could modulate the etiopathogenic process of obesity-associated hypertension.

References

1. Esler M, Kaye D. Increased sympathetic nervous system activity and its therapeutic reduction in arterial hypertension, portal hypertension and heart failure. J Auton Nerv Syst. 1998;72(2–3):210–9.
2. Ozel E, Tastan A, Ozturk A, Ozcan EE. Relationship between sympathetic Overactivity and left ventricular hypertrophy in resistant hypertension. Hellenic J Cardiol HJC Hellenike Kardiologike Epitheorese. 2015;56(6):501–6.
3. Tsioufis C, Kordalis A, Flessas D, Anastasopoulos I, Tsiachris D, Papademetriou V, et al. Pathophysiology of resistant hypertension: the role of sympathetic nervous system. Int J Hypertens. 2011;2011:642416.
4. Seravalle G, Dimitriadis K, Dell'Oro R, Grassi G. How to assess sympathetic nervous system activity in clinical practice. Curr Clin Pharmacol. 2013;8(3):182–8.

5. O'Callaghan EL, McBryde FD, Burchell AE, Ratcliffe LE, Nicolae L, Gillbe I, et al. Deep brain stimulation for the treatment of resistant hypertension. Curr Hypertens Rep. 2014;16(11):493.

6. Kawada T, Sugimachi M. Open-loop static and dynamic characteristics of the arterial baroreflex system in rabbits and rats. J Physiol Sci JPS. 2016;66(1):15–41.

7. Hering D, Schlaich M. The role of central nervous system mechanisms in resistant hypertension. Curr Hypertens Rep. 2015;17(8):58.

8. Morimoto S, Sasaki S, Miki S, Kawa T, Itoh H, Nakata T, et al. Pulsatile compression of the rostral ventrolateral medulla in hypertension. Hypertension. 1997;29(1 Pt 2):514–8.

9. Rumantir MS, Jennings GL, Lambert GW, Kaye DM, Seals DR, Esler MD. The 'adrenaline hypothesis' of hypertension revisited: evidence for adrenaline release from the heart of patients with essential hypertension. J Hypertens. 2000;18(6):717–23.

10. Presciuttini B, Duprez D, De Buyzere M, Clement DL. How to study sympatho-vagal balance in arterial hypertension and the effect of antihypertensive drugs? Acta Cardiol. 1998;53(3):143–52.

11. Perini R, Veicsteinas A. Heart rate variability and autonomic activity at rest and during exercise in various physiological conditions. Eur J Appl Physiol. 2003;90(3–4):317–25.

12. Clement DL, De Pue N, Jordaens LJ, Packet L. Adrenergic and vagal influences on blood pressure variability. Clin Exp Hypertens A Theory Practice. 1985;7(2–3):159–66.

13. Clement DL, Jordaens LJ, Heyndrickx GR. Influence of vagal nervous activity on blood pressure variability. J Hypertens Suppl Off J Int Soc Hypertens. 1984;2(3):S391–3.

14. Petkovich BW, Vega J, Thomas S. Vagal modulation of hypertension. Curr Hypertens Rep. 2015;17(4):532.

15. Plachta DT, Gierthmuehlen M, Cota O, Espinosa N, Boeser F, Herrera TC, et al. Blood pressure control with selective vagal nerve stimulation and minimal side effects. J Neural Eng. 2014;11(3):036011.

16. Lohmeier TE, Iliescu R. Lowering of blood pressure by chronic suppression of central sympathetic outflow: insight from prolonged baroreflex activation. J Appl Physiol (Bethesda, Md : 1985). 2012;113(10):1652–8.

17. Jordan J, Heusser K, Brinkmann J, Tank J. Electrical carotid sinus stimulation in treatment resistant arterial hypertension. Auton Neurosci Basic Clin. 2012;172(1–2):31–6.

18. Illig KA, Levy M, Sanchez L, Trachiotis GD, Shanley C, Irwin E, et al. An implantable carotid sinus stimulator for drug-resistant hypertension: surgical technique and short-term outcome from the multicenter phase II Rheos feasibility trial. J Vasc Surg. 2006;44(6):1213–8.

19. Kumar P, Prabhakar NR. Peripheral chemoreceptors: function and plasticity of the carotid body. Compr Physiol. 2012;2(1):141–219.

20. Iturriaga R, Del Rio R, Idiaquez J, Somers VK. Carotid body chemoreceptors, sympathetic neural activation, and cardiometabolic disease. Biol Res. 2016;49(1):13.

21. Katayama PL, Castania JA, Dias DP, Patel KP, Fazan R Jr, Salgado HC. Role of chemoreceptor activation in hemodynamic responses to electrical stimulation of the carotid sinus in conscious rats. Hypertension. 2015;66(3):598–603.

22. Ratcliffe LE, Pijacka W, McBryde FD, Abdala AP, Moraes DJ, Sobotka PA, et al. CrossTalk opposing view: which technique for controlling resistant hypertension? Carotid chemoreceptor denervation/modulation. J Physiol. 2014;592(18):3941–4.

23. Kopp UC. Role of renal sensory nerves in physiological and pathophysiological conditions. Am J Physiol Regul Integr Comp Physiol. 2015;308(2):R79–95.

24. Johns EJ. The neural regulation of the kidney in hypertension and renal failure. Exp Physiol. 2014;99(2):289–94.

25. Polimeni A, Curcio A, Indolfi C. Renal sympathetic denervation for treating resistant hypertension. Circ J Off J Jpn Circ Soc. 2013;77(4):857–63.

26. Volpe M, Rosei EA, Ambrosioni E, Cottone S, Cuspidi C, Borghi C, et al. Renal artery denervation for treating resistant hypertension : definition of the disease, patient selection and description of the procedure. High Blood Press Cardiovasc Prev Off J Ital Soc Hypertens. 2012;19(4):237–44.

27. Williams JM, Murphy S, Burke M, Roman RJ. 20-hydroxyeicosatetraeonic acid: a new target for the treatment of hypertension. J Cardiovasc Pharmacol. 2010;56(4):336–44.
28. Roman RJ. P-450 metabolites of arachidonic acid in the control of cardiovascular function. Physiol Rev. 2002;82(1):131–85.
29. Wainford RD, Carmichael CY, Pascale CL, Kuwabara JT. Galphai2-protein-mediated signal transduction: central nervous system molecular mechanism countering the development of sodium-dependent hypertension. Hypertension. 2015;65(1):178–86.
30. Santisteban MM, Ahmari N, Carvajal JM, Zingler MB, Qi Y, Kim S, et al. Involvement of bone marrow cells and neuroinflammation in hypertension. Circ Res. 2015;117(2):178–91.
31. Shi P, Diez-Freire C, Jun JY, Qi Y, Katovich MJ, Li Q, et al. Brain microglial cytokines in neurogenic hypertension. Hypertension. 2010;56(2):297–303.
32. Lazartigues E. Is microglia the new target for the treatment of resistant hypertension? Hypertension. 2015;66(2):265–6.
33. Shen XZ, Li Y, Li L, Shah KH, Bernstein KE, Lyden P, et al. Microglia participate in neurogenic regulation of hypertension. Hypertension. 2015;66(2):309–16.
34. Desir GV. Regulation of blood pressure and cardiovascular function by renalase. Kidney Int. 2009;76(4):366–70.
35. Desir GV. Role of renalase in the regulation of blood pressure and the renal dopamine system. Curr Opin Nephrol Hypertens. 2011;20(1):31–6.
36. Mell B, Jala VR, Mathew AV, Byun J, Waghulde H, Zhang Y, et al. Evidence for a link between gut microbiota and hypertension in the Dahl rat. Physiol Genomics. 2015;47(6):187–97.
37. Davern PJ, Chowdhury S, Jackson KL, Nguyen-Huu TP, Head GA. GABAA receptor dysfunction contributes to high blood pressure and exaggerated response to stress in Schlager genetically hypertensive mice. J Hypertens. 2014;32(2):352–62.
38. Brown NJ. This is not Dr. Conn's aldosterone anymore. Trans Am Clin Climatol Assoc. 2011;122:229–43.
39. Pitt B. "Escape" of aldosterone production in patients with left ventricular dysfunction treated with an angiotensin converting enzyme inhibitor: implications for therapy. Cardiovasc Drugs Ther Sponsored Int Soc Cardiovasc Pharmacother. 1995;9(1):145–9.
40. Duprez D, De Buyzere M, Rietzschel ER, Clement DL. Aldosterone and vascular damage. Curr Hypertens Rep. 2000;2(3):327–34.
41. Sato A, Saruta T. Aldosterone escape during angiotensin-converting enzyme inhibitor therapy in essential hypertensive patients with left ventricular hypertrophy. J Int Med Res. 2001;29(1):13–21.
42. Shamkhlova M, Trubitsyna NP, Katsaia GV, Goncharov NP, Malysheva NM, Il'in AV, et al. The angiotensin II inhibition escape phenomenon in patients with type 2 diabetes and diabetic nephropathy. Ter Arkh. 2008;80(1):49–52.
43. Jansen PM, Hofland J, van den Meiracker AH, de Jong FH, Danser AH. Renin and prorenin have no direct effect on aldosterone synthesis in the human adrenocortical cell lines H295R and HAC15. J Renin Angiotensin Aldosterone Syst JRAAS. 2012;13(3):360–6.
44. Athyros VG, Mikhailidis DP, Kakafika AI, Tziomalos K, Karagiannis A. Angiotensin II reactivation and aldosterone escape phenomena in renin-angiotensin-aldosterone system blockade: is oral renin inhibition the solution? Expert Opin Pharmacother. 2007;8(5):529–35.
45. Cherney DZ, Lai V, Miller JA, Scholey JW, Reich HN. The angiotensin II receptor type 2 polymorphism influences haemodynamic function and circulating RAS mediators in normotensive humans. Nephrol Dial, Transplant Off Publ Eur Dial Transplant Assoc Eur Renal Assoc. 2010;25(12):4093–6.
46. Cicoira M, Zanolla L, Rossi A, Golia G, Franceschini L, Cabrini G, et al. Failure of aldosterone suppression despite angiotensin-converting enzyme (ACE) inhibitor administration in chronic heart failure is associated with ACE DD genotype. J Am Coll Cardiol. 2001;37(7):1808–12.
47. Otani H, Otsuka F, Inagaki K, Suzuki J, Makino H. Roles of bone morphogenetic protein-6 in aldosterone regulation by adrenocortical cells. Acta Med Okayama. 2010;64(4):213–8.

48. Otani H, Otsuka F, Inagaki K, Suzuki J, Miyoshi T, Kano Y, et al. Aldosterone break-through caused by chronic blockage of angiotensin II type 1 receptors in human adrenocortical cells: possible involvement of bone morphogenetic protein-6 actions. Endocrinology. 2008;149(6):2816–25.
49. Rossi GP. Aldosterone breakthrough during RAS blockade: a role for endothelins and their antagonists? Curr Hypertens Rep. 2006;8(3):262–8.
50. Rossi GP, Cavallin M, Nussdorfer GG, Pessina AC. The endothelin-aldosterone axis and cardiovascular diseases. J Cardiovasc Pharmacol. 2001;38(Suppl 2):S49–52.
51. Turban S, Wang XY, Knepper MA. Regulation of NHE3, NKCC2, and NCC abundance in kidney during aldosterone escape phenomenon: role of NO. Am J Physiol Ren Physiol. 2003;285(5):F843–51.
52. Granger JP, Burnett JC Jr, Romero JC, Opgenorth TJ, Salazar J, Joyce M. Elevated levels of atrial natriuretic peptide during aldosterone escape. Am J Phys. 1987;252(5 Pt 2):R878–82.
53. Wang C, Chao J, Chao L. Adenovirus-mediated human prostasin gene delivery is linked to increased aldosterone production and hypertension in rats. Am J Physiol Regul Integr Comp Physiol. 2003;284(4):R1031–6.
54. Raizada V, Skipper B, Luo W, Griffith J. Intracardiac and intrarenal renin-angiotensin systems: mechanisms of cardiovascular and renal effects. J Invest Med Off Publ Am Fed Clin Res. 2007;55(7):341–59.
55. Grubler MR, Kienreich K, Gaksch M, Verheyen N, Hartaigh BO, Fahrleitner-Pammer A, et al. Aldosterone-to-renin ratio is associated with reduced 24-hour heart rate variability and QTc prolongation in hypertensive patients. Medicine. 2016;95(8):e2794.
56. Stowasser M. Aldosterone excess and resistant hypertension: investigation and treatment. Curr Hypertens Rep. 2014;16(7):439.
57. Sartori M, Calo LA, Mascagna V, Realdi A, Macchini L, Ciccariello L, et al. Aldosterone and refractory hypertension: a prospective cohort study. Am J Hypertens. 2006;19(4):373–9; discussion 380.
58. Shibata H, Itoh H. Mineralocorticoid receptor-associated hypertension and its organ damage: clinical relevance for resistant hypertension. Am J Hypertens. 2012;25(5):514–23.
59. Semplicini A, Strapazzon G, Papparella I, Sartori M, Realdi A, Macchini L, et al. RGS2 expression and aldosterone: renin ratio modulate response to drug therapy in hypertensive patients. J Hypertens. 2010;28(5):1104–8.
60. Gaddam KK, Nishizaka MK, Pratt-Ubunama MN, Pimenta E, Aban I, Oparil S, et al. Characterization of resistant hypertension: association between resistant hypertension, aldosterone, and persistent intravascular volume expansion. Arch Intern Med. 2008;168(11):1159–64.
61. Ames MK, Atkins CE, Lantis AC, Zum Brunnen J. Evaluation of subacute change in RAAS activity (as indicated by urinary aldosterone:creatinine, after pharmacologic provocation) and the response to ACE inhibition. J Renin Angiotensin Aldosterone Syst JRAAS. 2016;17(1). http://journals.sagepub.com/doi/abs/10.1177/1470320316633897?url_ver=Z39.88-2003&rfr_id=ori%3Arid%3Acrossref.org&rfr_dat=cr_pub%3Dpubmed
62. Ichihara A. (pro)renin receptor and vacuolar H(+)-ATPase. Keio J Med. 2012;61(3):73–8.
63. Oshima Y, Morimoto S, Ichihara A. Roles of the (pro)renin receptor in the kidney. World J Nephrol. 2014;3(4):302–7.
64. Shi P, Grobe JL, Desland FA, Zhou G, Shen XZ, Shan Z, et al. Direct pro-inflammatory effects of prorenin on microglia. PLoS One. 2014;9(10):e92937.
65. Nguyen G. Renin and prorenin receptor in hypertension: what's new? Curr Hypertens Rep. 2011;13(1):79–85.
66. Prieto MC, Botros FT, Kavanagh K, Navar LG. Prorenin receptor in distal nephron segments of 2-kidney, 1-clip goldblatt hypertensive rats. Ochsner J. 2013;13(1):26–32.
67. Ando T, Ichihara A. Novel approach to cardiovascular diseases: a promising probability of (pro)renin receptor [(P)RR]. Curr Pharm Des. 2014;20(14):2371–6.
68. Gonzalez AA, Womack JP, Liu L, Seth DM, Prieto MC. Angiotensin II increases the expression of (pro)renin receptor during low-salt conditions. Am J Med Sci. 2014;348(5):416–22.

69. Gonzalez AA, Green T, Luffman C, Bourgeois CR, Gabriel Navar L, Prieto MC. Renal medullary cyclooxygenase-2 and (pro)renin receptor expression during angiotensin II-dependent hypertension. Am J Physiol Ren Physiol. 2014;307(8):F962–70.
70. Wang F, Lu X, Peng K, Du Y, Zhou SF, Zhang A, et al. Prostaglandin E-prostanoid4 receptor mediates angiotensin II-induced (pro)renin receptor expression in the rat renal medulla. Hypertension. 2014;64(2):369–77.
71. Gonzalez AA, Prieto MC. Renin and the (pro)renin receptor in the renal collecting duct: role in the pathogenesis of hypertension. Clin Exp Pharmacol Physiol. 2015;42(1):14–21.
72. Li W, Peng H, Mehaffey EP, Kimball CD, Grobe JL, van Gool JM, et al. Neuron-specific (pro)renin receptor knockout prevents the development of salt-sensitive hypertension. Hypertension. 2014;63(2):316–23.
73. Bracquart D, Cousin C, Contrepas A, Nguyen G. The prorenin receptor. J Soc Biol. 2009;203(4):303–10.
74. Utsunomiya H, Nakamura M, Kakudo K, Inagami T, Tamura M. Angiotensin II AT2 receptor localization in cardiovascular tissues by its antibody developed in AT2 gene-deleted mice. Regul Pept. 2005;126(3):155–61.
75. Hsieh PS, Tai YH, Loh CH, Shih KC, Cheng WT, Chu CH. Functional interaction of AT1 and AT2 receptors in fructose-induced insulin resistance and hypertension in rats. Metab Clin Exp. 2005;54(2):157–64.
76. Strehlow K, Nickenig G, Roeling J, Wassmann S, Zolk O, Knorr A, et al. AT(1) receptor regulation in salt-sensitive hypertension. Am J Phys. 1999;277(5 Pt 2):H1701–7.
77. Harrison-Bernard LM, Schulman IH, Raij L. Postovariectomy hypertension is linked to increased renal AT1 receptor and salt sensitivity. Hypertension. 2003;42(6):1157–63.
78. Szombathy T, Szalai C, Katalin B, Palicz T, Romics L, Csaszar A. Association of angiotensin II type 1 receptor polymorphism with resistant essential hypertension. Clinica Chimica Acta Int J Clin Chem. 1998;269(1):91–100.
79. Hunyady L, Turu G. The role of the AT1 angiotensin receptor in cardiac hypertrophy: angiotensin II receptor or stretch sensor? Trends Endocrinol Metab TEM. 2004;15(9):405–8.
80. Liao Y, Husain A. The chymase-angiotensin system in humans: biochemistry, molecular biology and potential role in cardiovascular diseases. Can J Cardiol. 1995;11(Suppl F):13f–9f.
81. Mangiapane ML, Rauch AL, MacAndrew JT, Ellery SS, Hoover KW, Knight DR, et al. Vasoconstrictor action of angiotensin I-convertase and the synthetic substrate (Pro11,D-Ala12)-angiotensin I. Hypertension. 1994;23(6 Pt 2):857–60.
82. Nagata S, Varagic J, Kon ND, Wang H, Groban L, Simington SW, et al. Differential expression of the angiotensin-(1-12)/chymase axis in human atrial tissue. Ther Adv Cardiovasc Dis. 2015;9(4):168–80.
83. Park S, Bivona BJ, Ford SM Jr, Xu S, Kobori H, de Garavilla L, et al. Direct evidence for intrarenal chymase-dependent angiotensin II formation on the diabetic renal microvasculature. Hypertension. 2013;61(2):465–71.
84. Leckie BJ. Targeting the renin-angiotensin system: what's new? Curr Med Chem Cardiovasc Hematol Agents. 2005;3(1):23–32.
85. Leung PS. The peptide hormone angiotensin II: its new functions in tissues and organs. Curr Protein Pept Sci. 2004;5(4):267–73.
86. Re RN. The clinical implication of tissue renin angiotensin systems. Curr Opin Cardiol. 2001;16(6):317–27.
87. Zhuo JL, Li XC. New insights and perspectives on intrarenal renin-angiotensin system: focus on intracrine/intracellular angiotensin II. Peptides. 2011;32(7):1551–65.
88. Kumar R, Thomas CM, Yong QC, Chen W, Baker KM. The intracrine renin-angiotensin system. Clin Sci (London, England: 1979). 2012;123(5):273–84.
89. Re RN. Intracellular renin and the nature of intracrine enzymes. Hypertension. 2003;42(2):117–22.
90. De Mello WC, Danser AH. Angiotensin II and the heart : on the intracrine renin-angiotensin system. Hypertension. 2000;35(6):1183–8.

91. Singh VP, Le B, Khode R, Baker KM, Kumar R. Intracellular angiotensin II production in diabetic rats is correlated with cardiomyocyte apoptosis, oxidative stress, and cardiac fibrosis. Diabetes. 2008;57(12):3297–306.
92. Deliu E, Brailoiu GC, Eguchi S, Hoffman NE, Rabinowitz JE, Tilley DG, et al. Direct evidence of intracrine angiotensin II signaling in neurons. Am J Physiol Cell Physiol. 2014;306(8):C736–44.
93. Ellis B, Li XC, Miguel-Qin E, Gu V, Zhuo JL. Evidence for a functional intracellular angiotensin system in the proximal tubule of the kidney. Am J Physiol Regul Integr Comp Physiol. 2012;302(5):R494–509.
94. Ferrao FM, Lara LS, Lowe J. Renin-angiotensin system in the kidney: what is new? World J Nephrol. 2014;3(3):64–76.
95. Zhuo JL, Li XC. Novel roles of intracrine angiotensin II and signalling mechanisms in kidney cells. J Renin Angiotensin Aldosterone Syst JRAAS. 2007;8(1):23–33.
96. Haznedaroglu IC, Beyazit Y. Pathobiological aspects of the local bone marrow renin-angiotensin system: a review. J Renin Angiotensin Aldosterone Syst JRAAS. 2010;11(4):205–13.
97. Goker H, Haznedaroglu IC, Beyazit Y, Aksu S, Tuncer S, Misirlioglu M, et al. Local umbilical cord blood renin-angiotensin system. Ann Hematol. 2005;84(5):277–81.
98. Huang J, Hara Y, Anrather J, Speth RC, Iadecola C, Pickel VM. Angiotensin II subtype 1A (AT1A) receptors in the rat sensory vagal complex: subcellular localization and association with endogenous angiotensin. Neuroscience. 2003;122(1):21–36.
99. Glass MJ, Huang J, Speth RC, Iadecola C, Pickel VM. Angiotensin II AT-1A receptor immunolabeling in rat medial nucleus tractus solitarius neurons: subcellular targeting and relationships with catecholamines. Neuroscience. 2005;130(3):713–23.
100. Leung PS. The physiology of a local renin-angiotensin system in the pancreas. J Physiol. 2007;580(Pt 1):31–7.
101. Eggena P, Zhu JH, Sereevinyayut S, Giordani M, Clegg K, Andersen PC, et al. Hepatic angiotensin II nuclear receptors and transcription of growth-related factors. J Hypertens. 1996;14(8):961–8.
102. Carretero OA, Scicli AG. Local hormonal factors (intracrine, autocrine, and paracrine) in hypertension. Hypertension. 1991;18(3 Suppl):I58–69.
103. Wu Y, Takahashi H, Suzuki E, Kruzliak P, Soucek M, Uehara Y. Impaired response of regulator of Galphaq signaling-2 mRNA to angiotensin II and hypertensive renal injury in Dahl salt-sensitive rats. Hypertens Res Off J Jpn Soc Hypertens. 2016;39(4):210–6.
104. Muscogiuri G, Chavez AO, Gastaldelli A, Perego L, Tripathy D, Saad MJ, et al. The crosstalk between insulin and renin-angiotensin-aldosterone signaling systems and its effect on glucose metabolism and diabetes prevention. Curr Vasc Pharmacol. 2008;6(4):301–12.
105. Papparella I, Ceolotto G, Lenzini L, Mazzoni M, Franco L, Sartori M, et al. Angiotensin II-induced over-activation of p47phox in fibroblasts from hypertensives: which role in the enhanced ERK1/2 responsiveness to angiotensin II? J Hypertens. 2005;23(4):793–800.
106. Baritono E, Ceolotto G, Papparella I, Sartori M, Ciccariello L, Iori E, et al. Abnormal regulation of G protein alpha(i2) subunit in skin fibroblasts from insulin-resistant hypertensive individuals. J Hypertens. 2004;22(4):783–92.
107. Burns KD, Li N. The role of angiotensin II-stimulated renal tubular transport in hypertension. Curr Hypertens Rep. 2003;5(2):165–71.
108. Carey RM, Wang ZQ, Siragy HM. Role of the angiotensin type 2 receptor in the regulation of blood pressure and renal function. Hypertension. 2000;35(1 Pt 2):155–63.
109. Hilliard LM, Chow CL, Mirabito KM, Steckelings UM, Unger T, Widdop RE, et al. Angiotensin type 2 receptor stimulation increases renal function in female, but not male, spontaneously hypertensive rats. Hypertension. 2014;64(2):378–83.
110. Tallant EA, Diz DI, Ferrario CM. State-of-the-art lecture. Antiproliferative actions of angiotensin-(1-7) in vascular smooth muscle. Hypertension. 1999;34(4 Pt 2):950–7.
111. Meinert C, Gembardt F, Bohme I, Tetzner A, Wieland T, Greenberg B, et al. Identification of intracellular proteins and signaling pathways in human endothelial cells regulated by angiotensin-(1-7). J Proteome. 2016;130:129–39.

112. de Almeida PW, Melo MB, Lima Rde F, Gavioli M, Santiago NM, Greco L, et al. Beneficial effects of angiotensin-(1-7) against deoxycorticosterone acetate-induced diastolic dysfunction occur independently of changes in blood pressure. Hypertension. 2015;66(2):389–95.

113. Giani JF, Munoz MC, Mayer MA, Veiras LC, Arranz C, Taira CA, et al. Angiotensin-(1-7) improves cardiac remodeling and inhibits growth-promoting pathways in the heart of fructose-fed rats. Am J Physiol Heart Circ Physiol. 2010;298(3):H1003–13.

114. Katovich MJ, Grobe JL, Raizada MK. Angiotensin-(1-7) as an antihypertensive, antifibrotic target. Curr Hypertens Rep. 2008;10(3):227–32.

115. Singh N, Joshi S, Guo L, Baker MB, Li Y, Castellano RK, et al. ACE2/Ang-(1-7)/Mas axis stimulates vascular repair-relevant functions of CD34+ cells. Am J Physiol Heart Circ Physiol. 2015;309(10):H1697–707.

116. Dilauro M, Burns KD. Angiotensin-(1-7) and its effects in the kidney. ScientificWorldJournal. 2009;9:522–35.

117. Patel VB, Takawale A, Ramprasath T, Das SK, Basu R, Grant MB, et al. Antagonism of angiotensin 1–7 prevents the therapeutic effects of recombinant human ACE2. J Mol Med (Berlin, Germany). 2015;93(9):1003–13.

118. Tom B, Dendorfer A, Danser AH. Bradykinin, angiotensin-(1-7), and ACE inhibitors: how do they interact? Int J Biochem Cell Biol. 2003;35(6):792–801.

119. Bjorkholt Andersen L, Herse F, Christesen HT, Dechend R, Muller D. PP005. Vitamin D depletion aggravates hypertension in transgenic rats. Pregnancy Hypertens. 2013;3(2):69.

120. Garcia IM, Altamirano L, Mazzei L, Fornes M, Cuello-Carrion FD, Ferder L, et al. Vitamin D receptor-modulated Hsp70/AT1 expression may protect the kidneys of SHRs at the structural and functional levels. Cell Stress Chaperones. 2014;19(4):479–91.

121. Xue B, Pamidimukkala J, Lubahn DB, Hay M. Estrogen receptor-alpha mediates estrogen protection from angiotensin II-induced hypertension in conscious female mice. Am J Physiol Heart Circ Physiol. 2007;292(4):H1770–6.

122. Wei LH, Huang XR, Zhang Y, Li YQ, Chen HY, Heuchel R, et al. Deficiency of Smad7 enhances cardiac remodeling induced by angiotensin II infusion in a mouse model of hypertension. PLoS One. 2013;8(7):e70195.

123. Qiu Y, Tao L, Lei C, Wang J, Yang P, Li Q, et al. Downregulating p22phox ameliorates inflammatory response in angiotensin II-induced oxidative stress by regulating MAPK and NF-kappaB pathways in ARPE-19 cells. Sci Rep. 2015;5:14362.

124. Tain YL, Sheen JM, Yu HR, Chen CC, Tiao MM, Hsu CN, et al. Maternal melatonin therapy rescues prenatal dexamethasone and postnatal high-fat diet induced programmed hypertension in male rat offspring. Front Physiol. 2015;6:377.

125. Scholkens BA. Kinins in the cardiovascular system. Immunopharmacology. 1996; 33(1–3):209–16.

126. Natarajan AR, Eisner GM, Armando I, Browning S, Pezzullo JC, Rhee L, et al. The renin-angiotensin and renal dopaminergic systems interact in normotensive humans. J Am Soc Nephrol JASN. 2016;27(1):265–79.

127. Jose PA, Eisner GM, Felder RA. Dopaminergic defect in hypertension. Pediatr Nephrol (Berlin, Germany). 1993;7(6):859–64.

128. Sakamoto T, Chen C, Lokhandwala MF. Lack of renal dopamine production during acute volume expansion in Dahl salt-sensitive rats. Clin Exp Hypertens (New York, NY: 1993). 1994;16(2):197–206.

129. Armando I, Villar VA, Jose PA. Dopamine and renal function and blood pressure regulation. Compr Physiol. 2011;1(3):1075–117.

130. Choi MR, Kouyoumdzian NM, Rukavina Mikusic NL, Kravetz MC, Roson MI, Rodriguez Fermepin M, et al. Renal dopaminergic system: pathophysiological implications and clinical perspectives. World J Nephrol. 2015;4(2):196–212.

131. Sanada H, Jose PA, Hazen-Martin D, Yu PY, Xu J, Bruns DE, et al. Dopamine-1 receptor coupling defect in renal proximal tubule cells in hypertension. Hypertension. 1999;33(4):1036–42.

132. Hussain T, Kansra V, Lokhandwala MF. Renal dopamine receptor signaling mechanisms in spontaneously hypertensive and Fischer 344 old rats. Clin Exp Hypertens (New York, NY: 1993). 1999;21(1–2):25–36.

133. Yu P, Asico LD, Luo Y, Andrews P, Eisner GM, Hopfer U, et al. D1 dopamine receptor hyper-phosphorylation in renal proximal tubules in hypertension. Kidney Int. 2006;70(6):1072–9.
134. Yu P, Asico LD, Eisner GM, Hopfer U, Felder RA, Jose PA. Renal protein phosphatase 2A activity and spontaneous hypertension in rats. Hypertension. 2000;36(6):1053–8.
135. Salomone LJ, Howell NL, McGrath HE, Kemp BA, Keller SR, Gildea JJ, et al. Intrarenal dopamine D1-like receptor stimulation induces natriuresis via an angiotensin type-2 receptor mechanism. Hypertension. 2007;49(1):155–61.
136. Jose PA, Eisner GM, Drago J, Carey RM, Felder RA. Dopamine receptor signaling defects in spontaneous hypertension. Am J Hypertens. 1996;9(4 Pt 1):400–5.
137. Gurich RW, Beach RE. Abnormal regulation of renal proximal tubule Na(+)-K(+)-ATPase by G proteins in spontaneously hypertensive rats. Am J Phys. 1994;267(6 Pt 2):F1069–75.
138. Hussain T, Lokhandwala MF. Dopamine-1 receptor G-protein coupling and the involvement of phospholipase A2 in dopamine-1 receptor mediated cellular signaling mechanisms in the proximal tubules of SHR. Clin Exp Hypertens (New York, NY : 1993). 1997;19(1–2):131–40.
139. Yu PY, Eisner GM, Yamaguchi I, Mouradian MM, Felder RA, Jose PA. Dopamine D1A receptor regulation of phospholipase C isoform. J Biol Chem. 1996;271(32):19503–8.
140. Damasceno A, Santos A, Serrao P, Caupers P, Soares-da-Silva P, Polonia J. Deficiency of renal dopaminergic-dependent natriuretic response to acute sodium load in black salt-sensitive subjects in contrast to salt-resistant subjects. J Hypertens. 1999;17(12 Pt 2):1995–2001.
141. Mironova E, Boiko N, Bugaj V, Kucher V, Stockand JD. Regulation of Na+ excretion and arterial blood pressure by purinergic signalling intrinsic to the distal nephron: consequences and mechanisms. Acta Physiol (Oxf). 2015;213(1):213–21.
142. Drummond HA. Nontubular epithelial Na+ channel proteins in cardiovascular regulation. Phys Rep. 2015;3(5):e12404. doi:10.14814/phy2.12404.
143. Leenen FH, Hou X, Wang HW, Ahmad M. Enhanced expression of epithelial sodium channels causes salt-induced hypertension in mice through inhibition of the alpha2-isoform of Na+, K+−ATPase. Phys Rep. 2015;3(5):e12383. doi:10.14814/phy2.12383.
144. Hanukoglu I, Hanukoglu A. Epithelial sodium channel (ENaC) family: phylogeny, structure-function, tissue distribution, and associated inherited diseases. Gene. 2016;579(2):95–132.
145. Qadri YJ, Rooj AK, Fuller CM. ENaCs and ASICs as therapeutic targets. Am J Physiol Cell Physiol. 2012;302(7):C943–65.
146. Wang Q, Song B, Jiang S, Liang C, Chen X, Shi J, et al. Hydrogen sulfide prevents advanced glycation end-products induced activation of the epithelial sodium channel. Oxidative Med Cell Longev. 2015;2015:976848.
147. Mansley MK, Neuhuber W, Korbmacher C, Bertog M. Norepinephrine stimulates the epithelial Na+ channel in cortical collecting duct cells via alpha2-adrenoceptors. Am J Physiol Ren Physiol. 2015;308(5):F450–8.
148. Bao HF, Song JZ, Duke BJ, Ma HP, Denson DD, Eaton DC. Ethanol stimulates epithelial sodium channels by elevating reactive oxygen species. Am J Physiol Cell Physiol. 2012;303(11):C1129–38.
149. Snyder PM. Intoxicated Na(+) channels. Focus on "ethanol stimulates epithelial sodium channels by elevating reactive oxygen species". Am J Physiol Cell Physiol. 2012;303(11):C1125–6.
150. Pochynyuk O, Kucher V, Boiko N, Mironova E, Staruschenko A, Karpushev AV, et al. Intrinsic voltage dependence of the epithelial Na+ channel is masked by a conserved trans-membrane domain tryptophan. J Biol Chem. 2009;284(38):25512–21. Kashlan OB, Blobner BM, Zuzek Z, Tolino M, Kleyman TR. Na+ inhibits the epithelial Na+ channel by binding to a site in an extracellular acidic cleft. J Biol Chem. 2015;290(1):568–76.
151. Blaustein MP, Leenen FH, Chen L, Golovina VA, Hamlyn JM, Pallone TL, et al. How NaCl raises blood pressure: a new paradigm for the pathogenesis of salt-dependent hypertension. Am J Physiol Heart Circ Physiol. 2012;302(5):H1031–49.
152. Hamlyn JM, Linde CI, Gao J, Huang BS, Golovina VA, Blaustein MP, et al. Neuroendocrine humoral and vascular components in the pressor pathway for brain angiotensin II: a new axis in long term blood pressure control. PLoS One. 2014;9(9):e108916.

153. Fedorova OV, Agalakova NI, Talan MI, Lakatta EG, Bagrov AY. Brain ouabain stimulates peripheral marinobufagenin via angiotensin II signalling in NaCl-loaded Dahl-S rats. J Hypertens. 2005;23(8):1515–23.
154. Fedorova OV, Talan MI, Agalakova NI, Lakatta EG, Bagrov AY. Endogenous ligand of alpha(1) sodium pump, marinobufagenin, is a novel mediator of sodium chloride – dependent hypertension. Circulation. 2002;105(9):1122–7.
155. Gatti G, Lanzani C, Citterio L, Messaggio E, Carpini SD, Simonini M, et al. 6C.06: genes involved in blood pressure response to acute and chronic salt modifications: identification of a new pathway. J Hypertens. 2015;33(Suppl 1):e80–1.
156. Manunta P, Ferrandi M, Messaggio E, Ferrari P. A new antihypertensive agent that antagonizes the prohypertensive effect of endogenous ouabain and adducin. Cardiovasc Hematol Agents Med Chem. 2006;4(1):61–6.
157. Chen L, Song H, Wang Y, Lee JC, Kotlikoff MI, Pritchard TJ, et al. Arterial alpha2-Na+ pump expression influences blood pressure: lessons from novel, genetically engineered smooth muscle-specific alpha2 mice. Am J Physiol Heart Circ Physiol. 2015;309(5):H958–68.
158. Jin C, Sun J, Stilphen CA, Smith SM, Ocasio H, Bermingham B, et al. HV1 acts as a sodium sensor and promotes superoxide production in medullary thick ascending limb of Dahl salt-sensitive rats. Hypertension. 2014;64(3):541–50.
159. Touyz RM. The Neuroimmune Axis in the kidney: role in hypertension. Circ Res. 2015;117(6):487–9.
160. Pober JS. Is hypertension an autoimmune disease? J Clin Invest. 2014;124(10):4234–6.
161. Itani HA, Xiao L, Saleh MA, Wu J, Pilkinton MA, Dale BL, et al. CD70 exacerbates blood pressure elevation and renal damage in response to repeated hypertensive stimuli. Circ Res. 2016;118:1233–43.
162. Harrison DG. The immune system in hypertension. Trans Am Clin Climatol Assoc. 2014;125:130–8; discussion 138–40.
163. Harrison DG, Vinh A, Lob H, Madhur MS. Role of the adaptive immune system in hypertension. Curr Opin Pharmacol. 2010;10(2):203–7.
164. Kirabo A, Fontana V, de Faria AP, Loperena R, Galindo CL, Wu J, et al. DC isoketal-modified proteins activate T cells and promote hypertension. J Clin Invest. 2014;124(10):4642–56.
165. Traitanon O, Gorbachev A, Bechtel JJ, Keslar KS, Baldwin WM 3rd, Poggio ED, et al. IL-15 induces alloreactive CD28(−) memory CD8 T cell proliferation and CTLA4-Ig resistant memory CD8 T cell activation. Am J Transplant Off J Am Soc Transplant Am Soc Transplant Surg. 2014;14(6):1277–89.
166. Barbaro NR, Fontana V, Modolo R, De Faria AP, Sabbatini AR, Fonseca FH, et al. Increased arterial stiffness in resistant hypertension is associated with inflammatory biomarkers. Blood Press. 2015;24(1):7–13.
167. Barbaro NR, de Araujo TM, Tanus-Santos JE, Anhe GF, Fontana V, Moreno H. Vascular damage in resistant hypertension: TNF-alpha inhibition effects on endothelial cells. Biomed Res Int. 2015;2015:631594.
168. de La Sierra A, Larrousse M, Oliveras A, Armario P, Hernandez-Del Rey R, Poch E, et al. Abnormalities of vascular function in resistant hypertension. Blood Press. 2012;21(2):104–9.
169. Itani HA, Harrison DG. Memories that last in hypertension. Am J Physiol Ren Physiol. 2015;308(11):F1197–9.
170. Campbell DJ. Vaccination against high blood pressure. Curr Pharm Des. 2012;18(7):1005–10.
171. de Faria AP, Fontana V, Modolo R, Barbaro NR, Sabbatini AR, Pansani IF, et al. Plasma 8-isoprostane levels are associated with endothelial dysfunction in resistant hypertension. Clinica chimica acta. Int J Clin Chem. 2014;433:179–83.
172. Montezano AC, Touyz RM. Molecular mechanisms of hypertension – reactive oxygen species and antioxidants: a basic science update for the clinician. Can J Cardiol. 2012;28(3):288–95.
173. Montezano AC, Touyz RM. Reactive oxygen species and endothelial function – role of nitric oxide synthase uncoupling and Nox family nicotinamide adenine dinucleotide phosphate oxidases. Basic Clin Pharmacol Toxicol. 2012;110(1):87–94.

174. Virdis A, Bacca A, Colucci R, Duranti E, Fornai M, Materazzi G, et al. Endothelial dysfunction in small arteries of essential hypertensive patients: role of cyclooxygenase-2 in oxidative stress generation. Hypertension. 2013;62(2):337–44.
175. Magen E, Mishal J, Paskin J, Glick Z, Yosefy C, Kidon M, et al. Resistant arterial hypertension is associated with higher blood levels of complement C3 and C-reactive protein. J Clin Hypertens (Greenwich, Conn). 2008;10(9):677–83.
176. Ferri C, Croce G, Cofini V, De Berardinis G, Grassi D, Casale R, et al. C-reactive protein: interaction with the vascular endothelium and possible role in human atherosclerosis. Curr Pharm Des. 2007;13(16):1631–45.
177. Andrikou I, Tsioufis C, Dimitriadis K, Syrseloudis D, Valenti P, Almiroudi M, et al. Similar levels of low-grade inflammation and arterial stiffness in masked and white-coat hypertension: comparisons with sustained hypertension and normotension. Blood Press Monit. 2011;16(5):218–23.
178. Tan J, Hua Q, Xing X, Wen J, Liu R, Yang Z. Impact of the metalloproteinase-9/tissue inhibitor of metalloproteinase-1 system on large arterial stiffness in patients with essential hypertension. Hypertens Res Off J Jpn Soc Hypertens. 2007;30(10):959–63.
179. Dorr O, Liebetrau C, Mollmann H, Mahfoud F, Ewen S, Gaede L, et al. Beneficial effects of renal sympathetic denervation on cardiovascular inflammation and remodeling in essential hypertension. Clin Res Cardiol Off J German Cardiac Soc. 2015;104(2):175–84.
180. Eikelis N, Hering D, Marusic P, Sari C, Walton A, Phillips S, et al. The effect of renal denervation on endothelial function and inflammatory markers in patients with resistant hypertension. Int J Cardiol. 2015;188:96–8.
181. Xiao L, Kirabo A, Wu J, Saleh MA, Zhu L, Wang F, et al. Renal denervation prevents immune cell activation and renal inflammation in angiotensin II-induced hypertension. Circ Res. 2015;117(6):547–57.
182. El Rouby N, Cooper-DeHoff RM. Genetics of resistant hypertension: a novel pharmacogenomics phenotype. Curr Hypertens Rep. 2015;17(9):583.
183. Trotta R, Donati MB, Iacoviello L. Trends in pharmacogenomics of drugs acting on hypertension. Pharmacol Res. 2004;49(4):351–6.
184. Johnson JA. Advancing management of hypertension through pharmacogenomics. Ann Med. 2012;44(Suppl 1):S17–22.
185. Tabara Y, Kohara K, Miki T. Hunting for genes for hypertension: the millennium genome project for hypertension. Hypertens Res Off J Jpn Soc Hypertens. 2012;35(6):567–73.
186. Yugar-Toledo JC, Martin JF, Krieger JE, Pereira AC, Demacq C, Coelho OR, et al. Gene variation in resistant hypertension: multilocus analysis of the angiotensin 1-converting enzyme, angiotensinogen, and endothelial nitric oxide synthase genes. DNA Cell Biol. 2011;30(8):555–64.
187. Doris PA. Hypertension genetics, single nucleotide polymorphisms, and the common disease:common variant hypothesis. Hypertension. 2002;39(2 Pt 2):323–31.
188. Turner ST, Boerwinkle E, O'Connell JR, Bailey KR, Gong Y, Chapman AB, et al. Genomic association analysis of common variants influencing antihypertensive response to hydrochlorothiazide. Hypertension. 2013;62(2):391–7.
189. Johnson JA, Boerwinkle E, Zineh I, Chapman AB, Bailey K, Cooper-DeHoff RM, et al. Pharmacogenomics of antihypertensive drugs: rationale and design of the Pharmacogenomic evaluation of antihypertensive responses (PEAR) study. Am Heart J. 2009;157(3):442–9.
190. Fontana V, McDonough CW, Gong Y, El Rouby NM, Sa AC, Taylor KD, et al. Large-scale gene-centric analysis identifies polymorphisms for resistant hypertension. J Am Heart Assoc. 2014;3(6):e001398.
191. Lynch AI, Irvin MR, Davis BR, Ford CE, Eckfeldt JH, Arnett DK. Genetic and adverse health outcome associations with treatment resistant hypertension in GenHAT. Int J Hypertens. 2013;2013:578578.
192. Hirawa N, Fujiwara A, Umemura S. ATP2B1 and blood pressure: from associations to pathophysiology. Curr Opin Nephrol Hypertens. 2013;22(2):177–84.

193. Kato N. Ethnic differences in genetic predisposition to hypertension. Hypertens Res Off J Jpn Soc Hypertens. 2012;35(6):574–81.
194. Hong KW, Go MJ, Jin HS, Lim JE, Lee JY, Han BG, et al. Genetic variations in ATP2B1, CSK, ARSG and CSMD1 loci are related to blood pressure and/or hypertension in two Korean cohorts. J Hum Hypertens. 2010;24(6):367–72.
195. Cooper-DeHoff RM, Johnson JA. Hypertension pharmacogenomics: in search of personalized treatment approaches. Nat Rev Nephrol. 2016;12(2):110–22.
196. Bramlage P, Pittrow D, Wittchen HU, Kirch W, Boehler S, Lehnert H, et al. Hypertension in overweight and obese primary care patients is highly prevalent and poorly controlled. Am J Hypertens. 2004;17(10):904–10.
197. Isaksson H, Cederholm T, Jansson E, Nygren A, Ostergren J. Therapy-resistant hypertension associated with central obesity, insulin resistance, and large muscle fibre area. Blood Press. 1993;2(1):46–52.
198. Hall WD. Resistant hypertension, secondary hypertension, and hypertensive crises. Cardiol Clin. 2002;20(2):281–9.
199. Mancia G, Fagard R, Narkiewicz K, Redon J, Zanchetti A, Bohm M, et al. 2013 ESH/ESC guidelines for the Management of Arterial Hypertension: the task force for the management of arterial hypertension of the European Society of Hypertension (ESH) and of the European Society of Cardiology (ESC). Eur Heart J. 2013;34(28):2159–219.
200. Romero R, Bonet J, de la Sierra A, Aguilera MT. Undiagnosed obesity in hypertension: clinical and therapeutic implications. Blood Press. 2007;16(6):347–53.
201. Neter JE, Stam BE, Kok FJ, Grobbee DE, Geleijnse JM. Influence of weight reduction on blood pressure: a meta-analysis of randomized controlled trials. Hypertension. 2003;42(5):878–84.
202. Id D, Bertog SC, Ziegler AK, Hornung M, Hofmann I, Vaskelyte L, et al. Predictors of blood pressure response: obesity is associated with a less pronounced treatment response after renal denervation. Catheter Cardiovasc Interv Off J Soc Cardiac Angiography Interv. 2016;87:E30–8.
203. Stevens VJ, Obarzanek E, Cook NR, Lee IM, Appel LJ, Smith West D, et al. Long-term weight loss and changes in blood pressure: results of the trials of hypertension prevention, phase II. Ann Intern Med. 2001;134(1):1–11.
204. Redon J, Cifkova R, Laurent S, Nilsson P, Narkiewicz K, Erdine S, et al. The metabolic syndrome in hypertension: European society of hypertension position statement. J Hypertens. 2008;26(10):1891–900.
205. Simonenko VB, Goriutskii VN, Dulin PA. The role of insulin resistance in pathogenesis of arterial hypertension. Klin Med. 2014;92(9):27–33.
206. Redon J, Cifkova R, Laurent S, Nilsson P, Narkiewicz K, Erdine S, et al. Mechanisms of hypertension in the cardiometabolic syndrome. J Hypertens. 2009;27(3):441–51.
207. de Faria AP, Modolo R, Fontana V, Moreno H. Adipokines: novel players in resistant hypertension. J Clin Hypertens (Greenwich, Conn). 2014;16(10):754–9.
208. Yiannikouris F, Gupte M, Putnam K, Cassis L. Adipokines and blood pressure control. Curr Opin Nephrol Hypertens. 2010;19(2):195–200.
209. Bulcao C, Ferreira SR, Giuffrida FM, Ribeiro-Filho FF. The new adipose tissue and adipocytokines. Curr Diabetes Rev. 2006;2(1):19–28.
210. Sabbatini AR, Fontana V, Laurent S, Moreno H. An update on the role of adipokines in arterial stiffness and hypertension. J Hypertens. 2015;33(3):435–44.
211. Lago F, Dieguez C, Gomez-Reino J, Gualillo O. Adipokines as emerging mediators of immune response and inflammation. Nat Clin Pract Rheumatol. 2007;3(12):716–24.
212. Antuna-Puente B, Feve B, Fellahi S, Bastard JP. Adipokines: the missing link between insulin resistance and obesity. Diabete Metab. 2008;34(1):2–11.
213. Qi Y, Rathinasabapathy A, Huo T, Zhang J, Shang H, Katz A, et al. 7A.04: dl adipose stem cell is linked to obesity, elevated inflammatory cytokines and resistant hypertension. J Hypertens. 2015;33(Suppl 1):e90.

214. Cao Y, Tao L, Yuan Y, Jiao X, Lau WB, Wang Y, et al. Endothelial dysfunction in adiponectin deficiency and its mechanisms involved. J Mol Cell Cardiol. 2009;46(3):413–9.
215. Fantuzzi G. Adipose tissue, adipokines, and inflammation. J Allergy Clin Immunol. 2005;115(5):911–9; quiz 920.
216. Popko K, Gorska E, Stelmaszczyk-Emmel A, Plywaczewski R, Stoklosa A, Gorecka D, et al. Proinflammatory cytokines Il-6 and TNF-alpha and the development of inflammation in obese subjects. Eur J Med Res. 2010;15(Suppl 2):120–2.
217. Fain JN. Release of interleukins and other inflammatory cytokines by human adipose tissue is enhanced in obesity and primarily due to the nonfat cells. Vitam Horm. 2006;74:443–77.
218. How JM, Wardak SA, Ameer SI, Davey RA, Sartor DM. Blunted sympathoinhibitory responses in obesity-related hypertension are due to aberrant central but not peripheral signalling mechanisms. J Physiol. 2014;592(7):1705–20.
219. Nakamura M, Yamazaki O, Shirai A, Horita S, Satoh N, Suzuki M, et al. Preserved Na/HCO3 cotransporter sensitivity to insulin may promote hypertension in metabolic syndrome. Kidney Int. 2015;87(3):535–42.

Chapter 8
Pathophysiological Insights of Hypertension in Patients with Chronic Kidney Disease

Faruk Turgut, Mustafa Yaprak, and Faruk Tokmak

Hypertension is present in the vast majority of patients with chronic kidney disease (CKD) and constitutes a major cardiovascular risk factor for the excessive cardiovascular morbidity and mortality in this population [1, 2]. The prevalence of hypertension is progressively increasing with the severity of CKD, and control of blood pressure becomes more difficult with progression of CKD stage [3]. Hypertension is also extremely common among hemodialysis or peritoneal dialysis patients and those who have undergone renal transplantation. Moreover, resistant hypertension and nocturnal hypertension are observed at higher rates in CKD patients [4, 5]. Masked uncontrolled hypertension is also more prevalent among CKD patients [6]. Furthermore prevalence of hypertension varies with CKD etiology; strong association with hypertension was reported in patients with renal vascular disease (93%), established diabetic nephropathy (87%), polycystic kidney disease (74%), chronic pyelonephritis (63%), and glomerulonephritis (54%) [7]. However, patients with CKD caused by primary glomerular or vascular disease invariably have hypertension, whereas those with primary tubulointerstitial disease may be normotensive or, occasionally, salt losing.

Hypertension and CKD are closely associated with an overlapping and intermingled cause and effect relationship. Thus, control of hypertension does not only reduce cardiovascular risk but also represents an important modifiable factor in slowing further loss of kidney function. Understanding of the pathophysiology of

F. Turgut (✉) • M. Yaprak
Mustafa Kemal University, School of Medicine, Department of Internal Medicine,
Division of Nephrology, Antakya, Hatay, Turkey
e-mail: turgutfaruk@yahoo.com

F. Tokmak
Department of Nephrology, MVZ Gelsenkirchen-Buer, Gelsenkirchen, Germany

© Springer International Publishing AG 2017   127
A. Covic et al. (eds.), *Resistant Hypertension in Chronic Kidney Disease*,
DOI 10.1007/978-3-319-56827-0_8

hypertension is critical for the management of hypertension in CKD. However, there are large gaps in our understanding of pathogenesis and treatment of CKD-related hypertension.

Pathogenesis of Hypertension in CKD

The role of the kidney in CKD-related hypertension is complex because the kidney both contributes to hypertension and is damaged by hypertension. Blood pressure typically rises with declining kidney function, and sustained elevations in blood pressure accelerate the progression of kidney disease [8]. It is well established that hypertension improves after renal transplantation. In a series of patients with CKD due to histologically proven hypertensive nephrosclerosis, renal transplantation from normotensive donors resulted in the resolution of their hypertension [9].

Primary hypertension is the product of dynamic interactions between multiple genetic, physiological, environmental, and psychological factors. The kidneys play a pivotal role in long-term blood pressure regulation. The kidneys possess an enormous microvascular surface, which receives approximately 20–25% of cardiac output. Basically, high blood pressure is caused by an increase in cardiac output and/or increase of total peripheral resistance. Both can be deteriorated by a variety of different mechanisms in CKD (Fig. 8.1).

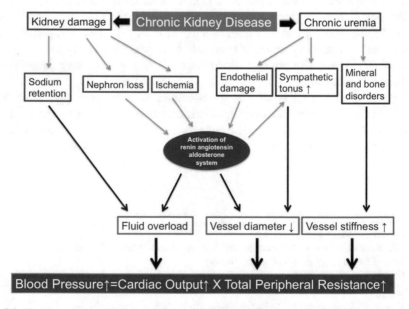

Fig. 8.1 Current concepts for the underlying mechanisms of hypertension in CKD

Table 8.1 Factors that may cause high blood pressure in chronic kidney disease

Well-known factors	Less-recognized factors	Plausible factors	Drugs
Sodium and volume excess	Mineral and bone disorders	Sleep apnea	ESAs
Activation of RAAS	Endothelins	Hyperuricemia	CNIs
SNS hyperactivity	Decreased NO	Inflammatory cytokines (i.e., TNF)	Steroids
Renovascular disease	Oxidative stress	Renalase	NSAIDs
Arterial stiffness			

RAAS renin-angiotensin-aldosterone system, *SNS* sympathetic nervous system, *NO* nitric oxide, *ESAs* erythropoietin-stimulating agents, *CNIs* calcineurin inhibitors, *NSAIDs* nonsteroid anti-inflammatory drugs

The kidney acts as an excretory organ, a component in the sympathetic axis, and a source of circulating constrictors and dilators. The traditional paradigm is that hypertension in CKD is due to either an excess of intravascular volume (volume dependent) or excessive activation of the renin-angiotensin-aldosterone system (RAAS) in relation to the state of sodium/volume balance (renin-dependent hypertension). However, numerous other factors of exogenous and endogenous nature can influence blood pressure in patients with CKD, including enhanced activity of the sympathetic nervous system, and factors influencing endothelial function. Table 8.1 shows a list of proposed factors in the pathophysiology of hypertension in CKD.

Role of Sodium Retention and Volume Overload

Sodium retention and consequent fluid overload have been well recognized in CKD-related hypertension. The normal kidneys are exquisitely sensitive to blood pressure. Acute rise in mean arterial pressure elicits a subtle increase in renal sodium and fluid excretion. This "pressure natriuresis" also runs contrary and retains sodium and fluid during decreases in blood pressure. The normal kidneys are also quite effective in balancing volume status so much so that extracellular fluid and blood volumes normally vary less than 10% with changes in salt intake. This delicate balance changes in a bad way with declining kidney function, and blood pressure often increases with excessive salt intake.

The regulation of sodium excretion is a highly complex process and is not still completely understood. There are so many regulatory pathways affecting sodium excretion by the kidney including the RAAS, the mineralocorticoid receptor, the endothelin system, and the nitric oxide (NO) [10]. The pathogenesis of hypertension is largely attributed to positive sodium balance in CKD patients. Many conditions are associated with impaired salt excretion in CKD, including reduced renal mass, the RAAS and sympathetic nervous system activation, and altered sodium chloride handling in the distal nephron.

A reduced number of nephrons have been proposed as one of the factors contributing to the development of primary hypertension. Autopsy series from victims of fatal accidents showed that hypertensive patients had fewer nephrons than matched normotensive controls [11]. With a decline in nephron numbers, abnormalities of sodium homeostasis are prominent, and prevalence of salt-sensitive hypertension increases in CKD patients. However, the exact nature of renal defect or defects responsible for inappropriate sodium excretion remains unclear.

Subtle renal defects associated with sodium excretion may underlie the pathophysiology of hypertension in CKD. It has been shown that normotensive subjects with family history of hypertension respond to salt loading with less natriuresis and higher blood pressure than those with no family history [12].

It is also theorized that sodium may elevate blood pressure through direct vasotoxic effects such as increased inflammation, oxidative stress, and arterial stiffness [13, 14]. High dietary salt intake exacerbates hypertension in patients with CKD, and dietary sodium restriction decreases extracellular volume and blood pressure in this patient group [15]. Chronic forms of glomerulonephritis nearly always show a mixture of volume-mediated and vasoconstrictor pathophysiology.

The Role of Volume Expansion

Rise in blood pressure is initially mediated by expansion of extracellular fluid volume, despite reduction in total peripheral vascular resistance. Renal salt and water retention is sufficient to increase the extracellular fluid and blood volume.

The critical role of volume expansion in hypertension due to CKD is underscored by the effect of ultrafiltration or diuretics on blood pressure. Patients with CKD have elevated extracellular fluid volume which can be corrected acutely with the help of loop diuretics. Persistent diuretic use results in dynamic changes in extracellular fluid volume that provides better blood pressure control in earlier stages of CKD [16]. In patients with ESRD, the role of extracellular fluid volume expansion is also apparent in the pathogenesis of hypertension. Inter-dialytic weight gain is associated with inter-dialytic increase in ambulatory blood pressure. It is reported that only a minority of patients undergoing better volume control with 8-h thrice-weekly or short daily hemodialysis require antihypertensive medications for blood pressure control in patients on maintenance hemodialysis [17, 18]. Similarly, better blood pressure control can be achieved by strict volume control in peritoneal dialysis patients [19].

Positive sodium balance and hypervolemia are the dominant but not sole factor in the pathogenesis of hypertension in CKD patients. Additional important volume-independent factors regulating blood pressure may also contribute to CKD-related hypertension. Some evidence suggests that there is an important sympathetic neural component for pathogenesis of hypertension.

The Central Role of the Renin-Angiotensin-Aldosterone System

The RAAS has powerful effects on control of the blood pressure and on target organ damage due to hypertension. It also controls fluid and electrolyte balance through coordinated effects on the heart, blood vessels, and kidneys. The system is largely mediated by kidneys, and abnormal activation of the RAAS plays a pivotal role in CKD-related hypertension.

In the classic pathway of the RAAS, renin release results in the subsequent generation of angiotensin II and aldosterone secretion. Angiotensin I has little effect on blood pressure and angiotensin II is the main effector of the RAAS. The activation of RAAS causes angiotensin II-mediated vasoconstriction as well as aldosterone-mediated salt retention, thus, resulting to increase both total peripheral resistance and blood volume. Angiotensin II can also potentiate sodium reabsorption and enhance sympathetic nervous system (SNS) activity.

While plasma renin activity is typically found to be markedly elevated only in patients with renal artery stenosis, many patients with CKD have "inappropriately normal" renin levels (i.e., lower levels would be expected, considering their degree of hypertension and fluid overload). There is also evidence of an intrarenal RAAS that is regulated independently of the systemic RAAS [20]. In the kidney, all of the RAAS components are present, and intrarenal angiotensin II is formed by independent multiple mechanisms. Inappropriate activation of the intrarenal RAAS is also an important contributor to the pathogenesis of CKD-related hypertension [20].

Markedly increased plasma renin activity has been well documented in hemodialysis patients with uncontrolled hypertension despite optimized ultrafiltration [21]. Treatment of such patients with bilateral nephrectomy or RAAS inhibitors has been shown to result in lowered blood pressure, suggesting the failing kidney as the source of excess renin activity [21, 22]. Increased renin activity occurs probably due to renin secretion in poorly perfused areas such as cysts and scars or after microangiopathic damage or tubulointerstitial inflammation.

A high incidence of hypertension (50–75%) occurs early in the course of autosomal polycystic kidney disease, and in this setting, activation of the RAAS is an important factor in the pathogenesis of hypertension. The release of excess renin is believed to be from renal ischemia due to compression of the renal vasculature by enlarging cysts in polycystic kidney disease.

Aldosterone not only potentiates sodium reabsorption in the distal nephron through the mineralocorticoid receptor but also directly affects vascular system by inducing oxidative stress, inflammation, hypertrophic remodeling, fibrosis, and endothelial dysfunction [23]. Aldosterone may play a significant role in the development in CKD-related hypertension [24, 25]. However, limited data from human studies suggest that aldosterone levels increase as kidney function declines.

Sympathetic Nervous System

Increased SNS activity is an important volume-independent cause in pathophysiology of hypertension in CKD patients. As the kidney is not only a part of excretory system but also a sensory organ, it is richly innervated with sensory and afferent nerves. In addition to being the target of SNS, the kidney may also be the origin and modulator of this activity. It is well established that renal denervation improves resistant hypertension in general population indicating the effect of renal sympathetic nerves on the pathogenesis of hypertension [26]. SNS hyperactivity leads to arterial blood pressure elevation and triggers arterial damage.

Increased SNS activity has been demonstrated in CKD patients [27, 28]. SNS overactivity is also a feature of renovascular hypertension. Although the underlying mechanisms of increased SNS activity are unclear, this overactivity in CKD may be caused by neurohormonal mechanisms arising from kidney damage. Chronic renal nerve activation stimulates renin along with its effects to modulate renal blood flow and tubular function. SNS has a modulatory role rather than primary role in the regulation of renin. Some studies have shown that plasma catecholamine levels are consistently increased in patients with end-stage renal disease (ESRD) [28]. Ischemic injury of kidney increases the activity of SNS. Furthermore, ischemic metabolites or uremic toxins may stimulate afferent nervous input to the central nervous system.

In addition to its direct pressor effect, it is possible that the activation of the RAAS may contribute to hypertension in CKD by stimulating the sympathetic nervous system. Moreover, locally released angiotensin II appears to mediate central activation of SNS activity [29]. Supporting this hypothesis, angiotensin-converting enzyme inhibition also reduces the SNS overactivity.

Patients with CKD also have inappropriately increased sympathetic activity for their effective volume status. Increased renal sympathetic nerve activity enhances the reabsorption of sodium chloride and fluid by the renal tubules, as well as the release of renin from the juxtaglomerular apparatus.

Other Humoral Factors

Manifold other humoral factors have been reported to contribute to elevation of blood pressure in CKD. The release of vasoconstrictors (thromboxane or endothelin) or deficiencies in the generation of vasorelaxant factors (nitric oxide, prostaglandins) at the level of the vascular endothelial cell may also participate in the elevation of blood pressure in CKD patients [30]. The increased levels of vasoconstrictor substances increasing peripheral resistance can be another predominant pathophysiologic factor in CKD-related hypertension. Imbalance between vasodilator and vasoconstrictor prostaglandins is also implicated in the pathogenesis of CKD-related hypertension [31].

Endothelins

Endothelins are produced primarily by cells of the vascular endothelium and collecting tubules. Endothelin-1 exerts a wide range of biologic effects in the kidney and is involved in normal renal function, modulating glomerular filtration rate, and solute and water reabsorption along the nephron. Besides these modulating effects, increased endothelin-1 levels are known to cause hypertension, inflammation, and glomerular and tubulointerstitial fibrosis [30]. During the course of CKD, the intrarenal synthesis of endothelin-1 is remarkably upregulated, and high level of endothelin-1 has been reported in both hypertensive and CKD patients [30]. Locally produced and released endothelin-1 not only causes constriction of most renal vessels but also causes inappropriate sodium and water retention. Impaired renal clearance of endothelin-1 may cause hypertension in CKD patients. In addition to its contractile actions on vascular smooth muscle, endothelins can also modulate SNS activity.

Nitric Oxide

NO plays a prominent role in the homeostatic regulation and integration of glomerular, vascular, and tubular function in the kidney [32]. Processes that can impair the release of NO or that reduce the bioavailability of NO impair an important vasodilatory response. CKD is a state of NO deficiency secondary to decreased NO production and/or increased bioinactivation of NO by reactive oxygen species [33]. Moreover, CKD leads to the accumulation of endogenous NO synthase inhibitors such as asymmetric dimethylarginine. Chronic inhibition of NO synthases promotes an increase in blood pressure and vasculopathy. Altered nitric oxide/endothelin balance further increases the blood pressure rising effects of these humoral factors.

Renalase

Renalase is the only known amine oxidase that metabolizes circulating catecholamines [34]. The kidney appears to be the major source of circulating renalase. Blood renalase concentration was found lower in patients with severe kidney disease, as compared with healthy subjects [34]. There may be a causal link between decreased renalase levels and increased dopamine and norepinephrine levels in patients with ESRD [34]. Recent evidences suggest that renalase lowers blood pressure and heart rate by metabolizing circulating catecholamines [35]. Abnormalities in the renalase pathway seem to contribute to the CKD-related hypertension.

Miscellaneous Other Non-humoral Factors

Mineral and Bone Disorders

The progression of CKD is associated with disorders of mineral metabolism (hyper-phosphatemia and hypocalcemia), leading to the development of secondary hyper-parathyroidism, which occurs even at early stages of CKD. Vascular stiffness is induced by altered mineral metabolism in CKD patients. Secondary hyperparathy-roidism may contribute to arterial stiffness and hypertension.

Hyperphosphatemia develops due to impaired renal phosphate excretion in advanced CKD patients. Hyperphosphatemia may directly induce vascular injury and indirectly stimulates osteoblastic differentiation of vascular smooth muscle cells. Vascular calcification or excessive collagen accumulation can further stiffen the arterial and/or arteriolar wall in patients with CKD. But decreased vascular compliance because of vascular calcification has a more pronounced effect on systolic pressure.

Fibroblast growth factor-23 (FGF-23), a hormone produced by osteoblasts, is involved in the regulation of phosphate and vitamin D metabolism. FGF-23 level rises in patients with CKD from early stages on. We still need to know more about the influence of FGF-23 on the pathogenesis of hypertension.

Uric Acid

Uric acid is the main urinary metabolite of purines. Hyperuricemia seems to be a cofactor in sodium-sensitive hypertension. It has been showed that circulating high uric acid levels were associated with increased prevalence of hypertension [36–38]. Potential mechanisms to account for this association are the activation of intrarenal RAAS, vascular smooth muscle cell proliferation, and impaired endothelial NO productions [39]. But the role of hyperuricemia in CKD-related hypertension is still a matter of controversy.

Oxidative Stress

Oxidative stress commonly accompanies both hypertension and CKD and is believed to contribute in part to their pathogenesis [40]. Oxidative stress occurs when generation of the reactive oxygen species (ROS) exceeds the natural antioxi-dant capacity of the organism. It is well known that uremia increases ROS activity and decreases antioxidant capacity. The exact mechanism through which oxidative stress may raise blood pressure has not been fully elucidated. Oxygen radicals and endogenous scavenging systems modulate vascular tone and function. ROS may stimulate vascular contraction directly through decreasing local NO production or modulate central SNS activation.

Drugs

Several drugs may contribute to hypertension in CKD patients (Table 8.1). Calcineurin inhibitors (CNIs) (cyclosporine and tacrolimus) are routinely used to prevent rejection after transplantation and occasionally to treat autoimmune disease. Hypertension induced by CNIs has been attributed to indirect vascular effects (vasoconstriction, impaired vasodilatation) and sodium retention by increasing endothelin-1, RAAS, and SNS activity and decreasing NO level [41, 42]. Tacrolimus appears to be less pro-hypertensive than cyclosporine. In addition to CNIs, glucocorticoids may also contribute to hypertension in kidney transplant recipients and patients with renal parenchymal disease. Glucocorticoids lead to fluid retention by their mineralocorticoid effect.

Erythropoiesis-stimulating agents (ESA) can worsen blood pressure control in CKD patients. The mechanisms responsible for ESA-induced hypertension have been attributed to increased blood viscosity, hypersensitivity to norepinephrine and angiotensin II, impaired endothelial relaxation or direct vasoconstrictor effect, increased cytosolic calcium, and increased blood serotonin or endothelin-1 levels [43].

Finally, independent of the organ system playing a role in high blood pressure, arterial hypertension may be considered a disease of vessels characterized by endothelial dysfunction, vascular remodeling, increased stiffness, and reduced distensibility [44]. It is clear that alterations in vascular function and structure are frequently observed in CKD. Processes that can stiffen the arterial or arteriolar wall, such as vascular calcification or excessive collagen accumulation, are both known to be more active in patients with CKD and contribute to an increase in blood pressure.

In conclusion, it is clear that hypertension in CKD is multifactorial; however, volume expansion by excessive salt intake and RAAS activation by several mechanisms are predominant factors contributing to hypertension in patients with CKD.

References

1. US Renal Data System USRDS 2010 Annual Data Report. Atlas of chronic kidney disease and end-stage renal disease in the United States. Bethesda: National Institutes of Health, National Institute of Diabetes and Digestive and Kidney Diseases; 2010.
2. Foley RN, Parfrey PS, Sarnak MJ. Clinical epidemiology of cardiovascular disease in chronic renal disease. Am J Kidney Dis. 1998;32(5 Suppl 3):S112–9.
3. USRD 2009. Atlas of Chronic Kidney Disease in the United States. Am J Kidney Dis. 2010;55(Suppl 1):S1–420.

4. Kanbay M, Turgut F, Uyar ME, Akcay A, Covic A. Causes and mechanisms of nondipping hypertension. Clin Exp Hypertens. 2008;30(7):585–97.
5. Borrelli S, De Nicola L, Stanzione G, Conte G, Minutolo R. Resistant hypertension in nondialysis chronic kidney disease. Int J Hypertens. 2013;2013:929183.
6. Bangash F, Agarwal R. Masked hypertension and white-coat hypertension in chronic kidney disease: a meta-analysis. Clin J Am Soc Nephrol. 2009;4(3):656–64.
7. Ridao N, Luño J, García de Vinuesa S, Gómez F, Tejedor A, Valderrábano F. Prevalence of hypertension in renal disease. Nephrol Dial Transplant. 2001;16(Suppl 1):70–3.
8. Muntner P, Anderson A, Charleston J, Chen Z, Ford V, Makos G, et al. Hypertension awareness, treatment, and control in adults with CKD: results from the Chronic Renal Insufficiency Cohort (CRIC) study. Am J Kidney Dis. 2010;55(3):441–51.
9. Curtis JJ, Luke RG, Dustan HP, Kashgarian M, Whelchel JD, Jones P, et al. Remission of essential hypertension after renal transplantation. N Engl J Med. 1983;309(17):1009–15.
10. Herrera M, Coffman TM. The kidney and hypertension: novel insights from transgenic models. Curr Opin Nephrol Hypertens. 2012;21(2):171–8.
11. Keller G, Zimmer G, Mall G, Ritz E, Amann K. Nephron number in patients with primary hypertension. N Engl J Med. 2003;348(2):101–8.
12. Widgren BR, Herlitz H, Hedner T, Berglund G, Wikstrand J, Jonsson O, et al. Blunted renal sodium excretion during acute saline loading in normotensive men with positive family histories of hypertension. Am J Hypertens. 1991;4(7 Pt 1):570–8.
13. Todd AS, Macginley RJ, Schollum JB, Johnson RJ, Williams SM, Sutherland WH, et al. Dietary salt loading impairs arterial vascular reactivity. Am J Clin Nutr. 2010;91(3):557–64.
14. Al-Solaiman Y, Jesri A, Zhao Y, Morrow JD, Egan BM. Low-Sodium DASH reduces oxidative stress and improves vascular function in salt-sensitive humans. J Hum Hypertens. 2009;23(12):826–35.
15. McMahon EJ, Bauer JD, Hawley CM, Isbel NM, Stowasser M, Johnson DW, et al. A randomized trial of dietary sodium restriction in CKD. J Am Soc Nephrol. 2013;24(12):2096–103.
16. Vasavada N, Agarwal R. Role of excess volume in the pathophysiology of hypertension in chronic kidney disease. Kidney Int. 2003;64(5):1772–9.
17. Saad E, Charra B, Raj DS. Hypertension control with daily dialysis. Semin Dial. 2004;17(4):295–8.
18. Ok E, Duman S, Asci G, Tumuklu M, Onen Sertoz O, Kayikcioglu M, et al. Comparison of 4- and 8-h dialysis sessions in thrice-weekly in-centre haemodialysis: a prospective, case-controlled study. Nephrol Dial Transplant. 2011;26(4):1287–96.
19. Günal AI, Duman S, Ozkahya M, Töz H, Asçi G, Akçiçek F, et al. Strict volume control normalizes hypertension in peritoneal dialysis patients. Am J Kidney Dis. 2001;37(3):588–93.
20. Kobori H, Nangaku M, Navar LG, Nishiyama A. The intrarenal renin-angiotensin system: from physiology to the pathobiology of hypertension and kidney disease. Pharmacol Rev. 2007;59(3):251–87.
21. Weidmann P, Maxwell MH, Lupu AN, Lewin AJ, Massry SG. Plasma renin activity and blood pressure in terminal renal failure. N Engl J Med. 1971;285(14):757–62.
22. Vaughan ED, Carey RM, Ayers CR, Peach MJ. Hemodialysis-resistant hypertension: control with an orally active inhibitor of angiotensin-converting enzyme. J Clin Endocrinol Metab. 1979;48(5):869–71.
23. Briet M, Schiffrin EL. Vascular actions of aldosterone. J Vasc Res. 2013;50(2):89–99.
24. Greene EL, Kren S, Hostetter TH. Role of aldosterone in the remnant kidney model in the rat. J Clin Invest. 1996;98(4):1063–8.
25. Ibrahim HN, Hostetter TH. The renin-aldosterone axis in two models of reduced renal mass in the rat. J Am Soc Nephrol. 1998;9(1):72–6.
26. Esler MD, Krum H, Sobotka PA, Schlaich MP, Schmieder RE, Böhm M, et al. Renal sympathetic denervation in patients with treatment-resistant hypertension (The Symplicity HTN-2 Trial): a randomised controlled trial. Lancet. 2010;376(9756):1903–9.

27. Converse RL, Jacobsen TN, Toto RD, Jost CM, Cosentino F, Fouad-Tarazi F, et al. Sympathetic overactivity in patients with chronic renal failure. N Engl J Med. 1992;327(27):1912–8.
28. Joles JA, Koomans HA. Causes and consequences of increased sympathetic activity in renal disease. Hypertension. 2004;43(4):699–706.
29. Ye S, Zhong H, Duong VN, Campese VM. Losartan reduces central and peripheral sympathetic nerve activity in a rat model of neurogenic hypertension. Hypertension. 2002;39(6):1101–6.
30. Richter CM. Role of endothelin in chronic renal failure—developments in renal involvement. Rheumatology (Oxford). 2006;45(Suppl 3):iii36–8.
31. Dunn MJ, Hood VL. Prostaglandins and the kidney. Am J Phys. 1977;233(3):169–84.
32. Kone BC, Baylis C. Biosynthesis and homeostatic roles of nitric oxide in the normal kidney. Am J Phys. 1997;272(5 Pt 2):F561–78.
33. Vaziri ND. Effect of chronic renal failure on nitric oxide metabolism. Am J Kidney Dis. 2001;38(4 Suppl 1):S74–9.
34. Xu J, Li G, Wang P, Velazquez H, Yao X, Li Y, et al. Renalase is a novel, soluble monoamine oxidase that regulates cardiac function and blood pressure. J Clin Invest. 2005;115(5):1275–80.
35. Desir GV. Regulation of blood pressure and cardiovascular function by renalase. Kidney Int. 2009;76(4):366–70.
36. Mellen PB, Bleyer AJ, Erlinger TP, Evans GW, Nieto FJ, Wagenknecht LE, et al. Serum uric acid predicts incident hypertension in a biethnic cohort: the atherosclerosis risk in communities study. Hypertension. 2006;48(6):1037–42.
37. Menè P, Punzo G. Uric acid: bystander or culprit in hypertension and progressive renal disease? J Hypertens. 2008;26(11):2085–92.
38. Kuriyama S, Maruyama Y, Nishio S, Takahashi Y, Kidoguchi S, Kobayashi C, et al. Serum uric acid and the incidence of CKD and hypertension. Clin Exp Nephrol. 2015;19(6):1127–34.
39. Feig DI, Kang DH, Johnson RJ. Uric acid and cardiovascular risk. N Engl J Med. 2008;359(17):1811–21.
40. Vaziri ND. Roles of oxidative stress and antioxidant therapy in chronic kidney disease and hypertension. Curr Opin Nephrol Hypertens. 2004;13(1):93–9.
41. Hoorn EJ, Walsh SB, McCormick JA, Zietse R, Unwin RJ, Ellison DH. Pathogenesis of calcineurin inhibitor-induced hypertension. J Nephrol. 2012;25(3):269–75.
42. Esteva-Font C, Ars E, Guillen-Gomez E, Campistol JM, Sanz L, Jiménez W, et al. Ciclosporin-induced hypertension is associated with increased sodium transporter of the loop of Henle (NKCC2). Nephrol Dial Transplant. 2007;22(10):2810–6.
43. Boyle SM, Berns JS. Erythropoietin and resistant hypertension in CKD. Semin Nephrol. 2014;34(5):540–9.
44. Touyz RM. New insights into mechanisms of hypertension. Curr Opin Nephrol Hypertens. 2012;21(2):119–21.

Chapter 9
Secondary Causes: Work-Up and Its Specificities in CKD: Influence of Arterial Stiffening

Antoniu Octavian Petriş

"First, the chicken or the egg" dilemma can be also identified in the relationship between hypertension (HTN) and chronic kidney disease (CKD), two growing worldwide health problems. In an epidemiological, cross-sectional, multicenter study (MULTIRISC) carried out in outpatient clinics belonging to cardiology, internal medicine, and endocrinology departments which defined CKD as an estimated glomerular filtration rate (eGFR) below 60 mL/min per 1.73 m^2, from 2608 patients 62.7% did not have CKD, 18.9% had "established" CKD (in addition, the serum creatinine level was ≥ 1.3 mg/dL in men or ≥ 1.2 mg/dL in women), and 18.4% had "occult" CKD (the creatinine level was lower) [1]. When the eGFR decreased below 45 mL/min/1.73m^2, mortality from cardiovascular disease increases more than threefold [2]. Within this binomial relationships has had to produce a significant change in mind-set for finding a solution to the problem how to motivate nephrologists to think more "cardiac" and cardiologists to think more "renal" this issue, making departmental barriers more permeable: the evaluation of renal function should be part of the work-up of patients with cardiovascular disease, and all patients with kidney disease should be assessed for cardiovascular disease [3].

Modern techniques to measure blood pressure (BP) were described more than 115 years ago starting with Scipione Riva Rocci mercury sphygmomanometer, but the features of the BP curve have highlighted other important goals, that is, the specific roles of pulse pressure (PP), arterial stiffness, pulse wave velocity (PWV), and wave reflections as potentially deleterious factors affecting the progression of HTN and CKD [4]. Furthermore, the level to which BP should be lowered is still controversial: below 125/7 5 mmHg among those with CKD and more than 1 g proteinuria (Joint National Commission-6 guidelines), below 130/80 mmHg among patients with CKD who are not on dialysis (Joint National Commission-7 guidelines), and a

A.O. Petriş (✉)
Cardiology Clinic, "St. Spiridon" County Emergency Hospital Iaşi, "Grigore T. Popa"
University of Medicine and Pharmacy, Iaşi, Romania
e-mail: antoniu.petris@yahoo.ro

© Springer International Publishing AG 2017
A. Covic et al. (eds.), *Resistant Hypertension in Chronic Kidney Disease*,
DOI 10.1007/978-3-319-56827-0_9

goal of less than 150/90 mmHg for hypertensive persons aged 60 years or older and for hypertensive persons 30–59 years of age to a diastolic goal of less than 90 mmHg with less evidence in hypertensive persons younger than 60 years for the systolic goal or in those younger than 30 years for the diastolic goal, a situation where the recommendation is BP of less than 140/90 mmHg (Joint National Commission-8 guidelines) [5, 6]. The same thresholds and goals are now recommended for hypertensive adults with diabetes or nondiabetic chronic kidney disease (CKD) as for the general hypertensive population younger than 60 years [6]. A full 60% of these recommendations were based on expert opinion, while just 10% were based on clinical trial evidence [7]. The available clinical trials targeted BP measured in the clinic but whose values are different from the real physiopathological changes: a meta-analysis using 24-h ambulatory BP monitoring shows that approximately 20% of patients with CKD have white-coat hypertension and about 5–10% have masked hypertension [8].

Surrogate markers of cardiovascular disease used in CKD work-up (mainly, for improvement of the risk stratification) include ankle–brachial index (clinical tool for gross estimation of obstruction in major-vessel lumen caliber), carotid ultrasound (assessing carotid intima-media thickness (IMT) and plaque – focal wall thickening by at least 50% of the surrounding IMT), aortic pulse wave velocity (reproducible evaluation of large-artery stiffness, using applanation tonometry, oscillometric pulse recognition algorithms, magnetic resonance imaging, or echo-tracking to measure diameter in end diastole and stroke change in diameter with a very high precision), and the echocardiography quantification of the subclinical hypertensive heart disease (e.g., left ventricular mass, diastolic dysfunction) [9].

Increased arterial stiffness is a major nontraditional cardiovascular risk factor in CKD reflecting the difficulty of the large arteries to convert flow oscillations into continuous blood flow due to fibroelastic intimal thickening, calcification of elastic lamellae, increased extracellular matrix, and extra collagen content [10]. Normally, by stretching, the arterial wall accumulates the elastic energy (aprox. 10% of the energy produced by the heart is stored in the large artery walls by their distension) that maintains the blood flow during diastole when the ejection phase is over ("Windkessel effect") [10].

Arteries become stiffer in physiological (aging) or pathological (hypertension, diabetes mellitus, and CKD) conditions. The "stiffness gradient" disappears, or a "stiffness mismatch" occurs (increased central elastic artery stiffness combined with a decrease in peripheral muscular artery stiffness) leading to the reversal of the physiological stiffness gradient and promoting end-organ damages through increased forward pressure wave transmission into the microcirculation [11]. Renal dysfunction has been shown to increase arterial stiffness via several mechanisms, including vascular calcification, chronic volume overload, inflammation, endothelial dysfunction (maladapted endothelial phenotype characterized by reduced nitric oxide (NO) bioavailability, increased oxidative stress, elevated expression of pro-inflammatory and prothrombotic factors, and reduced endothelial-derived vasodilation), oxidative stress (inducing vascular wall remodeling, intrinsic changes in SMC stiffness, and aortic SMC apoptosis), and overproduction of uric acid [12]. Increased T helper secretion of cytokines, chemokines, and growth factors leads to an inflammatory process and may lead to fragmentation of elastic membranes and destruction of cell-protective matrix layers. Decreased turnover of collagen and elastin, increased advanced glycation end products (AGEs), and matrix metallo-proteinase (MMP) (involved in the regulation of the structural integrity of the extracellular matrix – ECM) cross-links have been also demonstrated in vascular stiffening [12].

Noninvasive arterial testing for cardiovascular risk assessment providing a means for early detection of presymptomatic vascular disease that has been used to identify patients with subclinical atherosclerosis are arterial ultrasonography and measurements of arterial stiffness.

Flow-mediated dilatation (FMD) assessed by high-resolution ultrasonography of the brachial artery is considered a biomarker of endothelial function. Arterial vaso-dilatation in response to shear stress produced by increased flow is mediated predominantly by endothelium-derived nitric oxide. Impaired brachial artery dilatation to sublingually administered nitroglycerin is an "endothelium-independent" response that reflects arterial smooth muscle function. Relative disadvantages of this technique are that it is not easier to perform, requires a skilled operator with an appropriate training period, and these intrinsic difficulties make it more likely to be used in clinical research and not in individual evaluation [13].

Thickness of carotid artery intima and media (carotid IMT) can be measured optimally noninvasively by high-resolution ultrasonography with automated computerized edge-detection software and intravascular contrast agents that may decrease variability and improve precision [13].

Measurements of arterial stiffness include central pulse pressure/stroke volume index, pulse wave velocity (PWV), total arterial compliance, pulse pressure amplification, and augmentation index [14]. Two measures of arterial stiffness have been studied: the velocity of arterial pulse wave transmission across an arterial segment and the analysis of the arterial waveforms to estimate augmentation of systolic pressure by peripheral wave reflection [13]. As suggested by the European Society of Hypertension (ESH)/European Society of Cardiology (ESC) guidelines for the management of arterial hypertension, the measurement that is most widely used among the direct or indirect methods proposed to quantify arterial stiffness (as a tool for the assessment of subclinical target organ damage) is the propagative model based on PWV measurement, introduced in physiology (the "elastic" properties of the arterial wall determine the velocity of pulse wave propagation) by Bramwell and Hill (1922) [10, 12]. European Network for Non-invasive Investigation of Large Arteries position statement clarifies that arterial stiffness and central pressure measurements should be considered as recommended tests for the evaluation of cardiovascular risk, particularly in patients in whom target organ damage is not discovered by routine investigations [14]. Current methods for measuring arterial stiffness are carotid–femoral PWV (with predictive value for CV events and requires little technical expertise), central pulse wave analysis (with predictive value in patients with ESRD, hypertension, and CAD, provides additional information concerning wave reflections, and requires little technical expertise), and local arterial stiffness (with certain predictive value for CV events, is indicated for mechanistic analyses in research field, and requires a higher level of technical expertise) [14].

Typical values of PWV in the aorta range from approximately 5 to >15 m/s. A fixed threshold value (12 m/s) was proposed based on published epidemiological studies [15]. Aortic pulse wave velocity (PWV) is an estimate of the distance the pulse wave travels in the aorta and an estimate of the time that distance is traversed, the result (expressed in meters per second) being obtained by dividing the distance (usually expressed in millimeters) by the time (usually expressed in milliseconds) [9]. Three main arterial sites can be evaluated, mainly the aortic trunk (carotid–femoral) and the upper (carotid–brachial) and lower (femoral–dorsalis pedis) limbs. The "gold standard" method remains carotid–femoral PWV (cf-PWV) [14, 15]; brachial–ankle PWV (ba-PWV), a related technique based on oscillations in cuffs placed on the brachial artery and calf, is popular in Asia because it avoids exposing the groin, but the pulse wave pathway is still being discussed and its validity is still contested [12]. Indirect techniques use aortic characteristic impedance (the minimal impedance for higher frequencies of pressure-and-flow harmonics at the aortic root that is proportional to PWV, but its reliability is reduced due to the difficulty of obtaining trustworthy noninvasive data for aortic flow and pressure) and the rigidity estimates derived from BP measurement (e.g., ABPM-derived arterial stiffness index or crude brachial PP) [12].

Aortic PWV is a research tool useful as a marker of vascular risk when measured once in a population that is followed-up longitudinally and as outcome predictor when measuring longitudinal changes after intervention, showing the degree of loss of kidney function (stiffness of the aorta increases with decreasing kidney function) [9].

Several factors in addition to age, diabetes, and hypertension affect aortic PWV, including decreasing kidney function (microalbuminuria and proteinuria), glucose concentration, heart rate, sex, vascular calcification, and left ventricular hypertrophy (LVH). It has been already demonstrated that there is an independent association between arterial stiffness indices, PWV and augmentation index (Aix – % of pulse pressure), and severely increased albuminuria in nondiabetic, hypertensive patients with CKD stages 1–2 treated with renin–angiotensin–aldosterone system blockers [16]. The aortic–brachial arterial stiffness mismatch was strongly and independently associated with increased mortality in dialysis population, proving that arterial stiffness is also the strongest risk factor for cardiovascular disease in end-stage renal patients [17, 18].

We must be aware that the pulsatile nature of the central hemodynamics may have a deleterious impact on vital organs and increased aortic pulse pressure causes renal microvascular damage through altered renal hemodynamics resulting from increased peripheral resistance and/or increased flow pulsation, as indicated by the result from a study on 133 patients with hypertension where pressure waveforms were recorded on the radial, carotid, femoral, and dorsalis pedis arteries with applanation tonometry to estimate the aortic pressures and aortic (carotid–femoral) and peripheral (carotid–radial and femoral–dorsalis pedis) pulse wave velocities [19]. The renal resistive index, defined as [1 – (end-diastolic velocity/peak systolic velocity)], was strongly correlated with the aortic pulse pressure, incident pressure wave, augmented pressure, and aortic pulse wave velocity, although not with the mean arterial pressure or peripheral pulse wave velocities. Moreover, each 0.1 increase in renal resistive index was associated with a 5.4-fold increase in the adjusted relative risk of albuminuria [19].

Non-dipping nocturnal feature at 24-h ambulatory blood pressure monitoring (ABPM) (defined as a fall in nocturnal BP of <10%) is typically found in CKD and is associated with disease progression, but also as glomerular filtration rate declines, reverse dipping (nighttime BP readings that are higher than those during the day) becomes more apparent [20]. For renal protection there is a need for newer treatments in CKD (e.g., selective ETA blocking drugs) that will not only lower BP beyond the levels achieved with standard therapies but also favorably affect the 24-h profile of BP and arterial stiffness. To increase reproducibility of the results, the circadian BP pattern by 48-h ABPM was assessed in 10,271 hypertensive patients with and without CKD (5506 men/4765 women), 58.0 ± 14.2 years old, enrolled in the Hygia Project. The largest difference between groups was in the prevalence of the riser BP pattern (i.e., asleep SBP mean greater than awake SBP mean) in patients with and without CKD, respectively (17.6% vs. 7.1%; $p < 0.001$), significantly and progressively increased from 8.1% among those with stage 1 CKD to a very high 34.9% of those with stage 5 CKD. Prevalence of the riser BP pattern, associated with highest CVD risk among all possible BP patterns, was 2.5-fold more prevalent in CKD and up to fivefold more prevalent in end-stage renal disease. A blunted sleep-time BP decline, a characteristic of the non-dipping pattern, is common in patients with CKD. These findings indicate that CKD should be included among the clinical conditions for which ABPM is mandatory for proper diagnosis, CVD risk assessment, and the therapeutic regimen evaluation [21].

Ambulatory arterial stiffness index (AASI) is a parameter derived from the regression slope of the diastolic on systolic blood pressure, using all of the readings during ambulatory blood pressure monitoring (ABPM). AASI was significantly higher in CKD group, positively correlated to age and pulse pressure, and negatively correlated to nocturnal BP fall [22].

In hypertensive CKD patients, seric uric acid was correlated with the two indices of arterial stiffness, PWV and Aix (augmentation index adjusted for heart rate), with sex-specific variations. However, seric uric acid was associated independently with only Aix, but not with PWV, in the entire patient population and only in men [23].

Work-up for hypertension and CKD patient (Fig. 9.1) starts by identifying the concomitant conditions (age, diabetes mellitus, obesity) often associated with resistant hypertension. Older patients and patients with chronic kidney disease are particularly susceptible to salt intake; in diabetes the insulin resistance increases sympathetic nervous activity, vascular smooth muscle cell proliferation, and sodium retention; obesity is associated with an increased sympathetic activity, higher cardiac output, and a rise in peripheral vascular resistance due to reduced endothelium-dependent vasodilation; plasma aldosterone and endothelin are also increased, while excessive surrounding adipose tissue results in increased intrarenal pressures and changes in renal architecture [24]. We continue with the clinical evaluation and classification of each of these associate diseases: for hypertension based on ESH/ESC classification (blood pressure level and risk factors, asymptomatic organ damage or

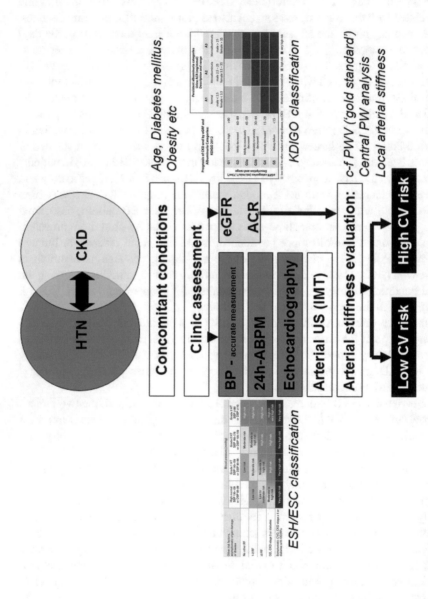

Fig. 9.1 Work-up for hypertension and CKD patient. *HTN* hypertension, *CKD* chronic kidney disease, *BP* blood pressure, *eGFR* estimated glomerular flow rate, *ACR* albumin/creatinine ratio, *ABPM* ambulatory blood pressure monitoring, *US* ultrasonography, *IMT* intima-media thickness, *PWV* pulse wave velocity, *CV* cardiovascular

disease) and for CKD on KDIGO (*Kidney Disease: Improving Global Outcomes*) classification based on estimated glomerular filtration rate (eGFR) and urine albumin/creatinine ratio (ACR) categories. These two simple tests allow asserting the diagnosis of CKD irrespective of the etiology: urinary albumin/creatinine ratio (ACR) more than 30 mg/g and eGFR, as measured by the Modification of Diet in Renal Diseases (MDRD) Study equation, less than 60 mL/min/1.73m² on at least two different occasions over 3 or more months. An accurate BP measurement is necessary and mandatory to avoid, for example, a "pseudoresistant hypertension" diagnosis: technical faults are related to not letting the patient rest at minimum of 5 min before measurement and using a small cuff (the cuff's air bladder must encircle at least 80% of the arm circumference); the average of two readings taken a minute apart represents the patient's blood pressure [24]. The correlation between BP level and target-organ damage, cardiovascular disease (CVD) risk, and long-term prognosis is greater for ambulatory than clinic BP. In addition to determining the usual mean BP values (awake, asleep, or 24 h), employed to diagnose hypertension based on ambulatory BP monitoring (ABPM), some specific features of the 24-h BP pattern have been assessed, among these is a blunted sleep-time BP decline, a characteristic of the non-dipping pattern, being common in patients with CKD [21]. Certainly, the target organs of hypertension are the three, well-known musketeers, the heart, brain, and kidneys, but we often forget the fourth musketeer, missing, by the way, from Dumas's book title too: the arteries. Identification of alterations in arterial function and structure may help refine cardiovascular risk assessment and labeling candidates for an aggressive therapy [13]. Ultrasound-derived carotid intima-media thickness (IMT) is considered a surrogate for systemic atherosclerotic disease burden, and carotid–femoral PWV (cf-PWV) is considered as the "gold standard" measurement of arterial stiffness, independently associated with glomerular filtration rate.

Further clinical trials are required for assessing the value of "destiffening" the aorta distinct from blood pressure reduction and to confirm the predictive value of arterial stiffness and wave reflection for the reduction in CV events in the long-term intervention studies [9].

Current data support the idea that the integration of demographic and clinical characteristics with information derived from arterial stiffness assessment may represent an accurate and cost-effective approach for individualizing CKD and HTN patients' care and treatment [25].

Agents that modulate mineral metabolism abnormalities (a noncalcium-containing phosphate binder – sevelamer, cinacalcet) and lipid-lowering agents (atorvastatin) may positively affect arterial stiffness [25].

Pharmacological strategies to date have included:

- Progressive withdrawal of alpha-blocking agents
- Efficacy of beta-blockers for coronary prevention
- The use of angiotensin blockade in HTN with glomerular injury, using angiotensin-converting enzyme inhibition or receptor blockade (first-line therapeutic intervention), as mono- but never double-blockade, to avoid major complications [7]

– Development of combination therapies with diuretics and/or calcium channel blockers [4]

Specific interventions, such as renin–angiotensin-system blockade, the use of statins, and decrease of calcium–phosphate product, may delay the progression of degeneration process in CKD patients.

Postural hypotension should be monitored closely, particularly in elderly, diabetics, and patients with arterial stiffness.

The level of albuminuria/proteinuria has become the principal criterion on which to stratify target blood pressure, irrespective of CKD stage.

Perspectives

Aortic stiffness is independently and significantly associated with progressive renal impairment in hypertensive patients with CKD irrespective of the stage, as a measure of arterial damage, and after the standardization of the measurement protocols and quality control procedures and risk-defining threshold values were established, this should be regarded as part of clinical cardiovascular risk stratification algorithms and target of future intervention studies.

References

1. Amenos AC, Gonzalez-Juanatey JR, Gutierrez PC, Gilarranz AM, Costae CG. Prevalence of chronic kidney disease in patients with or at a high risk of cardiovascular disease. Rev Esp Cardiol. 2010;63(2):225–8.
2. Hallan SI, Dahl K, Oien CM, et al. Screening strategies for chronic kidney disease in the general population: follow-up of cross sectional health survey. BMJ. 2006;333(7577):1047.
3. Kes P, Milicić D, Basić-Jukić N. How to motivate nephrologists to think more "cardiac" and cardiologists to think more "renal"? Acta Med Croatica. 2011;65(Suppl 3):85–9.
4. Kheder-Elfekih R, Yannoutsos A, Blacher J, London GM, Safar ME. Hypertension and chronic kidney disease: respective contribution of mean and pulse pressure and arterial stiffness. J Hypertens. 2015;31:[Epub ahead of print].
5. Agarwal R, Martinez-Castelao A, Wiecek A, Massy Z, Suleymanlar G, Ortiz A, Blankestijn PJ, Covic A, Dekker FW, Jager KJ, Lindholm B, Goldsmith D, Fliser D, London G, Zoccali C. EUropean REnal and CArdiovascular medicine working group of the European renal association–European dialysis and transplant association (ERA–EDTA). The lingering dilemma of arterial pressure in CKD: what do we know, where do we go? Kidney Int Suppl. 2011;1(1):17–20.
6. James PA, Oparil S, Carter BL, Cushman WC, Dennison-Himmelfarb C, Handler J, Lackland DT, LeFevre ML, MacKenzie TD, Ogedegbe O, Smith SC Jr, Svetkey LP, Taler SJ, Townsend RR, Wright JT Jr, Narva AS, Ortiz E, MD. 2014 evidence-based guideline for the management of high blood pressure in adults report from the panel members appointed to the eighth Joint National Committee (JNC 8). JAMA. 2014;311(5):507–20.

7. Covic A, Goldsmith D, Donciu M-D, Siriopol D, Popa R, Kanbay M, London G. From profusion to confusion: the Saga of managing hypertension in chronic kidney disease! J Clin Hypertens. 2015;17(6):421–7.
8. Bangash F, Agarwal R. Masked hypertension and white-coat hypertension in chronic kidney disease: a meta-analysis. Clin J Am Soc Nephrol. 2009;4(3):656–64.
9. Rubin MF, Rosas SE, Chirinos JA, Townsend RR. Surrogate markers of cardiovascular disease in CKD: what's under the hood? Am J Kidney Dis. 2011;57(3):488–97.
10. Covic A, Siriopol D. Pulse wave velocity ratio: the new "gold standard" for measuring arterial stiffness. Hypertension. 2015;65(2):289–90.
11. Boutouyrie P, Fliser D, Goldsmith D, Covic A, Wiecek A, Ortiz A, et al. Assessment of arterial stiffness for clinical and epidemiological studies: methodological considerations for validation and entry into the European renal and cardiovascular medicine registry. Nephrol Dial Transplant. 2014;29(2):232–9.
12. Jia G, Aroor AR, Sowers JR. Arterial stiffness: a nexus between cardiac and renal disease. Cardiorenal Med. 2014;4:60–71.
13. Kullo IJ, Malik AR. Arterial ultrasonography and tonometry as adjuncts to cardiovascular risk stratification. J Am Coll Cardiol. 2007;49(13):1413–26.
14. Laurent S, Cockcroft J, Van Bortel L, Boutouyrie P, Giannattasio C, Hayoz D, Pannier B, Vlachopoulos C, Wilkinson I, Struijker-Boudier H, on behalf of the European Network for Non-invasive Investigation of Large Arteries. Expert consensus document on arterial stiffness: methodological issues and clinical applications. Eur Heart J. 2006;27(21):2588–605.
15. Reference Values for Arterial Stiffness' Collaboration. Determinants of pulse wave velocity in healthy people and in the presence of cardiovascular risk factors: 'establishing normal and reference values'. Eur Heart J. 2010;31(19):2338–50.
16. Kalaitzidis RG, Karasavvidou DP, Tatsioni A, Pappas K, Katatsis G, Liontos A, Elisaf MS. Albuminuria as a marker of arterial stiffness in chronic kidney disease patients. World J Nephrol. 2015;4(3):406–14.
17. Fortier C, Mac-Way F, Desmeules S, Marquis K, De Serres SA, Lebel M, Boutouyrie P, Agharazii M. Aortic-brachial stiffness mismatch and mortality in dialysis population. Hypertension. 2015;65(2):378–84.
18. Ma Y, Zhou L, Dong J, Zhang X, Yan S. Arterial stiffness and increased cardiovascular risk in chronic kidney disease. Int Urol Nephrol. 2015;47(7):1157–64.
19. Hashimoto J, Ito S. Central pulse pressure and aortic stiffness determine renal hemodynamics. Pathophysiological implication for microalbuminuria in hypertension. Hypertension. 2011;58(5):839–46.
20. Dhaun N, Moorhouse R, MacIntyre IM, Melville V, Oosthuyzen W, Kimmitt RA, Brown KE, Kennedy ED, Goddard J, Webb DJ. Diurnal variation in blood pressure and arterial stiffness in chronic kidney disease. The role of endothelin-1. Hypertension. 2014;64(2):296–304.
21. Mojón A, Ayala D, Piñeiro L, Otero A, Crespo JJ, Moyá A, Bóveda J, de Lis JP, Fernández JR, Hermida RC, on behalf of the Hygia Project Investigators. Comparison of ambulatory blood pressure parameters of hypertensive patients with and without chronic kidney disease. Chronobiol Int. 2012;30(1–2):145–58.
22. Gismondi RA, Neves MF, Oigman W, Bregman R. Ambulatory arterial stiffness index is higher in hypertensive patients with chronic kidney disease. Int J Hypertens. 2012;2012:178078. doi:10.1155/2012/178078.
23. Elsurer R, Afsar B. Serum uric acid and arterial stiffness in hypertensive chronic kidney disease patients: sex-specific variations. Blood Press Monit. 2014;19(5):271–9.
24. Makris A, Seferou M, Papadopoulos DP. Resistant hypertension workup and approach to treatment. Int J Hypertens. 2011;2011:598694. doi:10.4061/2011/598694.
25. Bellasi A, Ferramosca E, Ratti C. Arterial stiffness in chronic kidney disease: the usefulness of a marker of vascular damage. Int J Nephrol. 2011;2011:734832. doi:10.4061/2011/734832.

Chapter 10
Secondary Causes: Work-Up and Its Specificities in CKD: Influence of Autonomic Dysfunction

Radu Iliescu and Dragomir Nicolae Şerban

The Kidney, Pressure Natriuresis and Long-Term Control of Blood Pressure

A thorough understanding of the mechanisms governing blood pressure regulation over long term and the influence of the sympathetic nervous system upon these mechanisms is necessary for the interpretation of clinical and experimental data documenting the role of sympathetic activation in resistant hypertension and kidney disease. While this and the following section provide only a brief overview, the expert reader may choose to focus on the more specific sections "Sympathetic Overactivation in Resistant Hypertension", "Non-pharmacological Suppression of Sympathetic Activity in Hypertension", and "Aspects of Sympathetic Activation in Resistant Hypertension Associated with CKD"

The relationship between renal perfusion pressure and the rate of sodium excretion by the kidneys plays a major role in the regulation of blood pressure and body fluid volume. If this relationship remains unchanged, any alteration in blood pressure induced by changes in cardiac output and/or the resistance of peripheral vasculature will lead to compensatory changes in renal sodium and water excretion and consequently extracellular fluid volume, with eventual return of blood pressure to normal levels. Therefore, any change in blood pressure would only be sustained over long term if the renal pressure natriuresis mechanism is impaired. Indeed, all forms of human or experimentally induced hypertension are associated with a resetting of the pressure natriuresis mechanism to higher blood pressure levels. In other

R. Iliescu (✉)
Department of Pharmacology, University of Medicine and Pharmacy "Gr. T. Popa" Iaşi, Iaşi, Romania
e-mail: radu.iliescu@umfiasi.ro; xiliescu@yahoo.com

D.N. Şerban
Department of Physiology, University of Medicine and Pharmacy "Gr. T. Popa" Iaşi, Iaşi, Romania

© Springer International Publishing AG 2017
A. Covic et al. (eds.), *Resistant Hypertension in Chronic Kidney Disease*,
DOI 10.1007/978-3-319-56827-0_10

words, a higher renal perfusion pressure becomes necessary for the kidneys to excrete the required amount of salt and water to precisely match the intake [1].

Under physiological circumstances, several neurohumoral mechanisms act in concert to amplify the effectiveness of the pressure natriuresis mechanism by directly increasing renal excretory capacity, before a measurable change in renal perfusion pressure becomes manifest. The major modulatory mechanism that determines the effectiveness of the pressure natriuresis is the renin-angiotensin-aldosterone system. Adequate suppression of the renin secretion by several-fold increases in sodium intake facilitates commensurate increases of the renal excretory capacity, so that blood pressure does not change chronically in the face of large variations of sodium input. Conversely, if the activity of the renin-angiotensin-aldosterone system cannot be adequately suppressed, proportional increases in blood pressure are required to allow the kidneys to excrete the additional salt and fluid and hypertension ensues. This situation is mimicked experimentally by continuous infusion of either angiotensin II or aldosterone in normal animals exposed to high salt intake [2]. Primary reductions in renal excretory capacity cause chronic increases in blood pressure owing to their effect of altering the pressure natriuresis relationship. Decreased glomerular filtration rate or increased tubular reabsorption would therefore initiate a compensatory increase in blood pressure that ultimately serves to maintain fluid balance.

Influence of Renal Sympathetic Nerve Activity on Blood Pressure Control by the Kidneys

The renal structures playing key roles in fluid homeostasis and control of blood pressure described above receive adrenergic innervation. Renal vascular innervation is distributed along the arterial segments in the cortex and outer medulla, including interlobar, arcuate, interlobular arteries, and afferent and efferent arterioles. Furthermore, adrenergic terminals to renal tubular epithelial cells are found along all segments of the nephron, including the proximal tubule, thick ascending limb of loop of Henle, distal convoluted tubule, and the collecting duct. Renin-secreting granular cells of the juxtaglomerular apparatus also receive direct sympathetic innervation [3].

In conjunction with the structural distribution, renal sympathetic nerve activity (RSNA) has effects that control the function of the different mechanisms involved in the modulation of the pressure natriuresis mechanism described above. Increased RSNA causes direct increases in tubular sodium reabsorption and renal vasoconstriction through activation of different subtypes of α-adrenergic receptors located on tubular and vascular smooth muscle cells of the kidney [4]. These direct effects of increased RSNA lead to a primary reduction of renal excretory capacity, commanding chronic alterations in the pressure natriuresis mechanism and ultimately chronic increases in BP. Furthermore, activation of β-adrenergic receptors located on the juxtaglomerular cells leads to increased renin secretion with attendant antin-atriuretic effects mediated by angiotensin II and aldosterone. Both the direct and indirect actions of renal adrenergic innervation provide the mechanistic basis for the idea that increased RSNA plays a causative role in the development of hypertension. Indeed, mounting evidence indicates that several forms of experimental and clinical hypertension are associated with increased RSNA and that complete removal of adrenergic influences on the kidneys by renal denervation attenuates or abolishes the hypertension [5].

Despite the clear role of RSNA in promoting and maintaining hypertension, the relative contribution of the renal mechanisms involved has been difficult to assess. Acute experimental studies where RSNA was progressively increased through direct electrical stimulation of renal sympathetic nerves indicated that the lowest levels of renal sympathetic nerve activation promote renin secretion, followed by reductions in sodium excretion and ultimately decreases in glomerular filtration rate (GFR) and renal blood flow (RBF), as the stimulation levels increase [3, 6]. These findings may suggest that relevant increases in RSNA that may be found chronically in undisturbed conditions would mainly promote antinatriuresis and hypertension by indirect effects on renin secretion and potentially direct tubular stimulation of sodium reabsorption, while direct vasoconstriction would occur only with supra-physiological levels of RSNA. Precise quantification of these mechanisms in the chronic setting is not only technically difficult but complicated by their interdependence. Experimental studies indicate that the acute effects of renal adrenergic stim-ulation are either not sustained over long term or eventually masked by compensatory mechanisms. Direct intrarenal infusion of norepinephrine (NE) in uninephrecto-mized dogs led acutely to a two- to threefold increase in plasma renin activity (PRA), accompanied by significant reductions in total and fractional sodium excre-tion, as well as GFR and renal plasma flow, consistent with the highest level of renal adrenergic activation, as mentioned above. However, although the same rate of NE infusion was maintained throughout 7 days, at the end of the study chronic hyper-tension was associated only with higher than normal levels of PRA, while all other renal functional alterations had waned off [6].

A thorough understanding of the complex interplay between the direct and indi-rect factors involved in the chronic control of renal function by RSNA is warranted in order to interpret the commonly used end points in experimental and clinical studies.

Increased renin secretion initiated by neural activation of juxtaglomerular cells leads to increased generation of Ang II, which promotes sodium reabsorption in the proximal tubule, mainly by reducing peritubular capillary hydrostatic pressure, owing to the prominent vasoconstriction of the efferent arterioles. In the absence of increased filtration, increased proximal tubular reabsorption would lower the amount of sodium delivered to the macula densa, which provides an additional drive for renin secretion. If increased RSNA includes direct tubular actions that increase sodium reabsorption, this effect would enhance the macula densa signal for renin secretion. However, as extracellular fluid volume accumulates due to impaired renal excretory capacity, blood pressure increases, which in turn activates the juxtaglomerular baroreceptor-mediated suppression of renin secretion. With high renal perfusion pressure and concomitant Ang II-mediated postglomerular vasocon-striction, GFR and filtration fraction would increase, and, despite high proximal tubular reabsorption, the net amount of sodium delivered to the macula densa returns to normal, eliminating the initial drive for renin secretion. Therefore, in the steady state, the initial neurally driven increase in renin secretion would be offset by the renin-suppressive factors including high blood pressure and normalization of the amount of sodium delivered to the macula densa, resulting in hypertension with a normal PRA. This time course is reflected in longitudinal measurements of PRA in a sympathetically mediated form of obesity hypertension in dogs [7]. Initial increases in sympathetic activation, reflected by increased plasma NE concentration associated with weight gain over the first 1–2 weeks, are paralleled by significant increases in PRA. Subsequently, as hypertension develops, PRA gradually returns to control levels by the fourth week. This study indicates that PRA levels may not reflect the importance of the chronic neural drive for RAS activation in mediating hypertension. As the RAS is the prominent modulator of pressure natriuresis, nor-mal PRA in the context of sympathetic activation and hypertension may rather indi-cate an inappropriate level of RAS activity. This contention is supported by studies showing that pharmacological suppression of RAS with an angiotensin converting enzyme (ACE) inhibitor effectively lowers blood pressure in established obesity hypertension despite apparently normal levels of PRA [8]. Furthermore, removal of the neural drive for renin secretion in obese hypertensive dogs by either global sup-pression of sympathetic activity via baroreflex activation therapy (BAT) or renal denervation (RDN) (these approaches are discussed below) lowers blood pressure to normal levels while significantly reducing PRA to below normal levels. In sum-mary, the neural drive for renin secretion and the consequent inability of the kidneys to maintain normal the normal pressure natriuresis by adequately suppressing RAS are paramount in mediating long-term hypertension in response to heightened RSNA.

Sympathetic Overactivation in Resistant Hypertension

Evidence of Sympathetic Activation in Resistant Hypertension

Mounting evidence indicates that excessive activation of the sympathetic nervous system is associated with both the development and progression of primary hyper-tension [5, 9, 10]. As compared to normotensive subjects, muscle sympathetic nerve traffic is higher in prehypertensive and borderline hypertensive subjects, indicating that sympathetic activation precedes and likely contributes to the pathogenesis of essential hypertension. Furthermore, for patients in the same age group the level of muscle sympathetic nerve activity parallels the severity of hypertension, such that resistant hypertensives display the strongest sympathetic activation [9], suggesting that while sympathetic overdrive directly contributes to the maintenance of hypertension, the degree of sympathetic activity dictates the prevailing levels of blood pressure. Excessive activation of the sympathetic nervous system in hypertension is highly inhomogeneous. Measurements of organ-specific norepinephrine spillover [11] and microneurographic nerve traffic recordings [5] revealed that hypertension-related increases in sympathetic neural drive appear to involve only some of the territories that receive sympathetic innervation, namely, the kidneys, heart, and muscle. The magnitude of sympathetic outflow to these organs is two- to threefold higher in hypertensive patients as compared to normotensives [11]. From a mechanistic point of view, the heightened renal sympathetic outflow likely plays a major role in the maintenance of high blood pressure levels through direct antinatriuretic actions on the renal tubules and tonic influences on the RAS. While a primary reduction in renal excretory capacity mediated by the increased RSNA would be sufficient to cause sustained hypertension, concomitant sympathetically mediated increases in total peripheral resistance and cardiac output may accelerate the progression of hypertension. In resistant hypertensive patients, renal sympathetic outflow is particularly enhanced, even more so than in untreated patients with mild-to-moderately severe hypertension [10]. Furthermore, the pattern of muscle sympathetic activation in these patients is characterized by increased frequency of single fiber firing, with burst activity frequently superimposed within the same cardiac cycle [12, 13]. This indicates that in resistant hypertension, the heightened sympathetic outflow relies not only on additional recruitment of individual fibers, as commonly found in essential hypertensives, but also to augmented firing frequency, suggesting specific mechanisms may be involved. While patients with resistant hypertension have several comorbidities with known contribution to sympathetic activation, such as obesity, sleep apnea, CKD or diabetes, the mechanisms implicated in drug resistance in these patients are not fully understood.

Mechanisms of Sympathetic Activation in Resistant Hypertension

The mechanisms leading to sympathoexcitation in essential hypertension are largely elusive and only seldom substantiated by experimental or clinical evidence [12]. The arterial baroreflex is a powerful controller of central sympathetic and parasympathetic outflow, and while its role in rapid buffering in blood pressure fluctuations via adjustments in autonomic function has been clearly recognized, its capacity to oppose sustained increases in blood pressure has long been dismissed based on experimental evidence of baroreceptor resetting to the prevailing blood pressure levels and transient hypertension following complete baroreceptor denervation [1]. However, recent experimental studies demonstrated sustained, baroreflex-mediated suppression of renal sympathetic outflow leading to increased renal excretory function in hypertensive dogs during chronic infusion of supraphysiological doses of angiotensin II [14]. These studies support the contention that during hypertension, baroreflex-mediated suppression of sympathetic outflow is a long-term compensatory mechanism, attenuating the severity of hypertension [15]. A corollary to this hypothesis is that the resetting of baroreflexes in hypertension may be incomplete. Furthermore, baroreflex dysfunction is one irrefutable abnormality commonly found in hypertension of primary origin [15]. Mounting evidence documented impaired (blunted) baroreflex control of heart rate in hypertensive patients. However, the efficacy of baroreflex buffering of sympathetic nerve traffic in response to pharmacologically induced, acute changes of blood pressure appears preserved in mild and even severe hypertension [16], indicative of resetting with normal dynamic function. While resetting would maintain the fundamental role of the baroreflex in the acute regulation of arterial pressure, it would also diminish its ability to chronically suppress sympathetic activity and counteract the severity of hypertension. To reconcile these apparently conflicting lines of evidence, a clear distinction should be made between the dynamic vs. the steady-state domains of operation of the baroreflex. Baroreflex-mediated acute responses of sympathetic outflow to a sudden change in blood pressure predominate in the arsenal of investigators assessing dynamic baroreflex function, but the long-term sympathetic modulation has not been easily amenable to investigation. Thus, if resetting of the baroreflex is complete, then it would be unlikely that dynamic baroreflex dysfunction could contribute to the sustained sympathoexcitation that plays a causal role in the pathogenesis of primary hypertension. On the other hand, if the baroreflex does not entirely adapt to long-term changes in arterial pressure, baroreflex dysfunction could play a role in the pathogenesis of primary hypertension.

Patients with resistant hypertension have inadequate blood pressure control despite treatment with multiple classes of drugs of which some were demonstrated to activate the sympathetic nervous system [17, 18], such as calcium channel blockers, diuretics, and even some sympatholytics. Thus, iatrogenically induced sympathetic activation may likely counteract the effects of antihypertensive medication and contribute to the intractable nature of hypertension in these patients. Peripherally acting sympatholytic agents such as $\alpha 1$- and β-adrenergic blockers could conceivably alleviate reflex sympathoexcitation but are rarely administered together and in concentrations sufficient to completely inhibit peripheral adrenergic responses. As increased renal sympathetic activity exerts its prohypertensive effects by stimulating renin and tubular reabsorption of sodium, which are dependent on the activation of $\alpha 1$- and β-adrenergic receptors, complete and concomitant blockade of these receptors is necessary in order to counteract neurally induced alterations in renal function that lead to increased arterial pressure. Centrally acting sympatholytic agents or non-pharmacological therapies (discussed below) capable of suppressing global sympathetic outflow, including RSNA, may thus provide an effective therapeutic tool to suppress sympathetically mediated increases in blood pressure. Recent experimental observations are relevant to this issue. Chronic lowering of blood pressure with a commonly used class of antihypertensive drugs, calcium channel blockers (amlodipine), was associated with marked sympathetic activation as revealed by several-fold increases in plasma NE concentration and profound activation of the renin-angiotensin system. Global sympathetic suppression by electrical activation of the carotid sinus (baroreflex activation therapy – discussed in detail below) completely abolished sympathoexcitation and lowered blood pressure further, while normalizing the activity of the RAS [19]. Furthermore, suppression of central sympathetic outflow by baroreflex activation has substantial chronic effects to lower arterial pressure by mechanisms independent of decreasing activation of $\alpha 1$- and β-adrenergic receptors. Blood pressure lowering in dogs receiving a combination of prazosin and propranolol in doses that abolished the cardiovascular responses to administration of $\alpha 1$- and β-adrenergic agonists was associated with activation of the sympathetic nervous system as reflected by a threefold increase in plasma NE concentration. Global suppression of sympathetic outflow by baroreflex activation reduced blood pressure further while returning plasma NE levels to control levels [20]. These studies indicate that baroreceptor unloading and attendant activation of the sympathetic nervous system are sustained responses to antihypertensive therapy and likely contribute to the difficulty to manage blood pressure in resistant hypertensive patients.

Resistant hypertensive patients are frequently obese, and this comorbidity adds a constellation of factors which could contribute to the sympathetic overdrive [21]. However, it is important to note that sympathetic activation in obesity often occurs in the absence of hypertension [5, 22]. A distinct pattern of sympathetic activation is present in obese hypertensives, as reflected by additional recruitment of fibers rather than increased firing rates of single fibers, as found in normotensive obese [23], suggestive of a particular mechanism of sympathetic activation in obesity when hypertension is associated. Furthermore, while cardiac sympathetic activity is only marginally elevated, renal sympathetic activity, although higher than in normotensive lean individuals, is similar in obese patients with or without hypertension [24]. Notwithstanding, pharmacological studies indicate that blood pressure of obese hypertensive humans depends to a greater extent on the renal sympathetic nervous system activation than in normotensive obese [25, 26].

Experimental and clinical studies have provided evidence for the involvement of several neurohumoral mechanisms in the sympathetic activation of obesity. Reflex control of sympathetic activity is impaired in obesity hypertension [27]. Whereas in lean hypertensive subjects only baroreflex control of heart rate is attenuated, baroreflex control of muscle sympathetic nerve activity is also blunted in obese hypertensive subjects [28]. If baroreceptors do not completely reset in obesity hypertension, dysfunctional baroreflex control of sympathetic activity may contribute to sustained sympathoactivation. In addition to the arterial baroreflex, peripheral chemoreflexes exert a powerful control over central sympathetic outflow such that activation of the carotid bodies leads to sympathoexcitation and attendant increases in blood pressure. Studies in the spontaneously hypertensive rat [29] and patients with primary hypertension [30] showed exaggerated sympathetic, pressor, and ventilator responses to chemoreflex activation by hypoxia and reversal of those variables by chemoreceptor deactivation in hyperoxic conditions. These observations raised the possibility that tonic chemoreceptor activation may contribute to sympathetically mediated hypertension and have led to development of current proof-of-concept trials designed to evaluate the antihypertensive efficacy of unilateral carotid body resection in resistant hypertensive patients [31]. However, the mechanism triggering sustained chemoreflex activation, especially in obesity hypertension, has remained elusive. Recent experimental evidence in a model of obesity-induced hypertension by administration of a high-fat diet provides support to the hypothesis that hypoxemia drives carotid body activation in obesity hypertension, with attendant sympathoexcitation. This canine model shares many of the metabolic, neurohumoral, and hemodynamic characteristics of human obesity hypertension [4, 15]. Furthermore, obesity is commonly characterized by high metabolic rate and oxygen consumption along with impaired ventilatory mechanics which may lead to chronic hypoxemia. Indeed, dogs fed with a high-fat diet for 4 weeks were hypoxemic, tachypneic, but eucapnic. Moreover, denervation of the carotid body by stripping the carotid sinus area resulted in a marked attenuation of obesity hypertension [31]. These data support the notion that in obesity hypertension, chronic hypoxemia provides the tonic drive for peripheral chemoreflex activation which results in sustained sympathoexcitation and hypertension.

Obstructive sleep apnea (OSA), common in obese and resistant hypertensive patients, has long been heralded as the major, if not the exclusive, cause of sympathetic activation in obesity. Obese hypertensive patients with OSA have sustained sympathetic activation beyond episodic occurrences during the nighttime. Although no mechanism has been proposed to explain this transition from acute to chronic and sustained sympathetic activation [24], the study in obese dogs [31] provides support for the concept that chronic intermittent hypoxemia (which is not routinely evaluated in clinical studies) may provide the tonic excitatory drive for chemoreflex activation resulting in sympathoexcitation in patients with OSA [32].

Several behavioral factors have been proposed to explain sympathetic activation in obesity-related hypertension, including overfeeding, sedentary lifestyle, or chronic mental stress [12]. Additionally, a plethora of experimental evidence suggested the role of humoral factors in mediated sympathoexcitation in hypertension, associated or not with obesity. These include hyperinsulinemia and associated insulin resistance, nitric oxide deficiency, endothelins, vasopressin natriuretic peptides, the renin-angiotensin system, and cytokines released from adipocytes such as tumor necrosis factor-α and interleukin-6 or leptin [9, 12, 24, 33]. While the role of leptin as a link between obesity, sympathoexcitation, and hypertension has been extensively documented in experimental studies in rodents [33], the data in humans is still scarce owing to methodological limitations [5]. Furthermore, although insulin-induced sympathoexcitation has been documented in human studies, the role of hyperinsulinemia in mediating obesity-hypertension has been questioned because insulin fails to increase blood pressure in humans and dogs [34]. Activation of the renin-angiotensin system may promote sympathetic nervous system activation by actions at the central nervous system level and peripheral nerve terminals. This notion is strongly supported by accumulating clinical data indicating that both angiotensin converting enzyme inhibitors and angiotensin II receptor blockers reduce central sympathetic outflow in hypertensive individuals [18]. However, due to the pleiotropic beneficial effects of these agents, especially upon comorbidities in resistant hypertension such as obesity, metabolic syndrome, and renal disease, a direct mechanistic link between the angiotensin II and sympathetic activation is not clear-cut. An emerging area of investigation is the activation of the central nervous system proopiomelanocortin-melanocortin 4 receptor (MC4R), a major regulator of appetite, energy expenditure, autonomic nervous system activity, and cardiovascular response to stress. In addition to mechanistic insight from experimental studies, the observation that MC4R deficiency in humans is associated with a lower prevalence of hypertension and lower blood pressure levels [35] provides support for the concept that the proopiomelanocortin-MC4R pathway may contribute to chronic sympathetic activation and hypertension [33, 35].

Non-pharmacological Suppression of Sympathetic Activity in Hypertension

Bearing on the relatively high, although not yet clearly established, incidence of resistant hypertension and the clear evidence of excessive sympathetic drive not only as powerful mediator of hypertension but also as mitigator of the antihypertensive effects of pharmacological therapies, intensive efforts have been recently directed toward the development of non-pharmacological sympathoinhibitory approaches. Of these, baroreflex activation therapy (BAT) and catheter-based radiofrequency renal nerve ablation have quickly reached technological maturity and stand nowadays the test of clinical efficacy [1, 4, 36].

Baroreflex Activation Therapy

The modern technology of BAT has overcome the limitations of the early attempts at electrical stimulation of the carotid baroreflex. The present system developed by CVRx Inc. has the capability of delivering electrical energy directly at the carotid sinus, through electrodes implanted in the perivascular space rather than the carotid sinus nerve, as in previous studies [4, 37]. This approach has the advantage of avoiding damage to the sinus nerve and also preventing concomitant activation of fibers carrying chemoreflex afferent signals from the carotid body. As noted above, activation of the carotid chemoreflex would provide a powerful sympathoexcitatory drive [31] thus limiting the efficacy of baroreflex activation. Furthermore, the electrode design of the current system virtually eliminates problems related to extraneous nerve and muscle stimulation seen in earlier studies, while the implantable miniature pulse generator allows externally programmable and controlled delivery of current throughout the day.

After a successful first-in-human proof-of-concept study of the first-generation Rheos (CVRx Inc.) system the Device-Based Therapy in Hypertension Trial

(DEBuT-HT) confirmed safety and efficacy of the BAT system in 45 resistant hypertensive patients who had significant reductions in blood pressure 3 months after the initiation of therapy which were sustained at 2 years of follow-up [38]. Following these promising results, the randomized, double-blind placebo controlled, Phase III Rheos pivotal trial in 265 patients with resistant hypertension was successful in meeting the predetermined sustained efficacy end point with 81% of the group having a reduction of systolic blood pressure of at least 10 mmHg at 12 months of the magnitude at least 50% of that obtained at month 6. However, the efficacy criterion remained unmet because the proportion of patients with blood pressure reduction at 6 months of at least 10 mmHg was only marginally greater in the BAT group as compared to placebo. This result was likely due to a less-than optimal trial design, as patients with inactive implants (placebo) had a larger reduction in systolic blood pressure than expected [39]. Notwithstanding, this trial emphasized the promise of BAT for the treatment of resistant hypertension as all patients receiving BAT had more than 30 mmHg reductions in their systolic blood pressure at 12 months, and this reduction was sustained for an average of 28 months follow-up [40]. Recent developments in the design and approach of BAT led to the Barostim neo, comprising a miniaturized electrode implanted unilaterally, with obvious benefits brought about by the reduction in the invasiveness of the implant procedure. The Barostim neo has demonstrated efficacy in significantly reducing systolic blood pressure by more than 25 mmHg in a trial on 30 resistant hypertensive patients at 6 months of follow-up and demonstrated a benign short- and long-term safety profile [41]. Stemming from this initial findings, a larger, FDA-approved multicenter randomized double-blind pivotal clinical trial is ongoing (The US Barostim Hypertension Pivotal Trial, NCT01679132), randomizing patients with resistant hypertension to receiving optimal medical management therapy with or without BAT.

The mechanisms involved in the blood pressure reduction by BAT have been explored in animal models and largely confirmed in humans. These studies suggest that global sympathoinhibition and concomitant suppression of renin secretion, likely mediated by reductions in renal sympathetic nerve activity, are the key mechanisms whereby BAT lowers blood pressure [4, 15]. Although the renal sympathetic nerves provide the apparent link between suppression of central sympathetic outflow and the reduction in blood pressure, experimental [42] and clinical [43] evidence indicate that BAT is capable of lowering blood pressure even when the renal nerves are not present. Although the mechanisms responsible for the blood pressure lowering effect of BAT in the absence of renal nerves are not evident and have not been explored to date, several mechanisms have been identified as potential candidates, including increased natriuretic peptides or renal interstitial pressure in an in silico study using a complex and established mathematical model of human physiology [44]. While these mechanisms warrant further investigation, it is conceivable that global sympathetic suppression by BAT may activate redundant natriuretic factors whose role only becomes apparent when sympathoinhibition does not include the renal nerves.

Renal Denervation

Since excessive renal sympathetic activation has been demonstrated to play a major role in promoting hypertension and sympathoexcitation is common in patients with resistant hypertension, renal denervation appeared as the logical therapeutic solution for those patients whose blood pressure cannot be controlled by medication. A novel catheter-based, radio-frequency ablation technique was designed to selectively eliminate renal innervation. Following successful proof-of-concept studies, the Symplicity device (Medtronic) was tested in two open label, uncontrolled trials in patients with resistant hypertension (SYMPLICITY HTN-1 and SYMPLICITY HTN-2). These studies have confirmed a significant reduction in systolic blood pressure of more than 30 mmHg which was sustained for as long as 3 years after the renal denervation [45]. The larger SYMPLICITY HTN-3 trial was designed to include a sham procedure, blinding, and more rigorous inclusion criteria for resistant hypertension. Although this trial met the safety end points, it however failed to achieve the primary end point, as patients with renal denervation had a reduction in systolic blood pressure of only 2 mmHg more pronounced than those who received pharmacological therapy alone [46]. The disappointing results of this last clinical trial have received numerous explanations including changes in medication and dosing, preferential use of classes of drugs in certain ethnic groups but were not found to be substantiated. Another possibility considered was that the extent of denervation was not uniform, a hypothesis difficult to assess since measurement of renal spillover of norepinephrine to quantitatively ascertain the degree of denervation has not been performed due to technical challenges [36]. However, the identification of those physiological factors that determine the blood pressure response to renal nerve ablation in the heterogeneous group of patients with resistant hypertension has remained unsolved. First of all, the iconoclastic contention that renal sympathetic activity is necessarily increased in all forms hypertension and that renal denervation invariably lowers blood pressure is challenged by multiple experimental studies which suggest that only those animal models where hypertension is sympathetically mediated respond to renal denervation. It is therefore unfortunate that the technology used to assess RSNA by renal norepinephrine spillover is not available for current clinical use since very little inference about the relationship between basal RSNA and the blood pressure response to renal denervation can be made in the absence of these measurements. Second, if the activity of the renin-angiotensin-aldosterone system escapes sympathetic modulation, such as would be the case during treatment with blockers of RAS [36] which may also lead to aldosterone breakthrough [47], or resistant hypertensive patients with CKD who may have normal aldosterone levels but increased sensitivity of the mineralocorticoid receptor [47], renal denervation would not be expected to cause sustained reductions in blood pressure [36]. Third, as volume expansion is a consistent pathological finding in patients with resistant hypertension, especially when CKD is a comorbid condition [48], experimental observations indicating that the renal nerves are not primary mediators of the modulation of renin secretion by dietary salt [49] suggest that the magnitude of blood pressure reduction following renal denervation may be independent of the level of salt intake. This possibility has not yet been tested in humans, however.

In addition to efferent sympathetic activity, the renal nerves also convey afferent signals from renal mechano- and chemoreceptors. Stimulation of renal chemoreceptors in response to ischemic metabolites and/or uremic toxins activates a sympathoexcitatory reflex. This reflex has been postulated to contribute to the excessive adrenergic drive found in several forms of hypertension, including resistant hypertension, and provided a conceptual basis for a putative effect of renal denervation to suppress sympathetic activity to other territories in addition to the kidneys [5]. However, clinical studies are inconsistent in ascertaining sustained reductions in muscle sympathetic nerve activity following renal denervation [33, 36]. Progressive renal injury in patients with CKD and resistant hypertension may however determine a more complete manifestation of this renal afferent sympathoexcitatory reflex, amenable to inhibition by renal denervation. This possibility remains unresolved since clinical trials of renal denervation have consistently excluded patients with overt impairment of renal function [36]. Thus, based on the currently available data, the antihypertensive effects of renal denervation are likely determined for the most part by interruption of efferent sympathetic traffic to the kidney.

Aspects of Sympathetic Activation in Resistant Hypertension Associated with CKD

Chronic kidney disease (CKD) is a complex pathological condition, whereby the vast majority of chronic renal failure cases evolve with chronic increase in arterial blood pressure (BP) in the systemic circulation, e.g., with hypertension. The latter favors multiple detrimental mechanisms, which ultimately lead to the various complications that define a global picture of chronic cardiovascular disease (CVD). This picture is superimposed over that of chronic renal failure, and there are various ways the involved pathological mechanisms are potentiating each other, by multiple vicious circles. Therefore, a major therapeutic aim in the evolution of CKD is to improve control of BP and hence to reduce CVD morbidity and mortality in this high-risk population, facing the frequent situation of hypertension resistant to classical antihypertensive drugs and their associations.

Due to such important issues, the complex relations involving CKD, hypertension, and autonomic dysfunction have been under increasingly intense investigation and debate over the last two decades. Quite many reviews have been published in this expanding area, including most recent ones focused right on the subject of this section, e.g., on CKD and specifically one of the following: resistant hypertension [50–52] sympathetic overactivity, including baroreflex dysfunction [53, 54]; arterial stiffness [55]; and clinical imaging of arterial calcification [56].

Resistant Hypertension and Chronic Kidney Disease

Ten years ago this issue was already thoroughly investigated, given that in CKD hypertension becomes more and more resistant to various treatments along the evolution of the pathogenic complex in each case. Because of the high complexity of the relation between CKD and hypertension, that we have just mentioned, hypertension in CKD has a very intricate pathogenesis [57]. Our understanding at that time was mainly based on a couple of traditional explanations (high volemia due to sodium and water retention; activation of the renin-angiotensin-aldosterone system (RAAS)), but other mechanisms were also considered, such as increased sympathetic activity, high endothelin production and/or decreased availability of endothelium-derived relaxing factors (EDRFs), arterial remodeling, renal ischemia, and sleep apnea [57]. Thus, autonomic dysfunction, with a focus on sympathetic overactivation, was already discussed at that time as possibly involved in hypertension pathogenesis, in general and in CKD in particular.

A rather simple terminological delineation helped in finding out that in CKD the pseudoresistance of hypertension to medication predicts renal outcome but is not associated with increased cardiorenal risk, while true resistance is prevalent and identifies patients with the highest CVD risk [58]. Here we use the term of resistant hypertension to generically designate a decreased efficiency of traditional antihypertensive remedies, but we emphasize the constant efforts of the medical community toward enhanced terminological precision in using such terms, e.g., resistant hypertension vs. refractory hypertension and controlled hypertension vs. uncontrolled hypertension [59]. Under such circumstances we consider that explicit reference to the antihypertensive scheme and to the determined vs. targeted ABP values should be made whenever appropriate in the context. We mention that hypertension control in CKD was found to be poor in the USA 10 years ago, mainly due to systolic hypertension [59].

Sympathetic Overactivation, Resistant Hypertension, and Chronic Kidney Disease

General aspects regarding sympathetic activity in hypertension have already been presented in this chapter (sections "Influence of Renal Sympathetic Nerve Activity on Blood Pressure Control by the Kidneys", "Sympathetic Overactivation in Resistant Hypertension", and "Non-pharmacological Suppression of Sympathetic Activity in Hypertension"), so here below we focus just on sympathetic overactivation in CKD (Fig. 10.1).

About 20 years ago the evidence for sympathetic overactivity in CKD started accumulating rather quickly, but it was still not clear if reducing sympathetic overactivity could be therapeutically relevant [57, 60]. Starting with the simple further reduction of glomerular filtration rate (GFR), by preferential constriction of afferent vs. efferent arterioles, various mechanisms were known by which chronic sympathetic

Fig. 10.1 The key role of sympathetic overactivation in the frame of pathogenic relations between chronic kidney disease (*CKD*) and hypertension

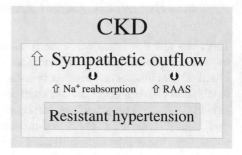

overactivity could be involved in CKD progression, such as facilitation of hypertension target organ damage, directly and/or mediated by angiotensin II [60]. Now we know that sympathetic activation and CKD go hand in hand, starting early in CKD evolution [61].

Mechanisms are far from elucidated, but now we do know that in CKD there is first a deficit in the baroreflex afferent component and then a gradual impairment of central control of renal sympathetic nerve activity and heart rate; both these earlier and later components are associated with serious baroreflex dysfunction [62]. A relevant study used the subtotal nephrectomy model and α2A-adrenoceptors knockout mice to investigate whether in renal failure the actual mechanism of increased noradrenaline release from renal sympathetic nerve endings involves altered intrinsic synaptic autoregulation [63]; the study revealed that those presynaptic adrenoceptors are less efficient in inhibiting noradrenaline release in renal failure. On the other side, it has been known for almost 40 years that reduced baroreflex sensitivity could contribute to hypertension in patients with end-stage chronic glomerulonephritis [64].

Baroreflex activation (discussed in some detail in the previous sections) has recently been shown to be effective in CKD with resistant hypertension, by decreasing ABP and proteinuria and by stabilizing estimated glomerular filtration rate (GFR) [65]. Baroreflex activation has also been shown to be a safe and effective therapy in end-stage renal disease (ESRD) [66]. Several small-scale studies investigated renal sympathetic denervation in CKD and, on purpose, the benefits of such procedures regarding resistant hypertension in CKD and, to some extent, the mechanisms involved.

Sympathetic vasoconstrictor tone itself can be more important as hypertensive mechanism than any "vascular amplifier effect," as shown in the Lewis polycystic kidney rat model of CKD [67]. It has been directly shown, by telemetry of ABP and of renal sympathetic nerve activity, that the increase in the latter could be a major hypertension mechanism in a rat model of genetic CKD [68].

Renal sympathetic denervation (by intravascular radiofrequency catheter), a safe and efficient remedy in hypertension resistant to antihypertensive drugs, possibly including hypertension in CKD [69, 70], does not affect patient adherence to the respective ongoing medication [71], while it was already known that renal denervation is more efficient in patients with resistant hypertension who also have impaired cardiac baroreflex sensitivity [72].

There are many different mechanisms by which vascular dysfunction contributes to the vicious circles discussed here, the ones involving the multiple relations between CKD, resistant hypertension, and autonomic dysfunction. In this highly complex context, it is known that deficit of nitric oxide (NO) and baroreflex dysfunction associate with various cardiovascular conditions. There is this interesting example of most recent finding with possible wide impact: sinocarotid baroreceptor artificial stimulation in rabbits enhanced the vasodilation induced by the NO donor sodium nitroprusside [73]. On the other side, one should keep in mind that autonomic dysfunction, as in sympathetic overactivation, could actually favor arterial dysfunction, as it has been shown that arterial baroreflex dysfunction promotes the development of atherosclerosis in rats and owing to inflammatory mechanisms [74].

Many studies, both in experimental models and in human subjects, have described the relation between hypertension and arterial stiffness, but connection to the arterial baroreflex has been more thoroughly addressed only recently, when it was shown, for example, that arterial stiffness, not strictly related to endothelial dysfunction, contributes to abnormal baroreflex in patients with hypertension [75]. Within this line of evidence it had been already suggested that reduced baroreflex sensitivity may be relevant for the pathophysiology of hemodialysis patients with vascular calcification [76], while one of our recent studies shows as well that volume overload in hemodialysis patients contributes to increased arterial stiffness but without affecting endothelium-independent or endothelium-dependent arterial reactivity [77].

We believe that, especially regarding such intricate mechanisms, careful results interpretation in the current knowledge context is crucial, as in the case of this study suggesting that "primary hypertension can be attributed to a mechanogenic etiology without challenging current conceptions of renal and sympathetic nervous system function" [78]. Refined multiparameter analysis indicates that estimation of baroreflex sensitivity using the causal method is the best marker for autonomic nervous system function [79].

Very fine control of intrarenal pressures and blood flow rate is ensured under normal conditions, while in CKD such regulatory mechanisms are progressively affected. So, there is a related substantial interest in the general features and mechanisms for vascular smooth muscle contractile activity and for the ways this is influenced by neural and humoral factors. But, aspects particular to the afferent and efferent arterioles are at least as important, if not even more, as suggested by an example of recent progress in understanding such differences based on the functional implications of certain subtypes of voltage-dependent calcium channels [80]. Peritoneal dialysis is useful in CKD, but it leads to a further increase of arterial stiffness together with a further decrease of baroreflex sensitivity [81]. Along with the various intended beneficial effects on renal and cardiovascular function, renal transplantation seems able to also normalize baroreflex sensitivity, and this occurs together with a decrease in the stiffness of central arteries [82]. Last but not least, spontaneous baroreflex indices correlate to local carotid mechanical properties, an aspect that should be considered when discussing baroreflex function in both pathological and normal conditions [83].

References

1. Lohmeier TE, Iliescu R. The baroreflex as a long-term controller of arterial pressure. Physiology (Bethesda). 2015;30:148–58. doi:10.1152/physiol.00035.2014.
2. Hall JE. Renal dysfunction, rather than nonrenal vascular dysfunction, mediates salt-induced hypertension. Circulation. 2016;133:894–906. doi:10.1161/CIRCULATIONAHA.115.018526.
3. Johns EJ, Kopp UC, DiBona GF. Neural control of renal function. Compr Physiol. 2011;1:731–67. doi:10.1002/cphy.c100043.
4. Iliescu R, Tudorancea I, Lohmeier TE. Baroreflex activation: from mechanisms to therapy for cardiovascular disease. Curr Hypertens Rep. 2014;16:453. doi:10.1007/s11906-014-0453-9.
5. Grassi G, Mark A, Esler M. The sympathetic nervous system alterations in human hypertension. Circ Res. 2015;116:976–90. doi:10.1161/CIRCRESAHA.116.303604.
6. Reinhart GA, Lohmeier TE, Hord CE. Hypertension induced by chronic renal adrenergic stimulation is angiotensin dependent. Hypertension. 1995;25:940–9.
7. Lohmeier TE, Dwyer TM, Irwin ED, Rossing MA, Kieval RS. Prolonged activation of the baroreflex abolishes obesity-induced hypertension. Hypertension. 2007;49:1307–14. doi:10.1161/HYPERTENSIONAHA.107.087874.
8. Robles RG, Villa E, Santirso R, Martínez J, Ruilope LM, Cuesta C, et al. Effects of captopril on sympathetic activity, lipid and carbohydrate metabolism in a model of obesity-induced hypertension in dogs. Am J Hypertens. 1993;6:1009–15.
9. Grassi G, Ram VS. Evidence for a critical role of the sympathetic nervous system in hypertension. J Am Soc Hypertens. 2016;10:457–66. doi:10.1016/j.jash.2016.02.015.
10. Esler M. The sympathetic nervous system in hypertension: back to the future? Curr Hypertens Rep. 2015;17:11. doi:10.1007/s11906-014-0519-8.
11. Esler M. The sympathetic nervous system through the ages: from Thomas Willis to resistant hypertension. Exp Physiol. 2011;96:611–22. doi:10.1113/expphysiol.2011.052332.
12. Parati G, Esler M. The human sympathetic nervous system: its relevance in hypertension and heart failure. Eur Heart J. 2012;33:1058–66. doi:10.1093/eurheartj/ehs041.
13. Hering D, Schlaich M. The role of central nervous system mechanisms in resistant hypertension. Curr Hypertens Rep. 2015;17:58. doi:10.1007/s11906-015-0570-0.
14. Lohmeier TE, Lohmeier JR, Reckelhoff JF, Hildebrandt DA. Sustained influence of the renal nerves to attenuate sodium retention in angiotensin hypertension. Am J Physiol Regul Integr Comp Physiol. 2001;281:R434–43.
15. Lohmeier TE, Iliescu R. Chronic activation of the baroreflex and the promise for hypertension therapy. Handb Clin Neurol. 2013;117:395–406. doi:10.1016/B978-0-444-53491-0.00032-8.
16. Grassi G, Cattaneo BM, Seravalle G, Lanfranchi A, Mancia G. Baroreflex control of sympathetic nerve activity in essential and secondary hypertension. Hypertension. 1998;31:68–72.
17. Calhoun DA, Jones D, Textor S, Goff DC, Murphy TP, Toto RD, et al. Resistant hypertension: diagnosis, evaluation, and treatment: a scientific statement from the American Heart Association Professional Education Committee of the Council for High Blood Pressure Research. Circulation. 2008;117:e510–26. doi:10.1161/CIRCULATIONAHA.108.189141.
18. Grassi G. Sympathomodulatory effects of antihypertensive drug treatment. Am J Hypertens. 2016;29:665–75. doi:10.1093/ajh/hpw012.
19. Iliescu R, Irwin ED, Georgakopoulos D, Lohmeier TE. Renal responses to chronic suppression of central sympathetic outflow. Hypertension. 2012;60:749–56. doi:10.1161/HYPERTENSIONAHA.112.193607.
20. Lohmeier TE, Hildebrandt DA, Dwyer TM, Iliescu R, Irwin ED, Cates AW, et al. Prolonged activation of the baroreflex decreases arterial pressure even during chronic adrenergic blockade. Hypertension. 2009;53:833–8. doi:10.1161/HYPERTENSIONAHA.109.128884.
21. Rao A, Pandya V, Whaley-Connell A. Obesity and insulin resistance in resistant hypertension: implications for the kidney. Adv Chronic Kidney Dis. 2015;22:211–7. doi:10.1053/j.ackd.2014.12.004.

22. Grassi G, Seravalle G, Brambilla G, Buzzi S, Volpe M, Cesana F, et al. Regional differences in sympathetic activation in lean and obese normotensive individuals with obstructive sleep apnoea. J Hypertens. 2014;32:383–8. doi:10.1097/HJH.0000000000000034.
23. Lambert E, Straznicky N, Schlaich M, Esler M, Dawood T, Hotchkin E, et al. Differing pattern of sympathoexcitation in normal-weight and obesity-related hypertension. Hypertension. 2007;50:862–8. doi:10.1161/HYPERTENSIONAHA.107.094649.
24. Esler M, Straznicky N, Eikelis N, Masuo K, Lambert G, Lambert E. Mechanisms of sympathetic activation in obesity-related hypertension. Hypertension. 2006;48:787–96. doi:10.1161/01.HYP.0000242642.42177.49.
25. Shibao C, Gamboa A, Diedrich A, Ertl AC, Chen KY, Byrne DW, et al. Autonomic contribution to blood pressure and metabolism in obesity. Hypertension. 2007;49:27–33. doi:10.1161/01.HYP.0000251679.87348.05.
26. Wofford MR, Anderson DC, Brown CA, Jones DW, Miller ME, Hall JE. Antihypertensive effect of alpha- and beta-adrenergic blockade in obese and lean hypertensive subjects. Am J Hypertens. 2001;14:694–8.
27. Thorp AA, Schlaich MP. Relevance of sympathetic nervous system activation in obesity and metabolic syndrome. J Diabetes Res. 2015;2015:341583. doi:10.1155/2015/341583.
28. Grassi G, Seravalle G, Dell'Oro R, Turri C, Bolla GB, Mancia G. Adrenergic and reflex abnormalities in obesity-related hypertension. Hypertension. 2000;36:538–42.
29. McBryde FD, Abdala AP, Hendy EB, Pijacka W, Marvar P, Moraes DJ, et al. The carotid body as a putative therapeutic target for the treatment of neurogenic hypertension. Nat Commun. 2013;4:2395. doi:10.1038/ncomms3395.
30. Somers VK, Mark AL, Abboud FM. Potentiation of sympathetic nerve responses to hypoxia in borderline hypertensive subjects. Hypertension. 1988;11:608–12.
31. Lohmeier TE, Iliescu R, Tudorancea I, Cazan R, Cates AW, Georgakopoulos D, et al. Chronic interactions between carotid baroreceptors and chemoreceptors in obesity hypertension. Hypertension 2016. doi:10.1161/HYPERTENSIONAHA.116.07232.
32. Mark AL, Somers VK. Obesity, hypoxemia, and hypertension: mechanistic insights and therapeutic implications. Hypertension. 2016; doi:10.1161/HYPERTENSIONAHA.116.07338.
33. Hall JE, do Carmo JM, da Silva AA, Wang Z, Hall ME. Obesity-induced hypertension: interaction of neurohumoral and renal mechanisms. Circ Res. 2015;116:991–1006. doi:10.1161/CIRCRESAHA.116.305697.
34. Brands MW, Hall JE, Keen HL. Is insulin resistance linked to hypertension? Clin Exp Pharmacol Physiol. 1998;25:70–6.
35. Greenfield JR, Miller JW, Keogh JM, Henning E, Satterwhite JH, Cameron GS, et al. Modulation of blood pressure by central melanocortinergic pathways. N Engl J Med. 2009;360:44–52. doi:10.1056/NEJMoa0803085.
36. Iliescu R, Lohmeier TE, Tudorancea I, Laffin L, Bakris GL. Renal denervation for the treatment of resistant hypertension: review and clinical perspective. Am J Physiol Renal Physiol. 2015;309:F583–94. doi:10.1152/ajprenal.00246.2015.
37. Schwartz SI, Griffith LSC, Neistadt A, Hagfors N. Chronic carotid sinus nerve stimulation in the treatment of essential hypertension. Am J Surg. 1967;114:5–15. doi:10.1016/0002-9610(67)90034-7.
38. Scheffers IJ, Kroon AA, Schmidli J, Jordan J, Tordoir JJ, Mohaupt MG, et al. Novel baroreflex activation therapy in resistant hypertension: results of a European multi-center feasibility study. J Am Coll Cardiol. 2010;56:1254–8. doi:10.1016/j.jacc.2010.03.089.
39. Bisognano JD, Bakris G, Nadim MK, Sanchez L, Kroon AA, Schafer J, et al. Baroreflex activation therapy lowers blood pressure in patients with resistant hypertension: results from the double-blind, randomized, placebo-controlled rheos pivotal trial. J Am Coll Cardiol. 2011;58:765–73. doi:10.1016/j.jacc.2011.06.008.
40. Bakris GL, Nadim MK, Haller H, Lovett EG, Schafer JE, Bisognano JD. Baroreflex activation therapy provides durable benefit in patients with resistant hypertension: results of long-term follow-up in the Rheos Pivotal Trial. J Am Soc Hypertens. 2012;6:152–8. doi:10.1016/j.jash.2012.01.003.

41. Hoppe UC, Brandt MC, Wachter R, Beige J, Rump LC, Kroon AA, et al. Minimally invasive system for baroreflex activation therapy chronically lowers blood pressure with pacemaker-like safety profile: results from the Barostim neo trial. J Am Soc Hypertens. 2012;6:270–6. doi:10.1016/j.jash.2012.04.004.
42. Lohmeier TE, Hildebrandt DA, Dwyer TM, Barrett AM, Irwin ED, Rossing MA, et al. Renal denervation does not abolish sustained baroreflex-mediated reductions in arterial pressure. Hypertension. 2007;49:373–9. doi:10.1161/01.HYP.0000253507.56499.bb.
43. Wallbach M, Halbach M, Reuter H, Passauer J, Lüders S, Böhning E, et al. Baroreflex activation therapy in patients with prior renal denervation. J Hypertens. 2016; doi:10.1097/HJH.0000000000000949.
44. Iliescu R, Lohmeier TE. Lowering of blood pressure during chronic suppression of central sympathetic outflow: insight from computer simulations. Clin Exp Pharmacol Physiol. 2010;37:e24–33. doi:10.1111/j.1440-1681.2009.05291.x.
45. Esler MD, Böhm M, Sievert H, Rump CL, Schmieder RE, Krum H, et al. Catheter-based renal denervation for treatment of patients with treatment-resistant hypertension: 36 month results from the SYMPLICITY HTN-2 randomized clinical trial. Eur Heart J. 2014; doi:10.1093/eurheartj/ehu209.
46. Bhatt DL, Kandzari DE, O'Neill WW, D'Agostino R, Flack JM, Katzen BT, et al. A controlled trial of renal denervation for resistant hypertension. N Engl J Med. 2014;370:1393–401. doi:10.1056/NEJMoa1402670.
47. Shibata H, Itoh H. Mineralocorticoid receptor-associated hypertension and its organ damage: clinical relevance for resistant hypertension. Am J Hypertens. 2012;25:514–23. doi:10.1038/ajh.2011.245.
48. Vemulapalli S, Tyson CC, Svetkey LP. Apparent treatment-resistant hypertension and chronic kidney disease: another cardiovascular-renal syndrome? Adv Chronic Kidney Dis. 2014;21:489–99. doi:10.1053/j.ackd.2014.08.006.
49. Hildebrandt DA, Irwin ED, Cates AW, Lohmeier TE. Regulation of renin secretion and arterial pressure during prolonged baroreflex activation: influence of salt intake. Hypertension. 2014;64:604–9. doi:10.1161/HYPERTENSIONAHA.114.03788.
50. Wolley MJ, Stowasser M. Resistant hypertension and chronic kidney disease: a dangerous liaison. Curr Hypertens Rep. 2016;18:36. doi:10.1007/s11906-016-0641-x.
51. Rossignol P, Massy ZA, Azizi M, Bakris G, Ritz E, Covic A, et al. The double challenge of resistant hypertension and chronic kidney disease. Lancet. 2015;386:1588–98. doi:10.1016/S0140-6736(15)00418-3.
52. Judd E, Calhoun DA. Management of hypertension in CKD: beyond the guidelines. Adv Chronic Kidney Dis. 2015;22:116–22. doi:10.1053/j.ackd.2014.12.001.
53. Kaur M, Chandran DS, Jaryal AK, Bhowmik D, Agarwal SK, Deepak KK. Baroreflex dysfunction in chronic kidney disease. World J Nephrol. 2016;5:53–65. doi:10.5527/wjn.v5.i1.53.
54. Thomas P, Dasgupta I. The role of the kidney and the sympathetic nervous system in hypertension. Pediatr Nephrol. 2015;30:549–60. doi:10.1007/s00467-014-2789-4.
55. Garnier AS, Briet M. Arterial stiffness and chronic kidney disease. Pulse (Basel, Switzerland). 2016;3:229–41. doi:10.1159/000443616.
56. Sag AA, Covic A, London G, Vervloet M, Goldsmith D, Gorriz JL, et al. Clinical imaging of vascular disease in chronic kidney disease. Int Urol Nephrol. 2016; doi:10.1007/s11255-016-1240-0.
57. Campese VM, Mitra N, Sandee D. Hypertension in renal parenchymal disease: why is it so resistant to treatment? Kidney Int. 2006;69:967–73. doi:10.1038/sj.ki.5000177.
58. De Nicola L, Gabbai FB, Agarwal R, Chiodini P, Borrelli S, Bellizzi V, et al. Prevalence and prognostic role of resistant hypertension in chronic kidney disease patients. J Am Coll Cardiol. 2013;61:2461–7. doi:10.1016/j.jacc.2012.12.061.
59. Siddiqui M, Dudenbostel T, Calhoun DA. Resistant and refractory hypertension: antihypertensive treatment resistance vs treatment failure. Can J Cardiol. 2016;32:603–6. doi:10.1016/j.cjca.2015.06.033.

60. Augustyniak RA, Tuncel M, Zhang W, Toto RD, Victor RG. Sympathetic overactivity as a cause of hypertension in chronic renal failure. J Hypertens. 2002;20:3–9.
61. Grassi G, Quarti-Trevano F, Seravalle G, Arenare F, Volpe M, Furiani S, et al. Early sympathetic activation in the initial clinical stages of chronic renal failure. Hypertension. 2011;57:846–51. doi:10.1161/HYPERTENSIONAHA.110.164780.
62. Salman IM, Hildreth CM, Ameer OZ, Phillips JK. Differential contribution of afferent and central pathways to the development of baroreflex dysfunction in chronic kidney disease. Hypertension. 2014;63:804–10. doi:10.1161/HYPERTENSIONAHA.113.02110.
63. Hoch H, Stegbauer J, Potthoff SA, Hein L, Quack I, Rump LC, et al. Regulation of renal sympathetic neurotransmission by renal α(2A)-adrenoceptors is impaired in chronic renal failure. Br J Pharmacol. 2011;163:438–46. doi:10.1111/j.1476-5381.2011.01223.x.
64. Tomiyama O, Shiigai T, Ideura T, Tomita K, Mito Y, Shinohara S, et al. Baroreflex sensitivity in renal failure. Clin Sci. 1980;58:21–7.
65. Wallbach M, Lehnig LY, Schroer C, Hasenfuss G, Müller GA, Wachter R, et al. Impact of baroreflex activation therapy on renal function—a pilot study. Am J Nephrol. 2014;40:371–80. doi:10.1159/000368723.
66. Beige J, Koziolek MJ, Hennig G, Hamza A, Wendt R, Müller GA, et al. Baroreflex activation therapy in patients with end-stage renal failure: proof of concept. J Hypertens. 2015;33:2344–9. doi:10.1097/HJH.0000000000000697.
67. Ameer OZ, Hildreth CM, Phillips JK. Sympathetic overactivity prevails over the vascular amplifier phenomena in a chronic kidney disease rat model of hypertension. Physiol Rep. 2014;2 doi:10.14814/phy2.12205.
68. Salman IM, Sarma Kandukuri D, Harrison JL, Hildreth CM, Phillips JK. Direct conscious telemetry recordings demonstrate increased renal sympathetic nerve activity in rats with chronic kidney disease. Front Physiol. 2015;6:218. doi:10.3389/fphys.2015.00218.
69. Ott C, Mahfoud F, Schmid A, Toennes SW, Ewen S, Ditting T, et al. Renal denervation preserves renal function in patients with chronic kidney disease and resistant hypertension. J Hypertens. 2015;33:1261–6. doi:10.1097/HJH.0000000000000556.
70. Kiuchi MG, Graciano ML, Carreira MA, Kiuchi T, Chen S, Lugon JR. Long-term effects of renal sympathetic denervation on hypertensive patients with mild to moderate chronic kidney disease. J Clin Hypertens (Greenwich). 2016;18:190–6. doi:10.1111/jch.12724.
71. Schmieder RE, Ott C, Schmid A, Friedrich S, Kistner I, Ditting T, et al. Adherence to antihypertensive medication in treatment-resistant hypertension undergoing renal denervation. J Am Heart Assoc. 2016;5 doi:10.1161/JAHA.115.002343.
72. Zuern CS, Eick C, Rizas KD, Bauer S, Langer H, Gawaz M, et al. Impaired cardiac baroreflex sensitivity predicts response to renal sympathetic denervation in patients with resistant hypertension. J Am Coll Cardiol. 2013;62:2124–30. doi:10.1016/j.jacc.2013.07.046.
73. Gmitrov J. Baroreceptor stimulation enhanced nitric oxide vasodilator responsiveness, a new aspect of baroreflex physiology. Microvasc Res. 2015;98:139–44. doi:10.1016/j.mvr.2014.11.004.
74. Cai GJ, Miao CY, Xie HH, Lu LH, Su DF. Arterial baroreflex dysfunction promotes atherosclerosis in rats. Atherosclerosis. 2005;183:41–7. doi:10.1016/j.atherosclerosis.2005.03.037.
75. Tomiyama H, Matsumoto C, Kimura K, Odaira M, Shiina K, Yamashina A. Pathophysiological contribution of vascular function to baroreflex regulation in hypertension. Circ J. 2014;78:1414–9.
76. Chesterton LJ, Sigrist MK, Bennett T, Taal MW, McIntyre CW. Reduced baroreflex sensitivity is associated with increased vascular calcification and arterial stiffness. Nephrol Dial Transplant. 2005;20:1140–7. doi:10.1093/ndt/gfh808.
77. Hogas S, Ardeleanu S, Segall L, Serban DN, Serban IL, Hogas M, et al. Changes in arterial stiffness following dialysis in relation to overhydration and to endothelial function. Int Urol Nephrol. 2012;44:897–905. doi:10.1007/s11255-011-9933-x.
78. Pettersen KH, Bugenhagen SM, Nauman J, Beard DA, Omholt SW. Arterial stiffening provides sufficient explanation for primary hypertension. PLoS Comput Biol. 2014;10:e1003634. doi:10.1371/journal.pcbi.1003634.

79. Lipponen JA, Tarvainen MP, Laitinen T, Karjalainen PA, Vanninen J, Koponen T, et al. Causal estimation of neural and overall baroreflex sensitivity in relation to carotid artery stiffness. Physiol Meas. 2013;34:1633–44. doi:10.1088/0967-3334/34/12/1633.
80. Thuesen AD, Andersen H, Cardel M, Toft A, Walter S, Marcussen N, et al. Differential effect of T-type voltage-gated Ca2+ channel disruption on renal plasma flow and glomerular filtration rate in vivo. Am J Physiol Renal Physiol. 2014;307:F445–52. doi:10.1152/ajprenal.00016. 2014.
81. Gupta A, Jain G, Kaur M, Jaryal AK, Deepak KK, Bhowmik D, et al. Association of impaired baroreflex sensitivity and increased arterial stiffness in peritoneal dialysis patients. Clin Exp Nephrol. 2016;20:302–8. doi:10.1007/s10157-015-1158-3.
82. Kaur M, Chandran D, Lal C, Bhowmik D, Jaryal AK, Deepak KK, et al. Renal transplantation normalizes baroreflex sensitivity through improvement in central arterial stiffness. Nephrol Dial Transplant. 2013;28:2645–55. doi:10.1093/ndt/gft099.
83. Lucini D, Palombo C, Malacarne M, Pagani M. Relationship between carotid artery mechanics and the spontaneous baroreflex: a noninvasive investigation in normal humans. J Hypertens. 2012;30:1809–16. doi:10.1097/HJH.0b013e3283568055.

Chapter 11
Secondary Causes: Work-Up and Its Specificities in CKD: Influence of Volume Overload, Excess Sodium Intake and Retention in CKD

Luminita Voroneanu, Dimitrie Siriopol, and Adrian Covic

Worldwide, it is estimated that more than 1 billion adults have hypertension; its prevalence is projected to climb to 1.5 billion by the year 2025 [1]; it is associated with premature death, stroke, and heart disease. The pathogenesis of hypertension is complex, involving increased systemic vascular resistance, arterial stiffening, cardiac output, excess salt intake, fluid retention, or a combination of all of these factors. The kidney plays an essential role in blood pressure (BP) pathogenesis, by appropriate renal adjustments of sodium balance and blood volume.

New Pathological Mechanisms Beyond Guyton's Theory

According to the classic concept of Guyton, high salt intake expands circulatory volume, which leads to an increase in perfusion pressure of the kidneys and in natriuresis that tends to restore the increased circulating volume to normal [2]. This pressure-natriuresis mechanism prevents the increase in BP that could arise from transient increase of circulating volume. In the context of induced renal dysfunction in animal experiments or in patients with chronic kidney disease (CKD), sodium loading causes extracellular volume expansion and volume loaded hypertension.

L. Voroneanu (✉) • D. Siriopol
Nephrology Clinic, Dialysis and Renal Transplant Center, 'C.I. PARHON' University Hospital, 'Grigore T. Popa', University of Medicine, Iași, Romania
e-mail: lumivoro@yahoo.com

A. Covic
Professor Internal Medicine & Nephrology, Grigore T. Popa University of Medicine, Iași, Romania
e-mail: lumivoro@yahoo.com

© Springer International Publishing AG 2017
A. Covic et al. (eds.), *Resistant Hypertension in Chronic Kidney Disease*,
DOI 10.1007/978-3-319-56827-0_11

169

According to this hypothesis, hypertension can develop only when the excretory ability of the kidney is impaired; in this context, the *kidney plays an essential role in BP regulation*. Moreover, it has been shown that mutations in a large number of genes related to the salt transport in the kidney determine monogenic forms of hypertension [3]. Fujita et al. recently identified two important signaling pathways in renal tubules that play key roles in electrolyte balance and the maintenance of normal BP: the β2-adrenergic stimulant-glucocorticoid receptor (GR)-with-no-lysine kinase (WNK)4-Na(+)-Cl(−) cotransporter pathway, which is active in the distal convoluted tubule (DCT) 1, and the Ras-related C3 botulinum toxin substrate (Rac)1-mineralocorticoid receptor (MR) pathway, which is active in DCT 2, connecting tubules, and collecting ducts. β2-Adrenergic stimulation due to increased renal sympathetic activity in obesity- and salt-induced hypertension suppresses histone deacetylase 8 activity via cAMP/PKA signaling, increasing the accessibility of GRs to the negative GR response element in the WNK4 promoter. This results in the suppression of WNK4 transcription followed by the activation of Na(+)-Cl(−) cotransporters in the DCT and elevated Na(+) retention and BP upon salt loading. The authors suggested that these new pathways might be novel therapeutic targets for the treatment of salt-sensitive hypertension and new diagnostic tools for determining the salt sensitivity of hypertensive patients [4].

However, in the last 15 years, the Guyton's traditional view was contradicted. In an elegant study, Heer et al. found that high sodium intake increases plasma volume in a dose-dependent manner, but not total body water. They concluded that in contrast to the traditional view, high sodium intake does not induce total body water storage but induces a relative fluid shift from the interstitial into the intravascular space [5]. More recently, Tietze et al. demonstrated that considerable quantities of nonosmotic sodium are accumulated in various tissues, such as skin, cartilage, bone, and muscle without water retention [6].

Experimental studies have shown that negatively charged glycosaminoglycans (GAG) in the skin interstitium are responsible for sodium storage. In rats, excess dietary sodium has been linked with (1) increased interstitial GAG content, (2) increased polymerization and sulfation of these GAGs, and (3) increased skin sodium concentrations (180–190 mmol/L) which exceed plasma sodium concentrations and was not accompanied by extracellular water retention.

It seems that nonosmotic sodium accumulation, which occurs acutely, is followed by amplified removal from skin via the newly developed lymphatics for ultimate renal excretion. In rats, a high-salt diet leads to interstitial hypertonic sodium accumulation in skin [7], resulting in increased density and hyperplasia of the lymph and capillary network. The mechanisms underlying these effects on lymphatics involve activation of tonicity-responsive enhancer binding protein (TonEBP) in mononuclear phagocyte system (MPS) cells infiltrating the interstitium of the skin. TonEBP binds the promoter of the gene encoding vascular endothelial growth factor C (VEGF-C) and causes VEGF-C secretion by macrophages [8] (Fig. 11.1). As a consequence, increased density and hyperplasia of the skin lymphocapillary network and increased endothelial nitric oxide synthesis is observed. MPS cell depletion or VEGF-C trapping by soluble VEGF receptor-3 blocks VEGF-C signaling, augments interstitial hypertonic volume retention, decreases endothelial nitric oxide synthase expression, and elevates BP in response to high-salt diet. The MPS cells act as onsite controllers of interstitial

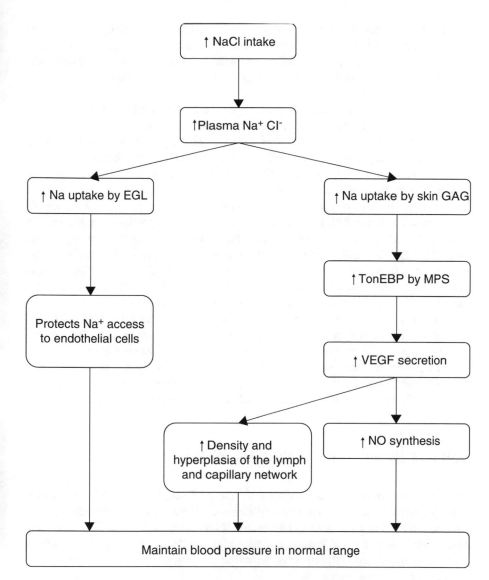

Fig. 11.1 Potential defensive mechanisms for high salt intake. *EGL* endothelial glycocalyx layer, *GAG* glycosaminoglycans, *MPS* mononuclear phagocyte system, *NO* nitric oxide, *TonEBP* tonicity-responsive enhancer binding protein, *VEGF* vascular endothelial growth factor

volume and BP homeostasis, providing a local regulatory salt-sensitive tonicity-responsive enhancer binding protein/vascular endothelial growth factor C-mediated mechanism in the skin to maintain normal blood pressure in states of interstitial Na(+) and Cl(−) accumulation. Failure of this physiological extrarenal regulatory mechanism leads to a salt-sensitive blood pressure response [7].

Another important player in this concept is the endothelial surface layer, a dynamic layer on the luminal side of the endothelium that is in continuous exchange with flowing blood. This soft surface layer, named endothelial glycocalyx layer

(EGL), is a negatively charged biopolymer known to preferentially bind sodium, because negatively charged GAG are abundantly present in this layer. Additionally, it is involved in regulating vascular permeability, has antiatherogenic and anti-inflammatory properties, and is an important mediator in shear-induced nitric oxide (NO) production.

At present, the sodium binding capacity of the EGL is not known. However, the sodium excess determines a reduction of heparin sulfate residues by 68%, which leads to destabilization and collapse of the EGL. Subsequently, sodium is bringing into the endothelial cells. Sodium overload transformed the endothelial cells from a sodium release into a sodium-absorbing state. These results might elucidate endothelial dysfunction and arterial hypertension associated with sodium abuse [9].

Additionally, in some pathological situation such as severe sepsis, CKD, or end-stage renal disease (ESRD), or during acute or chronic hyperglycemia, the EGL is perturbed, which is accompanied by an expanded extracellular volume, higher BP, or both, suggesting that variability in sodium homeostasis and salt sensitivity may be related to the quality of the EGL, in which endothelial GAGs act as an intravascular buffer compartment for sodium. For example, in 23 stable dialysis patients, the EGL alteration was associated with an increased need for ultrafiltration.

Endothelial surface layer has also been reported to influence the availability of NO production via mediating the epithelial sodium channel on the endothelial luminal surface (EnNaC). When the plasma sodium was increased, the density of EnNaC has been shown to be increased to leading to increasing sodium uptake, stiffen the endothelial cellular cortex, and diminishing NO production. Taken together, an increase of sodium delivery to the endothelial cell resulted in an increase in vascular tone [10].

Salt and Hypertension in the General Population

Alteration in dietary sodium determines different BP responses; if BP increases during a period of high dietary sodium or declines during a period of low sodium, these individuals have salt-sensitive hypertension. If there is no change in BP with sodium restriction, that individual has salt-resistant hypertension. Salt sensitivity in normotensives is associated with future hypertension; salt sensitivity hypertension is associated with increased mortality.

Salt sensitivity has been shown to be mainly prevalent in black, in obese, and in elderly hypertensive patients. It is frequently associated with diminished renal function and by a significantly enhanced cardiovascular risk. Furthermore, it is also associated with microalbuminuria, absence of the nocturnal decrease in arterial pressure, and absence of modulation of renal blood flow in response to sodium loading.

Excess salt intake is one of the most common and important risk factors involved in the pathogenesis of hypertension. Numerous animal studies [11–13] and clinical trials found a causal relation between salt intake and hypertension [14–19].

Additionally, data from epidemiological studies have shown a direct and positive association between excess salt intake and cardiovascular disease.

The INTERSALT Study engaged a standardized protocol with careful attention to the measurement of BP and collection of "gold standard" 24-h urinary Na estimates in 10,079 adults from 32 countries, providing a wide range in Na (the exposure variable). A significant positive relationship was shown between dietary Na and BP for both within- and across-population analyses. Recently, the Prospective Urban Rural Epidemiology (PURE) study provided new evidence about the association between sodium and potassium intake, estimated from morning urine specimens, BP, death, and major cardiovascular events [20]. In this study of 102,216 adults from 18 countries and 5 continents, the authors found a positive but heterogeneous association between estimated sodium excretion and BP. Approximately 90% of the participants had either a high (>5.99 g per day) or moderate (3.00–5.99 g per day) level of sodium excretion; approximately 10% excreted less than 3.00 g per day, and only 4% had sodium excretion in the range associated with current US guidelines for sodium intake (2.3 or 1.5 g per day). The authors found a steeper slope for this association among study participants with sodium excretion of more than 5 g per day, a modest association among those with sodium excretion of 3–5 g per day, and no significant association among those with sodium excretion of less than 3 g per day. The authors concluded from the findings that a very small proportion of the worldwide population consumes a low-sodium diet and that sodium intake is not related to BP in these persons, calling into question the feasibility and usefulness of reducing dietary sodium as a population-based strategy for reducing BP [20, 21]. Another very important finding of this study is the relation between sodium excretion and potassium excretion in regard to BP: high sodium excretion was more powerfully associated with increased BP in persons with lower potassium excretion; they proposed that the alternative approach of recommending high-quality diets rich in potassium might achieve greater health benefits, including blood pressure reduction, than aggressive sodium reduction alone. The major limitations of this study are (1) the absence of the direct measurements on 24-h urinary excretion on numerous occasions, which is the accepted model for evaluating electrolyte intake, and (2) the lack of an intervention component to assess the direct effects of altering sodium and potassium intake on blood pressure, thus making it unfeasible to establish causality.

On the other hand, sodium restriction determines a significant reduction in BP, with multiple meta-analysis and systematic reviews of randomized controlled trials showing this effect. The last one, published last year, from the Global Burden of Diseases Nutrition and Chronic Diseases Expert Group (NutriCode) including 107 randomized interventions in 103 trials, showed a linear dose–response relationship between reduced sodium intake and BP, jointly modified according to age, race, and the presence or absence of hypertension. The authors explained that larger effects in older adults and hypertensive persons would be consistent with decreasing vascular compliance and renal filtration; in blacks, larger effects would be consistent with differences in renal handling of sodium [22].

Salt and Hypertension in CKD

Evidence shows that almost all CKD patients are salt sensitive; in these patients, high salt intake is linked to risk factors for both heart disease and worsening kidney function, including high BP, excess proteinuria, and fluid overload. The effect of sodium intake on BP is traditionally thought to be driven primarily through changes in fluid volume, mediated by the renin-angiotensin-aldosterone system (RAAS), although recent research indicates that other mediators, like vascular stiffness or inflammation, may play an important role.

High sodium intake is thought to have direct toxic effects on blood vessels through mediating factors such as oxidative stress, inflammation, endothelial cell dysfunction, and vascular stiffness. High sodium intake enhances the generation of superoxide anion accompanied by enhanced renal expression and nicotinamide dehydrogenase activation. In addition, dietary salt increases the glomerular expression of TGF-β1 on renal tissue and also augments nitric oxide production. High salt intake also induces the intrarenal aldosterone receptor and promotes renal fibrotic injury; it might also determine tissue inflammation by triggering IL-17-producing CD4+ T cell development [23].

Moreover, the excess sodium intake abrogates the antiproteinuric effects of angiotensin converting enzyme inhibitors (ACEi) or angiotensin receptor blockers (ARBs), thereby exacerbating proteinuria. Sodium restriction amplifies the top of the dose response of RAAS-blockade for both blood pressure and proteinuria. The effect of moderate sodium restriction during RAAS-blockade on blood pressure and proteinuria is almost similar to the effect of adding a diuretic. In a recent systematic review and meta-analysis, including 11 studies and 516 participants, sodium intake reduction markedly reduces albumin excretion, more so during concomitant RAAS-blocking therapy and among patients with kidney damage. An average reduction in sodium intake of 92 mmol/d was associated with a 32.1% reduction in urinary albumin excretion. A greater reduction of urinary albumin excretion was associated with a higher decrease in BP during the intervention [24].

There were several short-term studies on the effect of restricting salt intake on BP levels in CKD patients. In a small prospective trial of patients with CKD, McMahon and colleagues determined that a low-sodium diet (60–80 mmol/d) resulted in a reduction of 10 mmHg systolic pressure compared with a high-sodium diet. The authors also demonstrated that the low-sodium diet in this trial reduced protein excretion by more than 300 mg/d and also the extracellular volume [25, 26]. In a recent Cochrane meta-analysis including 8 studies and 258 people (with early-stage CKD, renal transplantation, one study, and peritoneal dialysis, one study), reduced sodium intake significantly reduced BP and antihypertensive medication dosage [27]. However, the authors found a critical evidence gap in long-term effects of salt restriction in people with CKD; they were unable to determine the direct effects of sodium restriction on primary endpoints such as mortality and progression to ESRD.

Volume Overload and Hypertension

It is now recognized that unidentified, clinically unapparent volume expansion is an important cause for hypertension and resistance to antihypertensive treatment [28]. Several methods have been used for optimal determination of volemia, including clinical examination, measurement of inferior cave vein diameter using echocardiography, and the evaluation of cardiac biomarkers—mainly N-terminal prohormone brain natriuretic peptide (NT proBNP) or impedance measurements.

A positive correlation between measured plasma volume and systolic and diastolic BP was shown in several studies [29]; additionally, intensified diuretic treatment improved BP control via a quantifiable decrease in plasma volume [30, 31]. In the last 15 years, thoracic bioimpedance was used to evaluate hemodynamic status and to adjust complex antihypertensive treatment in general population. Taler et al. in a series of 104 patients with resistant hypertension randomized to hemodynamic guided treatment or specialist care showed that the patients treated according to hemodynamic measurements had an improved BP control rate (56% versus 33% in the control group, $P < 0.05$) and incremental reduction in systemic vascular resistance measurements compared with the group of patients treated as per clinical judgment alone. Higher doses of diuretics (not a greater prevalence of use) were prescribed for the hemodynamically managed group, leading to a greater blood pressure lowering [32]. Smith et al. investigated the role of hypertension therapy guided by impedance in 164 patients with uncontrolled hypertension and no significant accompanying diseases [33]. After 3 months of treatment, therapy based on hemodynamic evaluation was associated with considerably better BP control, including a significant decrease in average systolic and diastolic BP values. The hemodynamic arm achieved the BP goal (<140/90 mmHg) more frequently (77% versus 57% $P < 0.01$ and 55% versus 27% for a more aggressive BP control – at <130/85 mmHg $P < 0.0001$) compared with the control group. Similar results were obtained by Krzesinski et al. in 128 patients with uncontrolled hypertension [34]. Therapy based on impedance cardiography significantly increased the reduction in office systolic BP (11.0 vs. 17.3 mmHg; $p = 0.008$) and diastolic pressure (7.7 vs. 12.2 mmHg; $p = 0.0008$), as well as 24-h mean systolic BP (9.8 vs. 14.2 mmHg; $p = 0.026$), daytime systolic BP (10.5 vs. 14.8 mmHg; $p = 0.040$), and night-time systolic BP (7.7 vs. 12.2 mmHg; $p = 0.032$) [35].

Subclinical volume overload is present in more than 20% of CKD patients. In a prospective cohort study including 338 patients with CKD stage 3–5, fluid overload was associated with BP, proteinuria, renal inflammation with macrophage infiltration and tumor necrosis factor-α overexpression, glomerular sclerosis, and cardiac fibrosis [36]. Hung et al. used the body composition monitor, a multifrequency bioimpedance device, to measure the level of overhydration in CKD patients. Of the 338 patients with stages 3–5 CKD, included in this study, only 48% were euvolemic. Patients with volume overload were found to use significantly more antihypertensive medications and diuretics but had higher systolic BP and an increased arterial stiffness than patients without volume overload [37].

The value of guiding hypertension treatment based on subclinical extracellular fluid excess has been tested in one pilot study. Verdalles et al. used bioimpedance to assess fluid status and to guide diuretic therapy for treating hypertension in CKD patients [38]. They treated 30 patients with extracellular volume (ECV) expansion with a diuretic in contrast to 20 patients without ECV expansion who as an alternative received another additional antihypertensive medication. At 6 months of follow-up, systolic BP decreased by 21 mmHg in patients with expansion of ECV compared with 9 mmHg in patients without expansion of ECV ($P < 0.01$). In addition, nine of 30 patients with ECV expansion and two of 20 without ECV expansion achieved the target blood pressure of less than 140/90 mmHg at 6 months.

In hemodialysis, approximately 25% of the patients are overhydrated; based on bioimpedance and BP measurements, Wabel et al. described four distinct categories of individuals in dialysis: (i) normotensive, normovolemics; (ii) hypertensive, normovolemics; (iii) hypertensive, hypervolemics; and (iv) normotensive, hypervolemics. It is obvious that BP management by different classes of drugs could be tailored much easier and related to prevailing underlying pathophysiological mechanisms [39].

Furthermore, the impact of volume overload correction on BP management has been tested in several studies. In the DRIP study, Agarwal et al. included 150 patients without obvious volume overload; 50 patients were randomized to a control group and 100 patients randomized to ultrafiltration group, and all underwent interdialytic ambulatory BP monitoring three times (at baseline, 4 weeks, and 8 weeks). In the ultrafiltration group, the ambulatory BP was reduced within 4 weeks by 7/3 mmHg. This antihypertensive effect was sustained for 8 weeks of observation. Despite provoking occasional uncomfortable intradialytic symptoms, the quality of life was not impaired with reducing dry weight [40].

Additionally, bioimpedance-guided fluid management was associated with an improvement in BP control, intradialytic symptoms, left ventricular mass index, or arterial stiffness. Moissl et al. optimized the fluid status of 55 HD patients using a bioimpedance device over the course of 3 months. This active fluid management improved significantly the BP control; every 1 l change in fluid overload was accompanied by a 9.9 mmHg/L change in predialysis systolic BP [41].

Similar results were reported by Hur et al. in a prospective randomized trial including 156 hemodialysis patients; in the interventional group ($n = 78$), the fluid management was guided using bioimpedance; in the control group ($n = 78$), the fluid removal during dialysis was determined according to usual clinical practice. Pre- and post-dialysis systolic and diastolic BP significantly decreased in the intervention group compared with the control group. Moreover, a significant reduction in the left ventricular mass index was also observed in the intervention group as compared with the control group (mean difference between groups: -10.2; 95% CI -19.2 to -1.17; $p = 0.04$) [42]. Moreover, in another randomized trial, Onofriescu et al. showed that strict volume control guide by bioimpedance is associated with better survival rate ($P = 0.03$). After 2.5 years there was also an improvement arterial stiffness (measured with pulse wave velocity [m/s]) was significantly higher in the intervention group (-1.50 compared with 1.2; mean difference in change: -2.78; 95% CI -3.75 to 1.80; p < 0.001) [43].

In contrast, Ponce et al. founded that volume control was not associated with better BP control in 189 hemodialysis patients from 23 dialysis centers, although bioimpedance measurements provided a better volume control, BP, the number of hypotensive events, and hospitalizations were similar between the two groups [44].

Hypertension is also common in peritoneal dialysis; the presence of latent hypervolemia or insufficient patient compliance to salt and fluid retention might have a major role. Results of the recently published European Body Composition study showed that fluid overload is a frequent problem in this group of patients (severe fluid overload was present in 25.2% of 639 PD patients) [45]. Chen et al., in a prospective study including 121 HD and 84 PD patients, observed that all patients with overhydration had hypertension in both the hemodialysis and peritoneal dialysis groups [46]. Yilmaz et al. investigated the association between hydration status, measured with BIA methods and BP and left ventricular mass index (LVMI) in 43 HD and 33 PD patients. Systolic BP in both post-HD and PD groups and LVMI in the PD group were found to be significantly higher in overhydrated patients. In multiple linear regression analyses, fluid overload was independently associated with higher systolic BP and LVMI [47].

The impact of strict volume control on BP, LVMI, or mortality was evaluated in several studies. In 47 hypertensive PD patients, antihypertensive medications were discontinued, and salt restriction was initiated. In patients with persistent elevation of BP, enhanced peritoneal ultrafiltration was implemented by the use of a hypertonic dialysis solution (4.25% dextrose). Salt restriction alone or combined with ultrafiltration led to a decline in body weight by a mean of 2.8 kg, and BP decreased from a mean of 158.2 ± 17.0/95.7 ± 10.3 to 119.7 ± 16.0/779 ± 9.7 mmHg. Additionally, a significant decrease of the cardiothoracic index on the chest radiograph was also noted: from 48.0% ± 5.6% to 42.9% ± 4.5% [48].

In a randomized controlled study, Tang et al. used bioimpedance to improve the volume control and BP in 160 PD patients. The patients were randomly allocated to 2 groups: in Group 1 the patients and their primary nurses were informed of the overhydration values provided by bioimpedance spectroscopy, whereas in Group 2 the values were not revealed, and patients' volume was measured by the standard methods; the use of bioimpedance was associated with a better volume control and a significant improvement in systolic BP [49].

Another bedside method that received growing attention in recent years is lung ultrasonography (LUS) (Fig. 11.2). It determines the extravascular lung water, a small, but important component of total body fluids that represents the water content of lung interstitium and is strictly dependent on the filling pressure of the left ventricle. The comet-tail artifacts, also known as B-lines, are a type of reverberation phenomenon that occurs as a consequence of the mismatch between edematous septa and the overlying pleura [50, 51].

Although B-lines are a reliable diagnostic tool for the assessment and staging of the pulmonary congestion in heart failure patients, this method could be also of help in managing hypertension, especially in CKD patients. Several studies found a significant association between B-lines score and BP [52–55], but only in the simple correlation analysis. There was also observed an association between the B-lines score and bioimpedance parameters in some [57] but not all studies [52, 58].

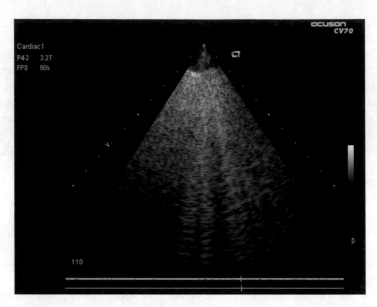

Fig. 11.2 B-lines by lung ultrasonography

In hemodialysis patients, the B-line score is associated with cardiovascular events [54] and all-cause mortality [54, 56, 59]. However, Siriopol et al. showed that only bioimpedance, and not lung ultrasonography, improves risk prediction for death, beyond classical and echocardiographic-based risk prediction scores/parameters [59]. Bioimpedance and lung ultrasonography may be complementary, providing different information, with bioimpedance being more specific to fluid status and lung ultrasonography to cardiac function. Although bioimpedance seems to possess more prognostic capabilities, in specific patients, a dry weight estimation based on lung ultrasonography could be considered. Currently, two randomized controlled trials regarding this approach are ongoing (ClinicalTrials. gov Identifiers: NCT01815762 and NCT02310061).

Conclusions

In conclusion, salt and volume matters. Maybe it is time to use individualized hemodynamic measures and individualized antihypertensive treatment in all patients. Although we have numerous drugs to lower BP, we have never aligned how we think they work with any phenotyping (or genotyping). So we have a "one size fits all" approach to raised BP. In CKD, we can see the folly of this all too clearly. Salt and water could make the difference. Given that we can now measure volume expansion reliably and noninvasively, and titrate BP treatment, why do we not bother, in all patients?

References

1. World Health Organization. A global brief on hypertension. WHO/DCO/WHD/2013.2. April 3, 2013 (http://apps.who.int/iris/bitstream/10665/79059/1/WHO_DCO_WHD_2013.2_eng. pdf).
2. Guyton AC, Coleman TG, Cowley AW, Scheel KW, Manning RD, Norman RA. Arterial pressure regulation. Overriding dominance of the kidneys in long-term regulation and in hypertension. Am J Med. 1972;52:584–94.
3. Lifton R, Gharavi AG, Geller DS. Molecular mechanisms of human hypertension. Cell. 2001;104:545–56.
4. Mu S, Shimosawa T, Ogura S, et al. Epigenetic modulation of the renal β-adrenergic-WNK4 pathway in salt-sensitive hypertension. Nat Med. 2011;17:573–80. Nishimoto M, Fujita T. Renal mechanisms of salt-sensitive hypertension: contribution of two steroid receptor-associated pathways. Am J Physiol Renal Physiol. 2015;308:F377–87.
5. Heer M, Baisch F, Kropp J, Gerzer R, Drummer C. High dietary sodium chloride consumption may not induce body fluid retention in humans. Am J Physiol Renal Physiol. 2000;278: F585–95.
6. Titze J, Maillet A, Lang R. Long-term sodium balance in humans in a terrestrial space station simulation study. Am J Kidney Dis. 2002;40:508–16. Rakova N, Jüttner K, Dahlmann A, Schröder A. Long-term space flight simulation reveals infradian rhythmicity in human Na(+) balance. Cell Metab. 2013;17:125–31.
7. Machnik A, Dahlmann A, Kopp C, et al. Mononuclear phagocyte system depletion blocks interstitial tonicity-responsive enhancer binding protein/vascular endothelial growth factor C expression and induces salt-sensitive hypertension in rats. Hypertension. 2010;55:755–61.
8. Machnik A, Neuhofer W, Jantsch J, et al. Macrophages regulate salt-dependent volume and blood pressure by a vascular endothelial growth factor-C-dependent buffering mechanism. Nat Med. 2009;15(5):545–52.
9. Oberleithner H, Peters W, Kusche-Vihrog K, et al. Salt overload damages the glycocalyx sodium barrier of vascular endothelium. Pflugers Arch. 2011;462:519–28.
10. Choi HY, Park HC, Ha SK. Salt sensitivity and hypertension: a paradigm shift from kidney malfunction to vascular endothelial dysfunction. Electrolyte Blood Press. 2015;13(1):7–16.
11. Ball OT, Meneely GR. Observations on dietary sodium chloride. J Am Diet Assoc. 1957; 33:366–70.
12. Dahl LK, Heine M, Tassinari L. Effects of chronic salt ingestion. Evidence that genetic factors play an important role in susceptibility to experimental hypertension. J Exp Med. 1962;115: 1173–90.
13. Denton D, Weisinger R, Mundy NI, et al. The effect of increased salt intake on blood pressure of chimpanzees. Nat Med. 1995;1:1009–16.
14. MacGregor GA, Markandu ND, Best FE, et al. Double-blind randomised crossover trial of moderate sodium restriction in essential hypertension. Lancet. 1982;1:351–5.
15. Intersalt Cooperative Research Group. Intersalt: an international study of electrolyte excretion and blood pressure. Results for 24 h urinary sodium and potassium excretion. BMJ. 1988; 297:319–28.
16. The Trials of Hypertension Prevention Collaborative Research Group. The effects of nonpharmacologic interventions on blood pressure and hypertension incidence in overweight people with high-normal blood pressure. JAMA. 1992;267:1213–20.
17. The Trials of Hypertension Prevention Collaborative Research Group. Effects of weight loss and sodium reduction intervention on blood pressure and hypertension incidence in overweight people with high-normal blood pressure: the trials of hypertension prevention, phase II. Arch Intern Med. 1997;157:657–66.
18. Whelton PK, Appel LJ, Espeland MA, et al. for the TONE Collaborative Research Group. Sodium reduction and weight loss in the treatment of hypertension in older persons. A random-

ized controlled trial of nonpharmacologic interventions in the elderly (TONE). JAMA. 1998; 279:839–46.

19. Sacks FM, Svetkey LP, Vollmer WM, et al; DASH-Sodium Collaborative Research Group. Effects on blood pressure of reduced dietary sodium and the Dietary Approaches to Stop Hypertension (DASH) diet. N Engl J Med. 2001;344:3–10.

20. Mente A, O'Donnell MJ, Rangarajan S, McQueen MJ, Poirier P, Wielgosz A, et al; PURE Investigators. Association of urinary sodium and potassium excretion with blood pressure. N Engl J Med. 2014;371(7):601–1.

21. Oparil S. Low sodium intake – cardiovascular health benefit or risk? N Engl J Med. 2014;371(7):677–9.

22. Mozaffarian D, Fahimi S, Singh GM, et al. for the Global Burden of Diseases Nutrition and Chronic Diseases Expert Group (NUTRICODE). Global Sodium Consumption and Death from Cardiovascular Causes. N Engl J Med. 2014; 371:624–34.

23. Hwang JH, Chin HJ, Kim S, Kim DK, Kim S, Park JH, Shin SJ, Lee SH, Choi BS, Lim CS. Effects of intensive low-salt diet education on albuminuria among nondiabetic patients with hypertension treated with olmesartan: a single-blinded randomized, controlled trial. Clin J Am Soc Nephrol. 2014;9(12):2059–69.

24. D'Elia L, Rossi G, Schiano di Cola M, Savino I, Galletti F, Strazzullo P. Meta-analysis of the effect of dietary sodium restriction with or without concomitant renin-angiotensin-aldosterone system-inhibiting treatment on albuminuria. Clin J Am Soc Nephrol. 2015;10(9):1542–52.

25. Middleton JP, Lehrich RW. Prescriptions for dietary sodium in patients with chronic kidney disease: how will this shake out? Kidney Int. 2014;86(3):457–9.

26. McMahon EJ, Bauer JD, Hawley CM, et al. A randomized trial of dietary sodium restriction in CKD. J Am Soc Nephrol. 2013;24:2096–103.

27. McMahon EJ, Campbell KL, Altered dietary salt for people with CKD. Nephrology. 2015;20:758–759.

28. Calhoun DA, Jones D, Textor S, Goff DC, Murphy TP, Toto RD, White A, Cushman WC, White W, Sica D, Ferdinand K, Giles TD, Falkner B, Carey RM. Resistant hypertension: diagnosis, evaluation, and treatment. A scientific statement from the American Heart Association Professional Education Committee of the Council for high blood pressure research. Hypertension. 2008;51(6):1403–19.

29. Dustan HP. Causes of inadequate response to antihypertensive drugs: volume factors. Hypertension. 1983;5:III-26–30.

30. Graves JW, Bloomfield RL, Buckalew VM. Plasma volume in resistant hypertension: guide to pathophysiology and therapy. Am J Med Sci. 1989;298:361–5.

31. Taler SJ. Individualizing antihypertensive combination therapies: clinical and hemodynamic considerations. Curr Hypertens Rep. 2014 Jul;16(7):451.

32. Taler SJ, Textor SC, Augustine JE. Resistant hypertension: comparing hemodynamic management to specialist care. Hypertension. 2002;39(5):982–8.

33. Smith R, Levy P, Ferrario C. for the Consideration of Noninvasive Hemodynamic Monitoring to Target Reduction of Blood Pressure Levels Study Group. Value of noninvasive hemodynamics to achieve blood pressure control in hypertensive subjects. Hypertension. 2006;47:771–7.

34. Krzesiński P, Gielerak G, Kowal J. A "patient-tailored" treatment of hypertension with use of impedance cardiography: a randomized, prospective and controlled trial. Med Sci Monit. 2013;19:242–50. The most recent randomized trial using hemodynamic measurements to guide hypertension treatment in patients with mild to moderate hypertension.

35. Krzesiński P, Gielerak G, Kowal J. A "patient-tailored" treatment of hypertension with use of impedance cardiography: a randomized, prospective and controlled trial. Med Sci Monit. 2013;19:242–50.

36. Hung SC, Lai YS, Kuo KL, Tarng DC. Volume overload and adverse outcomes in chronic kidney disease: clinical observational and animal studies. J Am Heart Assoc. 2015;4(5) doi:10.1161/JAHA.115.001918.

37. Hung SC, Kuo KL, Peng CH, Wu CH, Lien YC, Wang YC, Tarng DC. Volume overload correlates with cardiovascular risk factors in patients with chronic kidney disease. Kidney Int. 2014;85(3):703–9.
38. Verdalles U, de Vinuesa SG, Goicoechea M, et al. Utility of bioimpedance spectroscopy (BIS) in the management of refractory hypertension in patients with chronic kidney disease (CKD). Nephrol Dial Transplant. 2012;27(Suppl 4):iv31–5.
39. Wabel P, Moissl U, Chamney P, Jirka T, Machek P, Ponce P, Taborsky P, Tetta C, Velasco N, Vlasak J, Zaluska W, Wizemann V. Towards improved cardiovascular management: the necessity of combining blood pressure and fluid overload. Nephrol Dial Transplant. 2008;23(9): 2965–71.
40. Agarwal R, Alborzi P, Satyan S, Light RP. Dry-weight reduction in hypertensive hemodialysis patients (DRIP): a randomized, controlled trial. Hypertension. 2009;53:500–7.
41. Moissl U, Arias-Guillen M, Wabel P, Fontsere N, Carrera M, Campistol JM, Maduell F. Bioimpedance-guided fluid management in hemodialysis patients. Clin J Am Soc Nephrol. 2013;8(9):1575–82.
42. Hur E, Usta M, Toz H, Asci G, Wabel P, Kahvecioglu S, Kayikcioglu M, Demirci MS, Ozkahya M, Duman S, Ok E. Effect of fluid management guided by bioimpedance spectroscopy on cardiovascular parameters in hemodialysis patients: a randomized controlled trial. Am J Kidney Dis. 2013;61(6):957–65.
43. Onofriescu M, Hogas S, Voroneanu L, Apetrii M, Nistor I, Kanbay M, Covic AC. Bioimpedance-guided fluid management in maintenance hemodialysis: a pilot randomized controlled trial. Am J Kidney Dis. 2014;64(1):111–8.
44. Ponce P, Pham J, Gligoric-Fuerer O, Kreuzberg O. Fluid management in haemodialysis: conventional versus body composition monitoring (BCM) supported management of overhydrated patients. Port J Nephrol Hypert. 2014;28(3):239–48.
45. Van Biesen W, Williams JD, Covic AC, Fan S, Claes K, Lichodziejewska-Niemierko M, Verger C, Steiger J, Schoder V, Wabel P, Gauly A, Himmele R; EuroBCM Study Group. Fluid status in peritoneal dialysis patients: the European body composition monitoring (EuroBCM) study cohort. PLoS One. 2011;6(2):e17148.
46. Chen YC, Lin CJ, Wu CJ, Chen HH, Yeh JC. Comparison of extracellular volume and blood pressure in hemodialysis and peritoneal dialysis patients. Nephron Clin Pract. 2009; 113(2):c112–6.
47. Yılmaz Z, Yıldırım Y, Aydın FY, Aydın E, Kadiroğlu AK, Yılmaz ME, Acet H. Evaluation of fluid status related parameters in hemodialysis and peritoneal dialysis patients: clinical usefulness of bioimpedance analysis. Medicina (Kaunas). 2014;50(5):269–74.
48. Günal AI, Duman S, Ozkahya M, Töz H, Asçi G, Akçiçek F, Basçi A. Strict volume control normalizes hypertension in peritoneal dialysis patients. Am J Kidney Dis. 2001;37(3): 588–93.
49. Luo YJ, Lu XH, Woods F, Wang T. Volume control in peritoneal dialysis patients guided by bioimpedance spectroscopy assessment. Blood Purif. 2011;31(4):296–302.
50. Ziskin MC, Thickman DI, Goldenberg NJ, et al. The comet tail artifact. J Ultrasound Med. 1982;1:1–7.
51. Soldati G, Copetti R, Sher S. Sonographic interstitial syndrome: the sound of lung water. J Ultrasound Med. 2009;28:163–74.
52. Mallamaci F, Benedetto FA, Tripepi R, Rastelli S, Castellino P, Tripepi G, Picano E, Zoccali C. Detection of pulmonary congestion by chest ultrasound in dialysis patients. JACC Cardiovasc Imaging. 2010;3(6):586–94.
53. Panuccio V, Enia G, Tripepi R, Torino C, Garozzo M, Battaglia GG, Marcantoni C, Infantone L, Giordano G, De Giorgi ML, Lupia M, Bruzzese V, Zoccali C. Chest ultrasound and hidden lung congestion in peritoneal dialysis patients. Nephrol Dial Transplant. 2012;27(9):3601–5.
54. Zoccali C, Torino C, Tripepi R, Tripepi G, D'Arrigo G, Postorino M, Gargani L, Sicari R, Picano E, Mallamaci F; Lung US in CKD Working Group. Pulmonary congestion predicts cardiac events and mortality in ESRD. J Am Soc Nephrol. 2013;24(4):639–46.

55. Weitzel WF, Hamilton J, Wang X, Bull JL, Vollmer A, Bowman A, Rubin J, Kruger GH, Gao J, Heung M, Rao P. Quantitative lung ultrasound comet measurement: method and initial clinical results. Blood Purif. 2015;39(1–3):37–44.
56. Siriopol D, Hogas S, Voroneanu L, Onofriescu M, Apetrii M, Oleniuc M, Moscalu M, Sascau R, Covic A. Predicting mortality in haemodialysis patients: a comparison between lung ultrasonography, bioimpedance data and echocardiography parameters. Nephrol Dial Transplant. 2013;28(11):2851–9.
57. Basso F, Milan Manani S, Cruz DN, Teixeira C, Brendolan A, Nalesso F, Zanella M, Ronco C. Comparison and reproducibility of techniques for fluid status assessment in chronic hemodialysis patients. Cardiorenal Med. 2013;3(2):104–12.
58. Paudel K, Kausik T, Visser A, Ramballi C, Fan SL. Comparing lung ultrasound with bioimpedance spectroscopy for evaluating hydration in peritoneal dialysis patients. Nephrology (Carlton). 2015;20(1):1–5.
59. Siriopol D, Voroneanu L, Hogas S, Apetrii M, Gramaticu A, Dumea R, Burlacu A, Sascau R, Kanbay M, Covic A. Bioimpedance analysis versus lung ultrasonography for optimal risk prediction in hemodialysis patients. Int J Cardiovasc Imaging. 2016;32(2):263–70.

Chapter 12
Resistant Hypertension in Elderly People with Chronic Kidney Disease

Raúl Fernández-Prado, Esmeralda Castillo-Rodríguez, and Alberto Ortiz

Aging of the Population

Individuals over 60 years are usually considered elderly. Inside this group, two categories are recognized, those 60–80-year-olds and those aged over 80 years. It is likely that as the population ages, a new category of centenarians will be considered.

In recent decades, global life expectancy for both sexes increased from 65.3 years in 1990 to 71.5 years in 2013, and the trend is to a continuous increase. In 1950, the elderly were 8% of the world population; in 2000 they were 10%; and in 2050, according to United Nations projections, the proportion will reach 21% [1]. The issue is most pressing in most advanced economies (Fig. 12.1).

Reductions in the main causes of death are extending life expectancy. In high-income countries, age-adjusted death rates for cardiovascular diseases and cancers have decreased. In developing countries, child deaths from diarrhea, lower respiratory infections, and neonatal causes have also decreased. The reduction of the main causes of death and the aging of the population have resulted in an increase in other noncommunicable causes of death, like chronic kidney disease, which was the cause of death that increased the most in the past 20 years, after human immunodeficiency virus infection [2].

Raúl Fernández-Prado and Esmeralda Castillo Rodríguez contributed equally to this work.

R. Fernández-Prado
IIS-Fundación Jiménez Díaz-Universidad Autónoma de Madrid, Madrid, Spain

E. Castillo-Rodríguez
IIS-Fundacion Jimenez Diaz, Madrid, Spain

A. Ortiz (✉)
Unidad de Diálisis, IIS-Fundación Jiménez Díaz, Av Reyes Católicos 2, 28040 Madrid, Spain
e-mail: aortiz@fjd.es

© Springer International Publishing AG 2017   183
A. Covic et al. (eds.), *Resistant Hypertension in Chronic Kidney Disease*,
DOI 10.1007/978-3-319-56827-0_12

Fig. 12.1 Chronic kidney disease: underdiagnosed in the elderly (Elaborated from data obtained from Stevens et al. [4]). (**A**) Percentage of individuals with known CKD. (**B**) Percentage of individuals with undiagnosed CKD

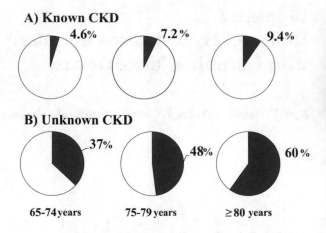

A) Known CKD

4.6%   7.2%   9.4%

B) Unknown CKD

37%   48%   60%

65-74 years   75-79 years   ≥80 years

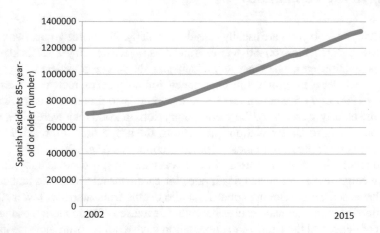

Fig. 12.2 The elderly population is rapidly increasing (Elaborated with official data from the Spanish National Statistics Institute (Instituto Nacional de Estadística, INE) [23])

Chronic Kidney Disease in the Elderly

Aging is associated with a progressive decrease in glomerular filtration rate. Indeed, the "physiological" loss of glomerular filtration rate has been quantified as a loss of 1 ml/min per year. However, the rate of loss of glomerular filtration rate is very variable: some individuals display stable glomerular filtration rate over the years, while some lose glomerular filtration rate at a faster rate and develop chronic kidney disease [3].

In this regard, the prevalence of chronic kidney disease increases with age (Fig. 12.2) [4]. Most elderly individuals with chronic kidney disease have not been diagnosed. However, the prevalence of chronic kidney disease is around 60% for those aged 80 years or older. Thus, population studies in such elderly individuals

Fig. 12.3 Mortality of older people according to glomerular filtration rate. (**a**) Mortality rate according to glomerular filtration rate and (**b**) mortality rate according to urinary albumin: creatinine ratio (Elaborated with data from Hallan et al. [5])

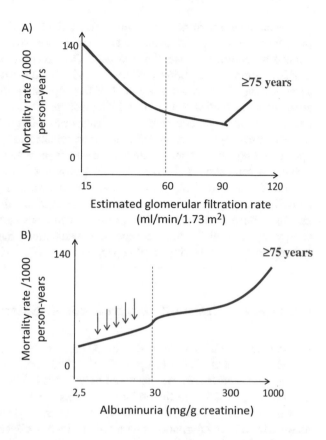

more probably reflect individuals with chronic kidney disease than not. While this has been characterized as the "physiological" decrease of glomerular filtration rate with age, a diagnosis of chronic kidney disease in the elderly has serious prognostic implications. Mortality of elderly individuals increases as glomerular filtration rate decreases, as in younger individuals (Fig. 12.3) [5]. However, while the relative increase in risk of death with decreasing glomerular filtration rate or increasing albuminuria may be higher in younger individuals, the absolute increase in risk is much higher in the elderly since their baseline risk is already higher than in younger population.

Blood Pressure Targets in the Elderly

During aging, both systolic blood pressure and pulse pressure progressively increase. It is important to note that there is no consensus among different guidelines for blood pressure targets in the elderly and even less in the elderly with chronic kidney disease. In part this is due to a scarce evidence base since the elderly and patients with chronic kidney disease are frequently excluded from clinical trials.

The table summarizes current and recent guidelines [6]. The definition of blood pressure targets is a key issue since treatment-resistant hypertension is usually defined as failure to reach those targets. The diversity of guidelines promotes a nihilistic approach to therapy of hypertension in the elderly. In this regard, and given the rapidly increasing segment of the population that is elderly (Fig. 12.1), adequately powered clinical trials with hard endpoints are urgently needed in elderly patients of different age ranges and categories of renal dysfunction. We must remember that aging is a process, and, thus, what is adequate for the 60–70 years age range may not be appropriate for the 80–90 years age range or for the growing number of centenarians. Conversely, a patient with chronic kidney disease and glomerular filtration rate category G1 and albuminuria category A2 may not benefit from the same approach as someone with glomerular filtration rate category G5. Health authorities should actively promote such trials since blood pressure can be adequately controlled with non-expensive medications, and pharma companies are unlikely to commit funding for this purpose.

Definition of Resistant Hypertension in Elderly People

Resistant hypertension is defined as blood pressure above goal despite adherence to a combination of at least three optimally dosed antihypertensive medications, one of which is a diuretic [6–9]. As discussed before, this is a nonspecific definition, since the precise goal is key to the definition. In this regard, the blood pressure goal for elderly individuals with chronic kidney disease ranges from 130/80 mmHg recommended by KDIGO for patients with chronic kidney disease and albuminuria, since no specification is made for the elderly, to <150/90 mmHg for those aged 80 years or older, without specification of exceptions for chronic kidney disease, as recommended by NICE and ESH/ESC (Table 12.1). Specifically, Eighth Joint National Committee (JNC 8) recommendations are as follows [10]:

Recommendation 1: In the general population aged ≥60 years, initiate pharmacologic treatment to lower blood pressure at systolic blood pressure (SBP) ≥150 mmHg or diastolic blood pressure (DBP) ≥90 mmHg, and treat to a goal SBP <150 mmHg and goal DBP <90 mmHg (strong recommendation – Grade A).

Recommendation 4: In the population aged ≥18 years with chronic kidney disease, initiate pharmacologic treatment to lower BP at SBP ≥140 mmHg or DBP ≥90 mmHg, and treat to goal SBP <140 mmHg and goal DBP <90 mmHg (expert opinion – Grade E).

Recommendation 5: In the population aged ≥18 years with diabetes, initiate pharmacologic treatment to lower BP at SBP ≥140 mmHg or DBP ≥90 mmHg, and treat to a goal SBP <140 mmHg and goal DBP <90 mmHg (expert opinion – Grade E).

Notice that while the goal for the elderly (aged ≥60 years) in the general population is <150/<90 mmHg and that this is a strong recommendation, no such age limit is provided for chronic kidney disease and diabetics, in whom based on expert

Table 12.1 Target blood pressure (BP) in chronic kidney disease and definition of resistant hypertension

	Target BP in chronic kidney disease	Target BP in chronic kidney disease with pathological albuminuria/proteinuria	Target BP in elderly persons	Definition of resistant hypertension
KDIGO	≤140/90	≤130/80	No specific targets	n. a.
CHEP	<140/90 in nondiabetic <130/80 in DM	As in chronic kidney disease	Age ≥80 years: Systolic BP <150[b]	n. a.
JNC 8	<140/90	As in chronic kidney disease	Age ≥60 years: <140/90 if DM and/or chronic kidney disease	n. a.
JNC 7	<130/80	As in chronic kidney disease	No specific targets	Failure to achieve goal BP in patients who are adhering to full doses of an appropriate three-drug regimen that includes a diuretic
ISH/ASH	<140/90	As in chronic kidney disease[a]	Age ≥80 years: <140/90 if DM and/or chronic kidney disease	BP ≥140/90 mmHg with use of three drugs (ACEi or ARB/CCB/diuretic) in full or maximally tolerated doses
NICE	<140/90 in nondiabetic <130/80 in DM	<130/80	Age ≥80 years: <150/90[b]	BP >140/90 mmHg after treatment with the optimal or best tolerated doses of an ACE inhibitor or an ARB plus a CCB plus a diuretic
NHFA	<130/80	<125/75	No specific targets	n. a.
ESC/ESH	Systolic BP <140	Systolic BP <130	Age ≥80 years: <150/90[b]	BP ≥140/90 mmHg with appropriate lifestyle measures and three drugs (a diuretic and two other drugs belonging to different classes, not necessarily including a MRA) at adequate doses

Adapted from [6]; with permission. BP expressed in mmHg

n. a. not addressed, *BP* blood pressure, *DM* diabetes mellitus, *ACE* angiotensin-converting enzyme, *ARB* angiotensin receptor blocker, *CCB* calcium channel blocker, *MRA* mineralocorticoid receptor antagonist

Note that BP targets apply to seated office BP measurements

[a]ISH/ASH generally recommend a < 140/90 mmHg BP target for chronic kidney disease but acknowledge that "some experts still recommend less than 130/80 mmHg" in albuminuria

[b]No specific recommendations are given for elderly persons with chronic kidney disease and/or DM

opinion a < 140/<90 mmHg goal is recommended. This variability contributes to further confusion about the epidemiology and consequences of treatment-resistant hypertension in the elderly.

Prevalence of Resistant Hypertension in Elderly People with Chronic Kidney Disease

A recent study found that 13% of hypertensive patients met the American Heart Association criteria for resistant hypertension [11]. However, the incidence markedly differed by age: 5.5% for those <50 years (8.5% men and 3.2% women) and 25% of those >80 years (16% of men and 31% of women). In patients <50 years, resistant hypertension was associated with male sex, obesity, and chronic kidney disease, while in those >80 years, resistant hypertension was associated with female sex diabetes mellitus, obesity, and chronic kidney disease. Chronic kidney disease was the common element. Resistant hypertension in chronic kidney disease has been recently reviewed in depth [6]. However this review raised more questions regarding this subject, especially in the elderly.

The prevalence of true resistant hypertension is unknown because most studies did not include key diagnostic criteria (e.g., antihypertensive medication doses, treatment adherence, and systematic exclusion of measurement artifacts) [6]. Estimates vary widely: 0.5–14% of people treated for hypertension have apparent treatment-resistant hypertension. However, this reflects apparent treatment-resistant hypertension since in the general population, only 50% of patients with apparent treatment-resistant hypertension have been prescribed optimum antihypertensive therapy. Moreover, 40% of apparent treatment-resistant hypertension could be white-coat hypertension or caused by medication nonadherence. Indeed, nonadherence is extremely hard to detect and even more so in large epidemiological study.

Etiology

The etiology of resistant hypertension in elderly patients with chronic kidney disease is most likely chronic kidney disease, the most frequent cause of secondary hypertension. It is still possible that elderly chronic kidney disease patients have a low frequency cause of secondary hypertension. However, in the context of chronic kidney disease and old age, most likely this will not be searched for in routine clinical settings. In this regard, three issues merit discussion: the cause and effect relationship between chronic kidney disease and hypertension, dietary habits, and noncompliance.

Hypertension is widely acknowledged to be the second major cause of end-stage renal disease after diabetes [12, 13]. However, recent genetic evidence has uncovered a mutation in the APOL1 gene as the cause of nephropathy in a majority of

African-American patients diagnosed as hypertensive nephropathy [14]. Since hypertensive nephropathy is most frequently diagnosed in African-Americans, this raises questions about any diagnosis of hypertensive nephropathy in other nephropathies. In this regard, hypertensive nephropathy is a frequent diagnosis in the elderly in whom no other cause of nephropathy is suspected not searched for. However most likely, hypertensive nephropathy represents a nephropathy of unknown cause that has slowly progressed under the radar since albuminuria is not routine assessed in nondiabetics, and the threshold to diagnose chronic kidney disease based on serum creatinine has been evolving over time. In this regard, chronic kidney disease is by far the most frequent cause of secondary hypertension in the elderly and, consequently, of treatment-resistant hypertension.

A high salt intake is, together with noncompliance, the most frequent cause of apparent treatment-resistant hypertension. There are some trends that may impact on both factors in elderly patients with chronic kidney disease. On one hand, both the elderly and patients with chronic kidney disease progressively decrease their dietary intake. A lower total dietary intake implies a low intake of most dietary components, including salt. This would suggest that excessive salt intake would not be expected to play a key role in apparent treatment-resistant hypertension in elderly patients with chronic kidney disease. However, chronic kidney disease may limit the ability of the kidney to excrete a salt load. In addition, it is difficult to start a low-sodium diet at age 80 when this has not been part of your lifestyle for eight decades. In this regard, malnutrition is a serious concern in elderly chronic kidney disease patients and may limit the possibility to reduce dietary salt.

Prescription of multiple medications is frequent in the elderly, especially if they have chronic kidney disease. This may negatively impact compliance. The problem is magnified in healthcare systems that do not cover the full cost of medication, since the elderly are frequently economically fragile.

Diagnostic Approach

The two essential steps in diagnosis treatment-resistant hypertension in the elderly are to confirm the presence of uncontrolled hypertension by a 24-h blood pressure monitoring to exclude white coat hypertension and a correct assessment of drug prescription and compliance.

Assessment of compliance in the elderly is difficult since they may need helpers that take care of the medication, and these helpers may not be present at the clinic visit. However, this is a key element of the diagnostic approach, as in the absence of compliance, blood pressure control will not improve despite multiple adjustments in medication. Exploration of noncompliance should be cautious, and respectful, otherwise we will get lies from the patient. The patient should perceive empathy and be offered the opportunity to acknowledge noncompliance without feeling guilty. If noncompliance is confirmed, a frank discussion should follow to understand the motives, since only by understanding these issues will help prescribe drugs that the patient will comply with. Specifically, the benefits of compliance should be emphasized and the motivation of the patient explored. This will save a lot of time and effort for both patient and doctor. In the past, the best way to explore noncompliance with diet or medication was to intern the patient. In our experience, most if not all patients became hypotensive within a week of in-hospital low-salt diet and direct observed of the intake of the medication that had been prescribed at home while "treatment resistant." The outcome was usually a reduction in the number of medications at discharge and improved compliance.

In addition, the physician should be alert to signs and symptoms of additional causes of secondary hypertension, atherosclerotic renal artery stenosis being one of the most common in this context.

Finally, a 24-h urine collection should be used to assess sodium intake, if feasible, since elderly patients may have difficulty collecting urine.

Twenty-four hour monitoring of blood pressure will allow exclusion of white-coat hypertension and disclose non-dipper night patterns characteristic of chronic kidney disease patients that might benefit from chronotherapy. Among hypertensive chronic kidney disease patients under nephrology care with a mean age of 65 years, 22% had true resistant hypertension patients (office blood pressure is $\geq$130/80 mmHg, despite adherence to $\geq$3 full-dose antihypertensive drugs including a diuretic agent or $\geq$4 drugs and ambulatory average blood pressure $\geq$ 125/75 mmHg) and 7% pseudoresistance (ambulatory average blood pressure < 125/75 mmHg). Pseudoresistance was not associated with an increased cardiorenal risk, while true resistance identified patients with the highest cardiovascular and renal risk [15].

A further concept is false isolated-office resistant hypertension (elevated clinic blood pressure, controlled awake blood pressure means, but elevated asleep systolic or diastolic blood pressure mean while treated with three hypertension medications in a non-dipper pattern) which was present in 9% of patients with a mean age of 65 years treated with $\geq$3 hypertension medications and evaluated by 48-h ambulatory blood pressure monitoring. These patients had higher prevalence of chronic kidney disease. Thus, the classification of resistant hypertension patients into categories of isolated-office resistant hypertension (i.e., with normal 24-h ambulatory blood pressure) masked resistant hypertension (i.e., normal office blood pressure and abnormal normal 24-h ambulatory blood pressure), and true resistant hypertension (i.e., both abnormal office blood pressure and abnormal normal 24-h ambulatory blood pressure) cannot be based on the comparison of clinic blood pressure with either daytime home blood pressure measurements or awake blood pressure mean from ambulatory blood pressure monitoring, especially in the elderly plus chronic kidney disease setting [16].

Therapeutic Approach

The therapeutic approach to the elderly patient with confirmed treatment-resistant hypertension and chronic kidney disease relies first on promoting compliance. While noncompliance associated apparent resistant hypertension is not really resistant hypertension, achieving compliance is the first step in clinical practice. The second step is to adjust the diuretic that patients should be taken before they are diagnosed of resistant hypertension. In this regard, in advance chronic kidney disease a loop diuretic may be needed, and low-dose thiazide from combination pills may be insufficient.

Once compliance has been achieved and diuretic therapy optimized, a next step may be the addition of low-dose mineralocorticoid receptor blocker, although potassium should be monitored and the patient provided with specific instructions to stop the medication if they develop risk factors for acute kidney injury or hyperkalemia such as dehydration. Special care is required for patients already under renin-angiotensin system blockade, as it is frequent among chronic kidney disease patients [17].

Emphasis should be made on avoiding hypotension, especially orthostatic hypotension, since it may result in falls that may bring the patient's demise. In this regard, 24-h blood pressure monitoring is underused in this age range and may allow the confirmation of hypotensive episodes that may not be reported by the patient.

Given the dismal outcome of patients with end-stage kidney disease [18], a careful correction of all cardiovascular risk factors since the earliest stage of disease is required to improve outcomes. In this regard, recognition and treatment of resistant hypertension in the elderly with chronic kidney disease, which is the fastest growing segment of chronic kidney disease patients, should be a key goal.

The Impact of SPRINT

The recently published Systolic Blood Pressure Intervention Trial (SPRINT) on patients at high risk for cardiovascular events but without diabetes observed that targeting a systolic blood pressure of less than 120 mmHg, as compared with less than 140 mmHg, resulted in lower rates of fatal and nonfatal major cardiovascular events and death from any cause, although significantly higher rates of some adverse events [19]. The reduction in major cardiovascular events and all-cause mortality with intensive blood pressure control was observed in older individuals, including patients with chronic kidney disease and mild proteinuria [20, 21]. This is likely to impact clinical practice in the near future.

While there were no significant interactions between treatment and subgroup with respect to the primary outcome, in subgroup analysis the elderly (≥75 years old) obtained clear benefit with regard to the primary outcome (hazard ratio (95% CI); 0.67 (0.51–0.86)). However, no significant benefit was observed in patients with chronic kidney disease (0.82 (0.63–1.07)), while benefit was observed for those without chronic kidney disease (0.70 (0.56–0.87)). Thus, it is unclear what the effect in elderly patients with kidney disease might be. This population might be more sensitive to certain adverse effects, such as acute kidney injury. In this regard, in the overall population, there was a higher rate (more than double) of acute kidney injury in the intensive-treatment group, which may be of particular concern for the chronic kidney disease and elderly population. Furthermore, there are two caveats. First, diabetics were excluded. Thus, results do not apply to the most frequent cause of chronic kidney disease. Second, patients with estimated glomerular filtration rate below 20 ml/min/1.7 m^2 were not included. Thus, results do not apply to subjects with advanced G4 or G5 chronic kidney disease categories.

In our opinion, at present there is no solid new evidence base from SPRINT to modify blood pressure targets for patients with chronic kidney disease, although expert opinion may extrapolate the results on secondary endpoints or benefits obtained in the overall population aged 75 years or more to the elderly chronic kidney disease population and support lower targets also for the nondiabetic elderly population with mild to moderate but not sever chronic kidney disease. In this regard, KDIGO will assess the impact of the SPRINT trial on its 2012 Blood Pressure Guideline [22]. A report on the outcomes of the specific elderly and chronic kidney disease population in SPRINT would be most welcomed.

Acknowledgments Grant support: ISCIII and FEDER funds CD14/00133, PI13/00047, Sociedad Española de Nefrologia, ISCIII-RETIC REDinREN/RD012/0021, and Comunidad de Madrid CIFRA S2010/BMD-2378. Salary support: FIS Miguel Servet to MDSN, ABS, and Joan Rodes to BFF. Programa Intensificación Actividad Investigadora (ISCIII/Agencia Laín-Entralgo/CM) to AO.

Conflict of interest statement None reported.

References

1. Izekenova AK, Kumar AB, Abikulova AK, Izekenova AK. Trends in ageing of the population and the life expectancy after retirement: a comparative country-based analysis. J Res Med Sci. 2015;20(3):250–2.
2. GBD 2013 Mortality and Causes of Death Collaborators. Global, regional, and national age–sex specific all-cause and cause-specific mortality for 240 causes of death, 1990–2013: a systematic analysis for the global burden of disease study 2013. Lancet. 2015;385:117–71.
3. Hemmelgarn BR, Zhang J, Manns BJ, Tonelli M, Larsen E, Ghali WA, Southern DA, McLaughlin K, Mortis G, Culleton BF. Progression of kidney dysfunction in the community-dwelling elderly. Kidney Int. 2006;69(12):2155–61.
4. Stevens LA, Li S, Wang C, Huang C, Becker BN, Bomback AS, Brown WW, Burrows NR, Jurkovitz CT, McFarlane SI, Norris KC, Shlipak M, Whaley-Connell AT, Chen SC, Bakris GL, McCullough PA. Prevalence of CKD and comorbid illness in elderly patients in the United States: results from the Kidney Early Evaluation Program (KEEP). Am J Kidney Dis. 2010;55(3 Suppl 2):S23–33.
5. Hallan SI, Matsushita K, Sang Y, Mahmoodi BK, Black C, Ishani A, Kleefstra N, Naimark D, Roderick P, Tonelli M, Wetzels JF, Astor BC, Gansevoort RT, Levin A, Wen CP, Coresh J; Chronic Kidney Disease Prognosis Consortium. Age and association of kidney measures with mortality and end-stage renal disease. JAMA. 2012;308(22):2349–60.
6. Rossignol P, Massy ZA, Azizi M, Bakris G, Ritz E, Covic A, et al; ERA-EDTA EURECA-m Working Group; Red de Investigación Renal (REDINREN) network; Cardiovascular and Renal Clinical Trialists (F-CRIN INI-CRCT) network. The double challenge of resistant hypertension and chronic kidney disease. Lancet. 2015;386(10003):1588–98.
7. Pickering TG, Hall JE, Appel LJ, et al. Recommendations for blood pressure measurement in humans and experimental animals: part 1: blood pressure measurement in humans: a statement for professionals from the Subcommittee of Professional and Public Education of the American Heart Association Council on high blood pressure research. Circulation. 2005;111(5):697–716.

8. Calhoun DA, Jones D, Textor S, et al. Resistant hypertension: diagnosis, evaluation, and treatment. A scientific statement from the American Heart Association Professional Education Committee of the Council for high blood pressure research. Hypertension. 2008;51(6):1403–19.
9. Sarafidis PA, Georgianos P, Bakris GL. Resistant hypertension – its identification and epidemiology. Nat Rev Nephrol. 2013;9(1):51–8.
10. James PA, Oparil S, Carter BL, Cushman WC, Dennison-Himmelfarb C, Handler J, Lackland DT, LeFevre ML, MacKenzie TD, Ogedegbe O, Smith SC Jr, Svetkey LP, Taler SJ, Townsend RR, Wright JT Jr, Narva AS, Ortiz E. 2014 evidence-based guideline for the management of high blood pressure in adults: report from the panel members appointed to the Eighth Joint National Committee (JNC 8). JAMA. 2014;311(5):507–20.
11. Gijón-Conde T, Graciani A, Banegas JR. Resistant hypertension: demography and clinical characteristics in 6,292 patients in a primary health care setting. Rev Esp Cardiol (Engl Ed). 2014;67(4):270–6.
12. U.S. Renal Data System Report. Available at: http://www.usrds.org/adr.aspx. Accessed 29 Feb 2016.
13. Pippias M, Jager KJ, Kramer A, Leivestad T, Sánchez MB, Caskey FJ, et al. The changing trends and outcomes in renal replacement therapy: data from the ERA-EDTA registry. Nephrol Dial Transplant. 2015;31(5):831–41. pii: gfv327 [Epub ahead of print].
14. Freedman BI, Cohen AH. Hypertension-attributed nephropathy: what's in a name? Nat Rev Nephrol. 2016;12(1):27–36.
15. De Nicola L, Gabbai FB, Agarwal R, Chiodini P, Borrelli S, Bellizzi V, Nappi F, Conte G, Minutolo R. Prevalence and prognostic role of resistant hypertension in chronic kidney disease patients. J Am Coll Cardiol. 2013;61(24):2461–7.
16. Ríos MT, Domínguez-Sardiña M, Ayala DE, et al. Prevalence and clinical characteristics of isolated-office and true resistant hypertension determined by ambulatory blood pressure monitoring. Chronobiol Int. 2013;30(1–2):207–20.
17. Esteras R, Perez-Gomez MV, Rodriguez-Osorio L, Ortiz A, Fernandez-Fernandez B. Combination use of medicines from two classes of renin-angiotensin system blocking agents: risk of hyperkalemia, hypotension, and impaired renal function. Ther Adv Drug Saf. 2015;6(4):166–76.
18. Ortiz A, Covic A, Fliser D, Fouque D, Goldsmith D, Kanbay M, et al. Board of the EURECA-m working group of ERA-EDTA. Epidemiology, contributors to, and clinical trials of mortality risk in chronic kidney failure. Lancet. 2014;383(9931):1831–43.
19. SPRINT Research Group, Wright JT Jr, Williamson JD, Whelton PK, Snyder JK, Sink KM, et al. A randomized trial of intensive versus standard blood-pressure control. N Engl J Med. 2015;373(22):2103–16.
20. Rocco MV, Cheung AK. A SPRINT to the finish, or just the beginning? Implications of the SPRINT results for nephrologists. Kidney Int. 2016;89(2):261–3.
21. Chertow GM, Beddhu S, Lewis JB, Toto RD, Cheung AK. Managing hypertension in patients with CKD: a Marathon, not a SPRINT. J Am Soc Nephrol. 2016;27(1):40–3.
22. SPRINT Trial News Release. 2015. Available at: http://www.kdigo.org/News%20Release/SPRINT%20Trial%20News%20Release%202015.pdf. Accessed 10 Mar 2016.
23 Instituto Nacional de Estadística. National Statistics Institute. Available at: www.ine.es/en/. Accessed 29 Feb 2016.

Chapter 13
Obstructive Sleep Apnea and Resistant Hypertension

Lauren A. Tobias and Francoise Roux

Introduction

Obstructive sleep apnea (OSA) is increasingly recognized as a modifiable contributor to systemic arterial hypertension. Patients with OSA have almost five times the risk of having resistant hypertension [1], and studies of patients with resistant hypertension demonstrate that a majority have OSA. Evidence suggests that treatment with positive airway pressure (PAP) therapy results in significant blood pressure reduction in these patients, supporting the need for accurate diagnosis and prompt treatment.

OSA is a very common disorder, estimated to affect approximately 20% of men and 10% of women, with increases seen in recent decades that likely relate to the increasing prevalence of obesity [2, 3]. OSA is characterized by repeated, intermittent episodes of upper airway collapse during sleep that result in recurrent breathing pauses. Pauses may cause either partial or complete obstruction of the upper airway during sleep and are terminated either hypopneas or apneas, respectively. Clinical consequences of OSA include loud snoring, transient oxygen desaturation, brain arousals from sleep, and disruptions in sleep causing poor sleep quality [4].

Daytime consequences of these events include hypersomnolence, impaired concentration, an increased risk of motor vehicle accidents [5, 6], and reductions in quality of life.

L.A. Tobias
Assistant Professor, Section of Pulmonary, Critical Care and Sleep Medicine,
Yale University School of Medicine, New Haven, CT, USA
e-mail: Lauren.Tobias@yale.edu

F. Roux (✉)
Pulmonary, Critical Care and Sleep Division, Starling Physicians, Hartford, CT, USA
e-mail: francoise.joelle.roux@gmail.com

© Springer International Publishing AG 2017
A. Covic et al. (eds.), *Resistant Hypertension in Chronic Kidney Disease*,
DOI 10.1007/978-3-319-56827-0_13

195

OSA and Hypertension

Studies have consistently supported a role for obstructive sleep apnea (OSA) as a risk factor for diurnal hypertension. A significant body of literature has now accumulated in both cross-sectional and prospective population-based epidemiologic studies to suggest a dose-response relationship between severity of OSA and likelihood of incident HTN that is independent of the risk factors common to both disorders such as obesity and metabolic syndrome [7, 8]. Both US and European guidelines for hypertension management recognize OSA as a frequent and modifiable contributor to systemic arterial hypertension [9].

Furthermore, in patients with preexisting hypertension as well as OSA, treatment of OSA may confer improvements in blood pressure control. Despite increasing evidence supporting that it is a major cause of refractory hypertension, OSA remains significantly underdiagnosed, particularly among women and nonobese patients [10].

While early studies of hemodynamics in patients with OSA relied on invasive blood pressure monitoring, more recent studies have employed ambulatory monitors with frequent sampling (e.g., every 15–30 min) in order to examine circadian variation in systolic and diastolic blood pressure. It is generally accepted that ambulatory blood pressure monitoring has greater prognostic value than office BP measurements.

OSA and Incident Hypertension

The prevalence of hypertension in patients with OSA ranges from 35 to 80% across studies [9], and the prevalence of resistant hypertension is expected to increase in the coming years [11]. Although some of the association between OSA and hypertension may be mediated by risk factors common to both disorders, such as obesity, a large body of evidence now supports an independent role of OSA in the pathogenesis of hypertension [7, 12–15].

The first prospective studies examined the relationship between OSA and the development of future hypertension in patients who were normotensive at baseline [7]. Early data came from the Wisconsin Sleep Cohort, an ongoing prospective longitudinal study of the causes and natural history of sleep disorders. Investigators found a significant dose-response relationship between sleep-disordered breathing at baseline and a diagnosis of new hypertension 4 years later, independent of potential confounding factors. Patients with even mild OSA were even at risk, with a twofold greater risk of becoming hypertensive, whereas those with moderate OSA had a threefold greater probability, compared with participants without OSA at baseline (AHI <1 event per hour) [7]. Another observational study by Marin and colleagues following nearly 2000 non-hypertensive subjects presenting to a sleep clinic over 10 years found an increased incidence of hypertension in patients with untreated OSA compared with controls [8].

Data from the Sleep Heart Health Study has been less conclusive. This multi-center longitudinal cohort study examining the cardiovascular consequences of sleep-disordered breathing in over 6000 individuals also found an increased odds of HTN in patients with sleep-disordered breathing in a dose-response manner [16, 17]. Although some of this relationship was explained by body mass index (BMI), the odds ratio for HTN after adjustment for possible confounders remained 1.37 comparing the highest and lowest categories of AHI ($\geq$30 versus <1.5). It has been postulated that the weaker association between obesity and HTN seen in this population as compared with the Wisconsin Sleep Cohort may be related to the older age of patients and the reference category of AHI 0–4.9, which may have included subjects with very mild OSA.

Taken together, these data suggest that CPAP can be expected to result in a modest reduction in blood pressure on the order of 2–3 mmHg for the population at large. However, this degree of reduction should be considered significant, as it has been shown to reduce cardiovascular mortality by 4–8% [18]. In patients with resistant hypertension, the magnitude of BP reduction attributable to CPAP appears to be even greater.

The strength of the association between OSA and hypertension may be modulated by other factors including age and somnolence status. For example, the association between OSA and hypertension appears to be stronger in young to middle-aged adults than older adults [17, 19]. Haas et al. conducted a large cross-sectional study of participants in the Sleep Heart Health Study stratified by age [20] and found that an association between systolic and diastolic hypertension existed only in those patients under the age of 60 years. However, it is possible that the higher medical comorbidity that accumulates with aging has obscured an independent association between OSA and HTN in such studies. Data are inconsistent regarding the role of sex in mediating the relationship between OSA and HTN [19, 21]. Nonetheless, given evidence that OSA is often underdiagnosed and undertreated in women, it is important to remain cognizant that the presence of OSA confers a likely similar risk of subsequent hypertension as it does in males [10].

Circadian Variability of BP in Patients with OSA

Most patients with OSA lack the normal physiological reduction in blood pressure ("nocturnal dipping") that occurs during sleep [22, 23]. The normal nocturnal dipping phenomenon is defined as a reduction in BP by at least 10% during the night as compared with the daytime. A "non-dipping" phenomenon has been observed commonly in both normotensive and hypertensive patients with OSA [24] and is thought to represent one mechanism by which OSA leads to an increased risk of target organ damage and cardiovascular events, as compared with subjects who experience the normal BP decline during sleep [22, 25, 26]. For example, left ventricular hypertrophy appears more closely linked to HTN during sleep than during wakefulness [27]. Data from the WSCS showed a dose-response relationship between the severity of baseline OSA and odds of developing an incident non-dipping profile in systolic blood pressure.

OSA and Resistant HTN

The prevalence of unsuspected OSA in patients with resistant hypertension is very high, estimated at 83% in one study [28, 29]. Refractory hypertension in patients with OSA is primary systolic rather than diastolic and is especially pronounced at night. This is particularly important given that systolic BP has stronger prognostic value for cardiovascular outcomes than does diastolic pressure [30].

One study of 125 patients with resistant hypertension was systematically evaluated for known secondary causes of hypertension including aortic coarctation, Cushing's syndrome, obstructive sleep apnea, drugs, pheochromocytoma, primary aldosteronism, renal parenchymal disease, renovascular hypertension, and thyroid disorders [31]. OSA (defined as an AHI of 15 or greater) emerged as by far the most common condition associated with resistant hypertension, seen in 64% of patients. Risk factors for the presence of OSA included age over 50 years, neck circumference $\geq$41 cm for women and $\geq$43 cm for men, and the presence of snoring in this population. Another smaller study evaluating patients with treatment-resistant hypertension found that 83% had unsuspected sleep apnea based on an apnea-hypopnea index $\geq$10 events/h [28].

There appears to be a dose-response relationship between the severity of OSA and the risk of resistant hypertension. Walia et al. recruited nearly 300 patients at high risk for cardiovascular disease despite medical management and found that patients with severe OSA had a fourfold higher adjusted odds of resistant hypertension (OR 4.1, 95% CI: 1.7–10.2) [32]. In addition, resistant hypertension was significantly more common in patients with untreated severe than moderate OSA (58% vs. 29%, respectively, $p = 0.01$).

Current guidelines on the management of resistant hypertension from the American Heart Association (2008) recommend screening for the presence of OSA in patients with resistant hypertension [33], and the seventh report of the Joint National Committee on Prevention, Detection, Evaluation, and Treatment of High Blood Pressure recognizes OSA as an identifiable cause of hypertension [18]. Joint recommendations from the European Respiratory Society and European Society of Hypertension echoed this recommendation in 2013, citing OSA as a "novel, frequent and modifiable cause of systemic arterial hypertension" [9].

Pathophysiologic Mechanisms Linking Hypertension and Sleep Apnea

A constellation of factors may underlie the relationship between HTN and OSA, including sympathetic activation, activation of the renin-angiotensin-aldosterone system, intermittent hypoxemia, inflammation, oxidative stress, and endothelial dysfunction. These are shown in Figs. 13.1, 13.2, and 13.3. Some of these mechanisms may act in a bidirectional manner.

Sympathetic Activation and Intermittent Hypoxia

Sympathetic activation is a key mechanism responsible for the resistant hypertension seen in patients with OSA. Several studies have demonstrated deranged autonomic function during both the night and day in patients with OSA, suggesting that the hypertension observed at night has a carryover effect that extends into the daytime hours and persists over time. The repetitive cessation of airflow during apneic and hypopneic episodes leads to recurrent hypoxemia and hypercapnia. This triggers chemoflex activation, resulting in stimulation of sympathetic activity. Studies of healthy human subjects have shown that periods of intermittent hypoxemia resulted in elevations in blood pressure and sympathetic activation [36, 37] that decreased with resumption of ventilation after apneic episodes. Interestingly, the frequency of hypoxic episodes, captured as an oxygen desaturation index, appears to be more important that the AHI in predicting the odds of OSA-related prevalent hypertension [38].

Activated Renin-Angiotensin-Aldosterone System

Aldosterone excess has also been hypothesized to play a role in the relationship between OSA and hypertension. Plasma aldosterone levels have been found to correlate strongly and significantly with AHI, a relationship seen in subjects with resistant hypertension but not in normotensive controls [29]. In support of the concept that fluid accumulation may worsen OSA, one study showed that drug-resistant hypertensive patients exhibited a great shift in the volume of fluid that migrated rostrally from the legs overnight and had a correspondingly higher AHI, than patients whose hypertension was well controlled [39]. A small but provocative study also suggested that anti-aldosteronic diuretics may reduce parapharyngeal edema and secondary upper airway obstruction, thereby improving both OSA severity and BP [40]. These data support the possibility of a bidirectional relationship between OSA and hypertension, whereby treatment of hypertension may improve OSA severity.

Inflammation and Oxidative Stress

The repeated cycles of deoxygenation and subsequent reoxygenation seen in OSA are associated with generation of reactive oxygen species and oxidative stress, with increases in levels of circulating adhesion molecules and inflammatory cytokines including TNF-alpha and IL-8.

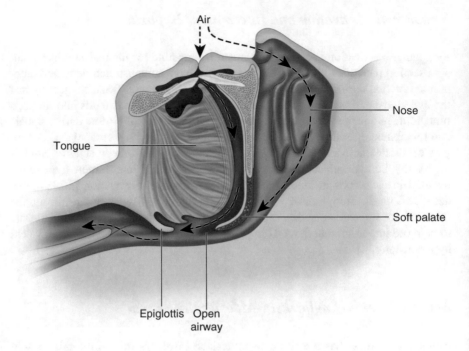

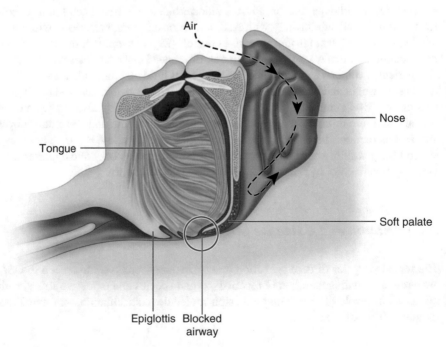

Fig. 13.1 Pathophysiology of obstructive sleep apnea (Data from Ref. [34])

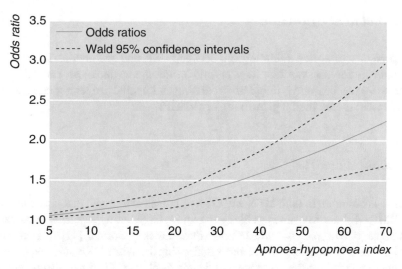

Fig. 13.2 Incidence of hypertension over time in patients without OSA and untreated patients with OSA of varying severities. Severity of OSA was defined by the apnea-hypopnea index (AHI) as mild OSA (AHI 5.0–14.9), moderate OSA (AHI 15.0–29.9), and severe OSA (AHI ≥ 30) (From Lavie et al. [14]; with permission)

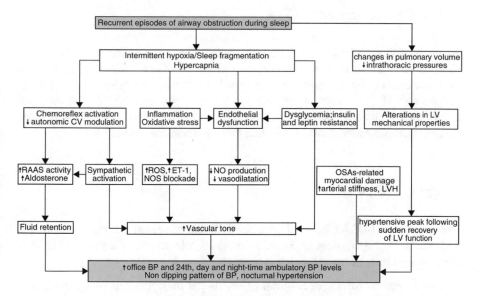

Fig. 13.3 Mechanisms by which obstructive sleep apnea syndrome (OSAS) may contribute to resistant hypertension (From Parati et al. [35]; with permission)

Endothelial Dysfunction

Research has supported a relationship between OSA and endothelial dysfunction as measured by forearm vascular flow, carotid intima-media thickness, carotid-femoral pulse-wave velocity and number of circulating endothelial progenitor cells, and levels of vascular endothelial growth factor (VEGF).

Metabolic Factors

Obesity is common to both HTN and OSA; studies have shown that obese individuals (BMI > 40) are five times as likely to require three antihypertensive medications as compared with patients whose body mass index is normal [41]. It is therefore crucial that any examination of the relationship between OSA and hypertension attempt to control for the presence and degree of obesity. OSA has also been linked to impaired glucose tolerance and prediabetes [42].

Other Consequences of OSA

Aside from its contribution to hypertension, OSA has been linked with other long-term health consequences and impairments in quality of life. Patients with OSA are also at increased risk of pulmonary arterial hypertension, coronary artery disease, cardiac arrhythmias, heart failure, stroke, insulin resistance, type 2 diabetes, and nonalcoholic fatty liver disease. Motor vehicle crashes are two to three times more common among patients with OSA than those without the disorder.

Diagnosis of OSA

The diagnosis of OSAS is based on a constellation of symptoms, clinical findings, and overnight sleep testing, as shown in Table 13.2. In adults, a diagnosis of OSA is made when either of the following is present:

- Five or more obstructive respiratory events per hour of sleep in a patient *with appropriate clinical symptoms* or medical comorbidities
- *Fifteen or more* obstructive respiratory events per hour of sleep regardless of associated symptoms or comorbidities

Qualifying clinical symptoms in the above diagnosis include excessive sleepiness, non-restorative sleep, fatigue, insomnia, habitual snoring, subjective nocturnal respiratory disturbance, and observed apneas, while comorbidities include HTN, mood disorder, cognitive dysfunction, coronary artery disease, stroke, congestive heart failure, atrial fibrillation, and type 2 diabetes.

Table 13.1 Diagnostic criteria for OSA. The presence either of *both* A and B, or of C alone, is needed for diagnosis

A. The presence of one or more of the following
1. The patient complains of sleepiness, non-restorative sleep, fatigue, or insomnia symptoms
2. The patient wakes with breath holding, gasping, or choking
3. The bed partner or other observer reports habitual snoring, breathing interruptions, or both during the patient's sleep
4. The patient has been diagnosed with hypertension, mood disorder, cognitive dysfunction, coronary artery disease, stroke, congestive heart failure, atrial fibrillation, or type 2 diabetes mellitus
B. Polysomnography (PSG) or out-of-center sleep testing (OCST) demonstrates
1. Five or more obstructive respiratory events (obstructive or mixed apneas, hypopneas, or respiratory effort-related arousals) per hour of sleep during PSG or per hour of monitoring (OCST)
C. PSG or OCST demonstrates
1. Fifteen or more obstructive respiratory events per hour of sleep during PSG or per hour of monitoring (OCST)

Adapted from American Academy of Sleep Medicine [43]

Respiratory events are characterized as either apneas (defined as a >90% reduction in tidal volume lasting ≥ 10 s) or hypopneas (defined as a $\geq 30\%$ reduction in airflow lasting ≥ 10 s and accompanied by either a $\geq 3\%$ reduction in oxygen saturation or an arousal from sleep as seen on electroencephalogram [44].

OSA severity is defined according to the apnea-hypopnea index (AHI), where mild OSA is defined by AHI 5–14 events/hour, moderate OSA by AHI 15–29 events/hour, and severe OSA by ≥ 30 or more events per hour. While somewhat clinically arbitrary, these thresholds have provided a structure for research purposes and may influence treatment decisions and in some cases insurance reimbursement for CPAP therapy.

Clinical Features of OSA

History and Risk Factors

Snoring and daytime sleepiness are common symptoms of OSA, but are not specific to the disorder. Nocturnal gasping or choking appears to be the most reliable indicator or sleep apnea [45]. Table 13.2 lists the varied clinical characteristics that may be seen in association with obstructive sleep apnea. While many patients may present with several of the features listed, some may have very few. It is common for a bedpartner's concerns to outweigh those of the patient. Risk factors for OSA include male gender, smoking, older age, larger neck circumference, and obesity.

Table 13.2 Clinical characteristics suggestive of obstructive sleep apnea (OSA)

Clinical characteristics
Male sex
Postmenopausal females
Overweight, especially if central adiposity
History of cardiovascular disease
Nighttime symptoms
Witnessed apneas
Loud, frequent snoring
Dry mouth
Nocturia
Awakening from sleep with choking, gasping, or dyspnea
Night sweats
Daytime symptoms
Excessive daytime sleepiness
Daytime fatigue
Concentration difficulties
Morning headaches
Physical examination
Neck circumference > 16″ in women and >17″ in men
Upper airway anatomic abnormalities (enlarged tonsils/uvula, macroglossia)
Retrognathia
Signs of right heart failure (lower extremity edema)

Screening Questionnaires

Several questionnaires and clinical prediction rules have been developed to aid in the diagnosis of OSA. The most commonly employed of these is the Epworth Sleepiness Scale (ESS) [46], an eight-item score in which patients rate their subjective sleepiness during everyday activities, with a score of 10 and above consistent with excessive sleepiness. Others include the Stanford Sleepiness Scale, the Berlin Questionnaire, and the STOP-BANG which was initially validated in perioperative patients. Although the ESS and other measures have been shown to correlate significantly with objective measures of sleepiness, test accuracy is variable across populations. Furthermore, their false-negative rates are unacceptably high, such that reliance on these tests alone is likely to lead to significant underdiagnosis of obstructive sleep apnea [47, 48].

Physical Examination

Examination may be normal, or may reveal obesity, a narrow oropharynx, or a large neck circumference, but no particular features on physical examination are sufficient to rule in or exclude the possibility of OSA.

Diagnostic Evaluation for OSA

Testing options for OSA include traditional laboratory polysomnography and out-of-center sleep testing (also referred to as ambulatory or OCST or home sleep apnea testing) [49]. While laboratory testing remains the "gold standard," OCST is an acceptable initial option for patients in whom there is a strong clinical suspicion of OSA. For many patients, OCST has the added benefits of convenience and improved tolerability, allowing patients to sleep in their habitual environment. It should be noted, however, that OCST often underestimates the frequency of respiratory events because recording time, rather than sleep time, is used as the denominator for the AHI [50]. Furthermore, OCST is intended only to evaluate for the presence of sleep-disordered breathing and should not be ordered if other sleep disorders including narcolepsy or periodic limb movements are suspected. Patients with comorbidities that increase the risk of additional or alternative sleep-related breathing disorders such as hypoventilation or central sleep apnea should also undergo laboratory testing rather than OCST. Nocturnal oximetry is not considered an adequate screening tool as it has poor sensitivity for detection of OSA.

Treatment Options for OSA

The goal of treating OSA is to reduce or ideally eliminate apneas, hypopneas, and oxygen desaturation during sleep and thereby improve sleep quality and daytime function and reduce medical comorbidities.

Weight Loss

Given the tight link between OSA and overweight/obesity, most patients warrant counseling on strategies for shedding excess body weight. There is evidence that bariatric surgery may improve OSA severity and blood pressure control [51]. Although it was initially hoped that CPAP might help patients to lose weight, subsequent data unfortunately has not supported this notion. Many of the studies examining the relationship between OSA and weight loss have been limited by small sample size, retrospective nature, lack of blinding, and imprecise measures of weight and/or adherence. However, a large multicenter double-blind, randomized study employing a sham-CPAP control group demonstrated a dose-response relationship between CPAP adherence and weight gain, with greater CPAP use associated with more weight gain over 6 months of follow-up [52]. One possible explanation for these results is greater energy expenditure due to increased work of breathing in those with untreated OSA.

CPAP

Nocturnal continuous positive airway pressure is considered first-line therapy for treating obstructive sleep apnea in the majority of patients. CPAP therapy involves a small device that delivers a set air pressure via a mask that fits over the patient's nose or nose and mouth in order to pneumatically stent open the airway, thereby eliminating the repetitive breathing pauses seen in OSA. CPAP is intended to be used during all hours of sleep, whether at night or during daytime naps. CPAP therapy effectively treats OSA in almost everyone and improves symptoms of OSA in many [53]. The more consistently a patient adheres to PAP therapy, the more likely he or she is to experience its benefits [54]. Greater hours of nightly PAP usage have been associated with several different clinical outcomes including quality of life and excessive daytime sleepiness [54]. Fortunately, all modern PAP devices come equipped with data chips and/or modems that enable providers to objectively monitor adherence and efficacy.

Effect of CPAP on Blood Pressure

Most trials suggest a modest but significant benefit of PAP on blood pressure reduction [55]. It is important to note that studies on PAP therapy are limited by several factors. First, it is difficult to establish the true impact of a therapy with which patients are variably and imperfectly adherent. Second, despite CPAP being, in practice, more often a lifelong therapy that may render its benefit over years rather than weeks, there are practical challenges with performing long-term studies in this area. Indeed, although early studies suggested more significant effect sizes of CPAP on BP, many of these were seen exclusively among PAP-compliant patients. Not surprisingly, the effect of CPAP on blood pressure reduction does appear to be modified by CPAP adherence [56]. Somnolence status also appears to contribute to the effect of CPAP on blood pressure, with sleepier patients gleaning more benefit from CPAP. Figure 13.4 shows one example of the beneficial effect of CPAP on mean arterial pressures in patients with OSA [57].

A prospective observational cohort study following patients with both OSA and hypertension for 2 years found an average decline by 4.9 mmHg in 24-h mean blood pressure after 6 months after PAP initiation [58]. Effects were greatest in patients reporting greater hypersomnolence and higher baseline BMI, suggesting that perhaps

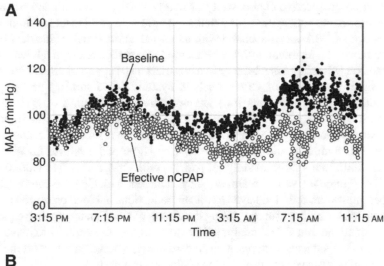

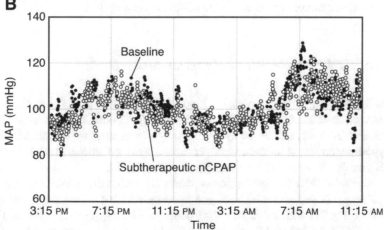

Fig. 13.4 Mean arterial pressures in patients with OSA before and after effective CPAP (**a**) and subtherapeutic CPAP (**b**). Substantial blood pressure reductions were seen in the group whose OSA was effectively treated with CPAP for 9 weeks. Mean arterial blood pressure decreased by 9.9 ± 11.4 mmHg with effective nCPAP treatment, whereas no relevant change occurred with subtherapeutic nCPAP ($P = 0.01$) (From Ref. [57]; with permission)

more obese and sleepier patients have more to gain as far as a BP reduction with CPAP use. Another study of non-sleepy patients with OSA found that the prescription of CPAP compared with usual care did not result in a significant reduction in the incidence of hypertension or cardiovascular events, lending further support to the greater effect of CPAP in sleepy patients, for reasons that are not fully understood [59].

In order to control for effects PAP might have on BP independent of its effect on sleep-disordered breathing, another group evaluated the effect of CPAP on blood pressure in hypertensive patients with and without OSA. They found that 3 weeks of CPAP resulted in a significant reduction in nocturnal blood pressure only in patients with underlying OSA (−10.3 mmHg systolic and −4.5 mmHg diastolic).

In a large prospective cohort study of nearly 2000 patients studied for over a decade, Marin and colleagues found that compared with participants without OSA, the presence of OSA was associated with increased adjusted risk of incident hypertension; however, treatment with CPAP therapy was associated with a lower risk of hypertension [8]. A large meta-analysis of 16 trials also supported a small but statistically significant effect of CPAP on both systolic (−2.5 mmHg) and diastolic (−1.8 mmHg) blood pressures [60] although the short duration of PAP therapy (<24 weeks across studies) may have led to an underestimate of its true impact. A more recent meta-analysis of 28 trials showed similar results, with reductions in systolic (−2.58 mmHg) and diastolic (−2.01 mmHg) blood pressures favoring PAP treatment [60]. In a long-term study of patients with OSA and HTN randomized to either CPAP or conservative treatment, those adherent with CPAP usage for at least 5.6 h per night were found to have significant reductions in blood pressure at 1-year follow-up [61]. Another trial examining the effects of CPAP in hypertensive patients over a year found that CPAP facilitated de-escalation of the antihypertensive treatment in 71% of subjects with resistant hypertension, but had no effect on the number of antihypertensives required by the controlled group [62].

Effect of CPAP on Resistant Hypertension

Studies suggest that CPAP may affect blood pressure more strongly in those OSA patients with resistant hypertension than in the general population of hypertensive patients. For instance, a meta-analysis focusing specifically on patients with resistant hypertension found an even stronger effect, with reductions in systolic BP by 3 mmHg and in diastolic BP by 5 mmHg on average [63].

The recent HIPARCO trial further supports the notion that CPAP may be especially effective in patients with resistant hypertension [64]. This multicenter randomized controlled trial of nearly 200 patients with OSA of at least moderate severity (AHI ≥ 15 using 4% hypopnea criteria) was randomized to 12 weeks of CPAP versus no CPAP. Patients were taking an average of 3.8 antihypertensive drugs per patient and had a mean AHI of 40 events/hr. In an intention-to-treat analysis, those who used CPAP regularly experienced statistically significant reductions in 24-h mean blood pressure by 4.4 mmHg, respectively, in a per-protocol analysis and a 14% increase in the percentage of patients with a normal nocturnal blood pressure dipper pattern at 12 weeks. There was a dose-response relationship between the hours of CPAP use and the degree of 24-h mean blood pressure reduction, whereby each additional hour of CPAP use translated into a 2 mmHg reduction in systolic and 1 mmHg reduction in diastolic blood pressure. It is notable that since patients with a history of poor antihypertensive medication adherence were excluded from this study, these results may have magnified the benefits of CPAP relative to the general population.

Another small randomized study of patients with resistant hypertension and at least moderate OSA randomized to either CPAP or sham-CPAP for 8 weeks found the CPAP promoted a 5 mmHg greater reduction in systolic blood pressure [65].

Table 13.3 Nocturnal blood pressure reduction with CPAP use in patients with resistant hypertension

	No. of studies	Mean change (mmHg)	95% CI, P value
Mean difference in SBP after CPAP	5	−6.79	−13.86 to 0.26, P = 0.05
Mean difference in DBP after CPAP	5	−3.67	−8.05 to 0.71, P = 0.10
Mean net change in SBP between CPAP and control	3	−2.08	−4.33 to 0.16, P = 0.06
Mean net change in DBP between CPAP and control	3	−1.47	−3.22 to 0.28, P = 0.10

From reference Iftikhar et al. [66]; with permission

Additionally, recent meta-analyses have provided further support for the therapeutic benefit of CPAP therapy specifically on resistant hypertension [66]. Table 13.3 shows the magnitude of blood pressure reduction across the six studies included in this meta-analysis. CPAP was found to have a greater effect on blood pressure reduction in patients with resistant hypertension than those without resistant hypertension, with average reductions of 6–7 and 5–6 mmHg in ambulatory systolic and diastolic blood pressures.

Taken together, these studies suggest that CPAP can be expected to result in a modest, favorable effect on blood pressure reduction, on the order of 2–3 mmHg for the population at large. However, this degree of reduction should be considered significant, as it has been shown to reduce cardiovascular mortality by 4–8%. In patients with severe and resistant hypertension, the magnitude of BP reduction attributable to CPAP appears to be even more significant.

CPAP vs. Antihypertensives for Blood Pressure Control

The effect of CPAP on blood pressure does not appear to be as potent as that of antihypertensives, albeit from the limited direct comparisons that exist. An important clinical question, and one likely of interest to patients, is how CPAP impacts blood pressure relative to that obtained with standard antihypertensive medications. The first such trial randomized patients to receive either CPAP or an antihypertensive regimen with valsartan using a crossover design [67]. Valsartan was found to be superior to CPAP, with patients on valsartan experiencing a fourfold greater reduction in 24-h mean blood pressure than those on CPAP alone (11 mmHg vs. 3 mmHg) over an 8-week time period. Another study sought to evaluate the blood pressure response to CPAP as "add-on" therapy in patients already taking losartan [68]. They found that losartan resulted in blood pressure reductions but to a lesser degree in patients with OSA than those without OSA.

Although CPAP can be expected to achieve a lesser magnitude of blood pressure reduction than antihypertensive medications, the effect of both therapies may be additive. It may be prudent to manage patients' expectations about CPAP therapy for OSA by explaining that it is unlikely to produce blood pressure reduction sufficient to allow discontinuation of antihypertensive therapy. Figure 13.5 shows one proposed algorithm for the diagnostic management of patients with hypertension and suspected OSA.

Mandibular Advancement Devices

Despite its established effectiveness and recent technological advances in the device, many patients still have difficulty tolerating CPAP therapy and exhibit suboptimal compliance. CPAP intolerance can affect a large number of OSA patients [70], and additional interventions, such as group education, generally fail to increase compliance to a level that would prevent the development of comorbidities [71]. Long-term CPAP adherence rates vary widely across studies but have been as low as 30% after 6 months of treatment [72]. In patients unable or unwilling to tolerate CPAP, mandibular advancement devices (MADs) represent the best therapeutic alternative [73, 74].

Efficacy of MADs on OSA

MADs are indicated for the treatment of mild-to-moderate OSA (AHI of 5–29.9) in patients intolerant of CPAP therapy or a rescue therapy in severe OSA patients who are unable to achieve regular CPAP adherence. MADs advance the mandible forward relative to the maxilla, thereby increasing the upper airway volume by widening the lateral dimensions of the velopharyngeal space [75]. Randomized controlled trials and crossover studies have confirmed the efficacy of the MADs in reducing snoring, the AHI, and the arousal index and in improving oxygenation compared to control oral devices that do not advance the lower jaw, but there is high interindividual variability in the response to MAD therapy [76–79].

A parallel randomized controlled trial in mild-to-moderate OSA patients found that MAD therapy was as effective as CPAP therapy when polysomnography-controlled titration was done for both treatment modalities and superior to placebo in mild-to-moderate OSA patients [80].

Several studies have shown that MADs are more successful in patients with milder OSA, positional OSA, and lower BMI and in females [76, 77, 81–83]. However, other studies have reported superior efficacy of CPAP compared to MADs in treating OSA [82], and a recent review of all the studies comparing the effectiveness of the MADs to CPAP confirmed that CPAP therapy has a superior therapeutic success rate than the MADs even in mild-to-moderate OSA [84]. Given that adherence is at the crux of both therapies, the superior efficacy of CPAP may not translate into better clinical outcomes if CPAP patients are less compliant than those using MADs.

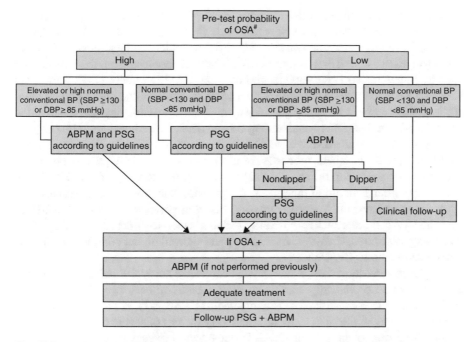

Fig. 13.5 Proposed algorithm for the diagnostic management of patients with hypertension associated with obstructive sleep apnea (OSA). *BP* blood pressure, *SBP* systolic BP, *DBP* diastolic BP, *ABPM* ambulatory BP monitoring, *PSG* polysomnography. # denotes according to clinical evaluation and questionnaires, for example, Epworth and Berlin; z indicates hypertension guidelines recommend the use of home BP monitoring in most hypertensive patients (Reproduced with permission of the European Respiratory Society © [69])

Effect of MADs on Blood Pressure

A few studies have demonstrated a favorable effect of MADS on blood pressure reduction in patients with OSA. A prospective randomized, controlled crossover study found that 4 weeks of MAD therapy resulted in a 24-h ambulatory blood pressure reduction of ±1.1 mmHg for systolic blood pressure and 3.4 ± 0.9 mmHg for diastolic blood pressure compared with the control group. The magnitude of blood pressure reduction with MADs has been overall similar to that seen with CPAP therapy, despite MAD therapy's less potent effect on AHI reduction [85]. It is noteworthy that many studies have quoted longer durations of MAD usage than are typically seen in studies of CPAP.

Another randomized, crossover trial evaluated patients with mild-to-moderate OSA assigned to 3 months of MAD versus CPAP therapy versus no therapy [86] and found that CPAP therapy was more effective in improving sleep-disordered breathing than MAD and placebo. However, MAD treatment was effective in decreasing nocturnal diastolic blood pressure and in restoring the physiologic nocturnal dipping in blood pressure among OSA patients in contrast to CPAP therapy.

Self-reported compliance with MAD was greater than the objectively measured one with CPAP therapy, raising the possibility that OSA was better treated with MADs. Another case series study showed that MAD treatment led to blood pressure declines in OSA patients over a 3-year period [87]. A more recent trial from the same author among hypertensive OSA patients showed that MAD treatment could reduce the 24-h mean systolic blood pressure compared to the controls and with a greater magnitude of decrease in the subgroup of patients with a baseline daytime mean blood pressure higher than 135/85 and among OSA patients with a baseline AHI > 15 [88]. A meta-analysis confirmed that MADs can decrease systolic, diastolic, and nocturnal blood pressure, albeit, modestly, in mild-to-moderate OSA [89]. A large randomized crossover controlled trial [90] comparing the efficacy of MAD to CPAP found that, after 1 month of therapy, blood pressure reductions among patients with moderate-to-severe OSA were equivalent between patients on CPAP and MAD, despite CPAP more effectively treating patients' sleep-disordered breathing. Most patients preferred MAD over CPAP therapy and showed higher compliance with the MAD compared to CPAP therapy.

As far as long-term data, a randomized controlled study following patients over 2 years found no clinically significant difference in efficacy in mild-to-moderate OSA patients treated with MADs compared to CPAP [91]. A cohort study found that the efficacy of the MADs on the respiratory indices of severe OSA patients was slightly inferior to the one of CPAP therapy over a 5-year period but was non-inferior to CPAP in reducing the cardiovascular risks associated with OSA [92]. A single study has provided evidence for reduced cardiovascular mortality in severe OSA patients using MADs compared to controls, in a manner non-inferior to the efficacy of CPAP [93].

In summary, the beneficial effects of MAD treatment on blood pressure parameters in patients with OSA appear to be modest but likely sustained over the long term [87], perhaps in part due to higher adherence with the therapy than is typically seen with CPAP.

Other Therapies

Nocturnal supplemental oxygen therapy has been proposed as another possible alternative for patients unable to tolerate CPAP. Based on the results of a study of patients with cardiovascular disease or risk factors in whom treatment of obstructive sleep apnea with CPAP—but not oxygen—resulted in significant blood pressure reductions, we cannot recommend this as an acceptable first-line therapy [94].

Other alternative therapies include upper airway surgeries (e.g., uvulopalatopharyngoplasty), nasal expiratory resistance devices, or implantation of a hypoglossal nerve stimulator, but none of these therapies is as effective as CPAP in treating OSA [95, 96]. A small group of carefully selected patients may be appropriate candidates for more invasive options including maxillomandibular advancement surgery or tracheostomy.

Conclusions

A large body of evidence supports the role of OSA as an independent factor in the pathogenesis of daytime hypertension and appears to represent the single greatest modifiable factor in patients with resistant hypertension specifically. The relationship between OSA and hypertension persists even after controlling for obesity as a modifier of the OSA-hypertension association. CPAP reduces blood pressure to a modest degree in patients with resistant hypertension but has a more potent effect in this population than the more general population of hypertensive individuals. Greater CPAP adherence may be expected to result in larger BP reductions in a dose-response fashion. Given that even mild reductions in blood pressure may result significant reductions in cardiovascular risk, we recommend aggressive screening for OSA in all patients with resistant hypertension, including the elderly. Sleep centers should generally have a low threshold for testing such patients, even in the presence of minimal daytime symptoms, since treatment is generally well tolerated.

References

1. Gonçalves SC, Martinez D, Gus M, de Abreu-Silva EO, Bertoluci C, Dutra I, et al. Obstructive sleep apnea and resistant hypertension: a case-control study. Chest. 2007;132(6):1858–62.
2. Peppard PE, Young T, Barnet JH, Palta M, Hagen EW, Hla KM. Increased prevalence of sleep-disordered breathing in adults. Am J Epidemiol. 2013;177(9):1006–14.
3. Young T, Peppard PE, Gottlieb DJ. Epidemiology of obstructive sleep apnea: a population health perspective. Am J Respir Crit Care Med. 2002;165(9):1217–39.
4. Jordan AS, McSharry DG, Malhotra A. Adult obstructive sleep apnoea. Lancet (Lond Engl). 2014;383(9918):736–47.
5. Howard ME, Desai AV, Grunstein RR, Hukins C, Armstrong JG, Joffe D, et al. Sleepiness, sleep-disordered breathing, and accident risk factors in commercial vehicle drivers. Am J Respir Crit Care Med. 2004;170(9):1014–21.
6. Terán-Santos J, Jiménez-Gómez A, Cordero-Guevara J. The association between sleep apnea and the risk of traffic accidents. Cooperative Group Burgos-Santander. N Engl J Med. 1999;340(11):847–51.
7. Peppard PE, Young T, Palta M, Skatrud J. Prospective study of the association between sleep-disordered breathing and hypertension. N Engl J Med. 2000;342(19):1378–84.
8. Marin JM, Agusti A, Villar I, Forner M, Nieto D, Carrizo SJ, et al. Association between treated and untreated obstructive sleep apnea and risk of hypertension. JAMA. 2012;307(20): 2169–76.
9. Parati G, Lombardi C, Hedner J, Bonsignore MR, Grote L, Tkacova R, et al. Recommendations for the management of patients with obstructive sleep apnoea and hypertension. Eur Respir J. 2013;41(3):523–38.
10. Kapur V, Strohl KP, Redline S, Iber C, O'Connor G, Nieto J. Underdiagnosis of sleep apnea syndrome in U.S. communities. Sleep Breath Schlaf Atm. 2002;6(2):49–54.
11. Daugherty SL, Powers JD, Magid DJ, Tavel HM, Masoudi FA, Margolis KL, et al. Incidence and prognosis of resistant hypertension in hypertensive patients. Circulation. 2012; 125(13):1635–42.

12. Cano-Pumarega I, Durán-Cantolla J, Aizpuru F, Miranda-Serrano E, Rubio R, Martínez-Null C, et al. Obstructive sleep apnea and systemic hypertension: longitudinal study in the general population: the Vitoria sleep cohort. Am J Respir Crit Care Med. 2011;184(11):1299–304.
13. Goff EA, O'Driscoll DM, Simonds AK, Trinder J, Morrell MJ. The cardiovascular response to arousal from sleep decreases with age in healthy adults. Sleep. 2008;31(7):1009–17.
14. Lavie P, Herer P, Hoffstein V. Obstructive sleep apnoea syndrome as a risk factor for hypertension: population study. BMJ. 2000;320(7233):479–82.
15. Grote L, Hedner J, Peter JH. Sleep-related breathing disorder is an independent risk factor for uncontrolled hypertension. J Hypertens. 2000;18(6):679–85.
16. Nieto FJ, Young TB, Lind BK, Shahar E, Samet JM, Redline S, et al. Association of sleep-disordered breathing, sleep apnea, and hypertension in a large community-based study. Sleep heart health study. JAMA. 2000;283(14):1829–36.
17. O'Connor GT, Caffo B, Newman AB, Quan SF, Rapoport DM, Redline S, et al. Prospective study of sleep-disordered breathing and hypertension: the sleep heart health study. Am J Respir Crit Care Med. 2009;179(12):1159–64.
18. Chobanian AV, Bakris GL, Black HR, et al. The seventh report of the joint national committee on prevention, detection, evaluation, and treatment of high blood pressure: the JNC 7 report. JAMA. 2003;289(19):2560–71.
19. Bixler EO, Vgontzas AN, Lin HM, Ten Have T, Leiby BE, Vela-Bueno A, et al. Association of hypertension and sleep-disordered breathing. Arch Intern Med. 2000;160(15):2289–95.
20. Haas DC, Foster GL, Nieto FJ, Redline S, Resnick HE, Robbins JA, et al. Age-dependent associations between sleep-disordered breathing and hypertension: importance of discriminating between systolic/diastolic hypertension and isolated systolic hypertension in the sleep heart health study. Circulation. 2005;111(5):614–21.
21. Drager LF, Pereira AC, Barreto-Filho JA, Figueiredo AC, Krieger JE, Krieger EM, et al. Phenotypic characteristics associated with hypertension in patients with obstructive sleep apnea. J Hum Hypertens. 2006;20(7):523–8.
22. Wolf J, Hering D, Narkiewicz K. Non-dipping pattern of hypertension and obstructive sleep apnea syndrome. Hypertens Res Off J Jpn Soc Hypertens. 2010;33(9):867–71.
23. Narkiewicz K, Kato M, Phillips BG, Pesek CA, Davison DE, Somers VK. Nocturnal continuous positive airway pressure decreases daytime sympathetic traffic in obstructive sleep apnea. Circulation. 1999;100(23):2332–5.
24. Hla KM, Young T, Finn L, Peppard PE, Szklo-Coxe M, Stubbs M. Longitudinal association of sleep-disordered breathing and nondipping of nocturnal blood pressure in the Wisconsin sleep cohort study. Sleep. 2008;31(6):795–800.
25. Parati G, Valentini M. Prognostic relevance of blood pressure variability. Hypertension. 2006;47(2):137–8.
26. Ohkubo T, Hozawa A, Yamaguchi J, Kikuya M, Ohmori K, Michimata M, et al. Prognostic significance of the nocturnal decline in blood pressure in individuals with and without high 24-h blood pressure: the Ohasama study. J Hypertens. 2002;20(11):2183–9.
27. Verdecchia P, Schillaci G, Guerrieri M, Gatteschi C, Benemio G, Boldrini F, et al. Circadian blood pressure changes and left ventricular hypertrophy in essential hypertension. Circulation. 1990;81(2):528–36.
28. Logan AG, Perlikowski SM, Mente A, Tisler A, Tkacova R, Niroumand M, et al. High prevalence of unrecognized sleep apnoea in drug-resistant hypertension. J Hypertens. 2001;19(12):2271–7.
29. Pratt-Ubunama MN, Nishizaka MK, Boedefeld RL, Cofield SS, Harding SM, Calhoun DA. Plasma aldosterone is related to severity of obstructive sleep apnea in subjects with resistant hypertension. Chest. 2007;131(2):453–9.
30. Schillaci G, Pirro M, Mannarino E. Assessing cardiovascular risk should we discard diastolic blood pressure? Circulation. 2009;119(2):210–2.

31. Pedrosa RP, Drager LF, Gonzaga CC, Sousa MG, de Paula LKG, Amaro ACS, et al. Obstructive sleep apnea: the most common secondary cause of hypertension associated with resistant hypertension. Hypertension. 2011;58(5):811–7.
32. Walia HK, Li H, Rueschman M, Bhatt DL, Patel SR, Quan SF, et al. Association of severe obstructive sleep apnea and elevated blood pressure despite antihypertensive medication use. J Clin Sleep Med JCSM Off Publ Am Acad Sleep Med. 2014;10(8):835–43.
33. Calhoun DA, Jones D, Textor S, Goff DC, Murphy TP, Toto RD, et al. Resistant hypertension: diagnosis, evaluation, and treatment a scientific statement from the American Heart Association Professional Education Committee of the Council for high blood pressure research. Circulation. 2008;117(25):e510–26.
34. Tobias L. "PocketDoktor" patient information booklet on Obstructive Sleep Apnea, 2014, Pelz Verlag GmbH, Germany.
35. Parati G, Ochoa JE, Bilo G, Mattaliano P, Salvi P, Kario K, et al. Obstructive sleep apnea syndrome as a cause of resistant hypertension. Hypertens Res Off J Jpn Soc Hypertens. 2014;37(7):601–13.
36. Foster GE, Brugniaux JV, Pialoux V, Duggan CTC, Hanly PJ, Ahmed SB, et al. Cardiovascular and cerebrovascular responses to acute hypoxia following exposure to intermittent hypoxia in healthy humans. J Physiol. 2009;587(Pt 13):3287–99.
37. Tamisier R, Pépin JL, Rémy J, Baguet JP, Taylor JA, Weiss JW, et al. 14 nights of intermittent hypoxia elevate daytime blood pressure and sympathetic activity in healthy humans. Eur Respir J. 2011;37(1):119–28.
38. Tkacova R, McNicholas WT, Javorsky M, Fietze I, Sliwinski P, Parati G, et al. Nocturnal intermittent hypoxia predicts prevalent hypertension in the European Sleep Apnoea Database cohort study. Eur Respir J. 2014;44(4):931–41.
39. Friedman O, Bradley TD, Chan CT, Parkes R, Logan AG. Relationship between overnight rostral fluid shift and obstructive sleep apnea in drug-resistant hypertension. Hypertension. 2010;56(6):1077–82.
40. Gaddam K, Pimenta E, Thomas SJ, Cofield SS, Oparil S, Harding SM, et al. Spironolactone reduces severity of obstructive sleep apnoea in patients with resistant hypertension: a preliminary report. J Hum Hypertens. 2010;24(8):532–7.
41. Sharma AM, Wittchen H-U, Kirch W, Pittrow D, Ritz E, Göke B, et al. High prevalence and poor control of hypertension in primary care: cross-sectional study. J Hypertens. 2004;22(3):479–86.
42. Rasche K, Keller T, Tautz B, Hader C, Hergenç G, Antosiewicz J, et al. Obstructive sleep apnea and type 2 diabetes. Eur J Med Res. 2010;15(Suppl 2):152–6.
43. American Academy of Sleep Medicine. International Classification of Sleep Disorders. 3rd ed. Darien: American Academy of Sleep Medicine; 2014.
44. Berry RB, Budhiraja R, Gottlieb DJ, Gozal D, Iber C, Kapur VK, et al. Rules for scoring respiratory events in sleep: update of the 2007 AASM manual for the scoring of sleep and associated events. Deliberations of the sleep apnea definitions task force of the American Academy of Sleep Medicine. J Clin Sleep Med JCSM Off Publ Am Acad Sleep Med. 2012;8(5):597–619.
45. Myers KA, Mrkobrada M, Simel DL. Does this patient have obstructive sleep apnea?: the rational clinical examination systematic review. JAMA. 2013;310(7):731–41.
46. Johns MW. A new method for measuring daytime sleepiness: the Epworth sleepiness scale. Sleep. 1991;14(6):540–5.
47. Ramachandran SK, Josephs LA. A meta-analysis of clinical screening tests for obstructive sleep apnea. Anesthesiology. 2009;110(4):928–39.
48. Qaseem A, Dallas P, Owens DK, Starkey M, Holty J-EC, Shekelle P. Diagnosis of obstructive sleep apnea in adults: a clinical practice guideline from the American college of physicians diagnosis of obstructive sleep apnea in adults. Ann Intern Med. 2014;161(3):210–20.

49. Epstein LJ, Kristo D, Strollo PJ, Friedman N, Malhotra A, Patil SP, et al. Clinical guideline for the evaluation, management and long-term care of obstructive sleep apnea in adults. J Clin Sleep Med JCSM Off Publ Am Acad Sleep Med. 2009;5(3):263–76.
50. Collop NA, Tracy SL, Kapur V, Mehra R, Kuhlmann D, Fleishman SA, et al. Obstructive sleep apnea devices for out-of-center (OOC) testing: technology evaluation. J Clin Sleep Med JCSM Off Publ Am Acad Sleep Med. 2011;7(5):531–48.
51. Buchwald H, Avidor Y, Braunwald E, Jensen MD, Pories W, Fahrbach K, et al. Bariatric surgery: a systematic review and meta-analysis. JAMA. 2004;292(14):1724–37.
52. Quan SF, Budhiraja R, Clarke DP, Goodwin JL, Gottlieb DJ, Nichols DA, et al. Impact of treatment with continuous positive airway pressure (CPAP) on weight in obstructive sleep apnea. J Clin Sleep Med JCSM Off Publ Am Acad Sleep Med. 2013;9(10):989–93.
53. Antic NA, Catcheside P, Buchan C, Hensley M, Naughton MT, Rowland S, et al. The effect of CPAP in normalizing daytime sleepiness, quality of life, and neurocognitive function in patients with moderate to severe OSA. Sleep. 2011;34(1):111–9.
54. Weaver TE, Maislin G, Dinges DF, Bloxham T, George CFP, Greenberg H, et al. Relationship between hours of CPAP use and achieving normal levels of sleepiness and daily functioning. Sleep. 2007;30(6):711–9.
55. Wang AY-M. Sleep-disordered breathing and resistant hypertension. Semin Nephrol. 2014;34(5):520–31.
56. Campos-Rodriguez F, Perez-Ronchel J, Grilo-Reina A, Lima-Alvarez J, Benitez MA, Almeida-Gonzalez C. Long-term effect of continuous positive airway pressure on BP in patients with hypertension and sleep apnea. Chest. 2007;132(6):1847–52.
57. Becker HF, Jerrentrup A, Ploch T, Grote L, Penzel T, Sullivan CE, et al. Effect of nasal continuous positive airway pressure treatment on blood pressure in patients with obstructive sleep apnea. Circulation. 2003;107(1):68–73.
58. Robinson GV, Langford BA, Smith DM, Stradling JR. Predictors of blood pressure fall with continuous positive airway pressure (CPAP) treatment of obstructive sleep apnoea (OSA). Thorax. 2008;63(10):855–9.
59. Barbé F, Durán-Cantolla J, Sánchez-de-la-Torre M, Martínez-Alonso M, Carmona C, Barceló A, et al. Effect of continuous positive airway pressure on the incidence of hypertension and cardiovascular events in nonsleepy patients with obstructive sleep apnea: a randomized controlled trial. JAMA. 2012;307(20):2161–8.
60. Bazzano LA, Khan Z, Reynolds K, He J. Effect of nocturnal nasal continuous positive airway pressure on blood pressure in obstructive sleep apnea. Hypertension. 2007;50(2):417–23.
61. Barbé F, Durán-Cantolla J, Capote F, de la Peña M, Chiner E, Masa JF, et al. Long-term effect of continuous positive airway pressure in hypertensive patients with sleep apnea. Am J Respir Crit Care Med. 2010;181(7):718–26.
62. Dernaika TA, Kinasewitz GT, Tawk MM. Effects of nocturnal continuous positive airway pressure therapy in patients with resistant hypertension and obstructive sleep apnea. J Clin Sleep Med JCSM Off Publ Am Acad Sleep Med. 2009;5(2):103–7.
63. Varounis C, Katsi V, Kallikazaros IE, Tousoulis D, Stefanadis C, Parissis J, et al. Effect of CPAP on blood pressure in patients with obstructive sleep apnea and resistant hypertension: a systematic review and meta-analysis. Int J Cardiol. 2014;175(1):195–8.
64. Martínez-García M-A, Capote F, Campos-Rodríguez F, Lloberes P, Díaz de Atauri MJ, Somoza M, et al. Effect of CPAP on blood pressure in patients with obstructive sleep apnea and resistant hypertension: the HIPARCO randomized clinical trial. JAMA. 2013;310(22):2407–15.
65. de Oliveira AC, Martinez D, Massierer D, Gus M, Gonçalves SC, Ghizzoni F, et al. The antihypertensive effect of positive airway pressure on resistant hypertension of patients with obstructive sleep apnea: a randomized, double-blind, clinical trial. Am J Respir Crit Care Med. 2014;190(3):345–7.
66. Iftikhar IH, Valentine CW, Bittencourt LRA, Cohen DL, Fedson AC, Gíslason T, et al. Effects of continuous positive airway pressure on blood pressure in patients with resistant hyperten-

sion and obstructive sleep apnea: a meta-analysis. J Hypertens. 2014;32(12):2341–50; discussion 2350.
67. Pépin J-L, Tamisier R, Barone-Rochette G, Launois SH, Lévy P, Baguet J-P. Comparison of continuous positive airway pressure and valsartan in hypertensive patients with sleep apnea. Am J Respir Crit Care Med. 2010;182(7):954–60.
68. Thunström E, Manhem K, Rosengren A, Peker Y. Blood pressure response to losartan and continuous positive airway pressure in hypertension and obstructive sleep apnea. Am J Respir Crit Care Med. 2016;193(3):310–20.
69. Gianfranco P, Lombardi C, Hedner J, Bonsignore MR, Grote L, Tkacova R, Lévy P, Riha R, Bassetti C, Narkiewicz K, Mancia G, McNicholas WT. Recommendations for the management of patients with obstructive sleep apnoea and hypertension. Eur Respir J. 2013; 41(3): 523–38
70. Weaver TE, Grunstein RR. Adherence to continuous positive airway pressure therapy: the challenge to effective treatment. Proc Am Thorac Soc. 2008;5(2):173–8.
71. Weaver TE. Don't start celebrating – CPAP adherence remains a problem. J Clin Sleep Med JCSM Off Publ Am Acad Sleep Med. 2013;9(6):551–2.
72. Lindberg E, Berne C, Elmasry A, Hedner J, Janson C. CPAP treatment of a population- based sample—what are the benefits and the treatment compliance? Sleep Med. 2006;7(7):553–60.
73. Ramar K, Dort LC, Katz SG, Lettieri CJ, Harrod CG, Thomas SM, et al. Clinical practice guideline for the treatment of obstructive sleep apnea and snoring with oral appliance therapy: an update for 2015. J Clin Sleep Med JCSM Off Publ Am Acad Sleep Med. 2015;11(7):773–827.
74. Kushida CA, Morgenthaler TI, Littner MR, Alessi CA, Bailey D, Coleman J, et al. Practice parameters for the treatment of snoring and obstructive sleep apnea with oral appliances: an update for 2005. Sleep. 2006;29(2):240–3.
75. Chan ASL, Sutherland K, Schwab RJ, Zeng B, Petocz P, Lee RWW, et al. The effect of mandibular advancement on upper airway structure in obstructive sleep apnoea. Thorax. 2010;65(8):726–32.
76. Johnston CD, Gleadhill IC, Cinnamond MJ, Gabbey J, Burden DJ. Mandibular advancement appliances and obstructive sleep apnoea: a randomized clinical trial. Eur J Orthod. 2002;24(3):251–62.
77. Mehta A, Qian J, Petocz P, Darendeliler MA, Cistulli PA. A randomized, controlled study of a mandibular advancement splint for obstructive sleep apnea. Am J Respir Crit Care Med. 2001;163(6):1457–61.
78. Petri N, Svanholt P, Solow B, Wildschiødtz G, Winkel P. Mandibular advancement appliance for obstructive sleep apnoea: results of a randomised placebo controlled trial using parallel group design. J Sleep Res. 2008;17(2):221–9.
79. Bartolucci ML, Bortolotti F, Raffaelli E, D'Antò V, Michelotti A, Bonetti GA. The effectiveness of different mandibular advancement amounts in OSA patients: a systematic review and meta-regression analysis. Sleep Breath. 2016;20(3):911–9.
80. Aarab G, Lobbezoo F, Hamburger HL, Naeije M. Oral appliance therapy versus nasal continuous positive airway pressure in obstructive sleep apnea: a randomized, placebo-controlled trial. Respir Int Rev Thorac Dis. 2011;81(5):411–9.
81. Ferguson KA, Ono T, Lowe AA, al-Majed S, Love LL, Fleetham JA. A short-term controlled trial of an adjustable oral appliance for the treatment of mild to moderate obstructive sleep apnoea. Thorax. 1997;52(4):362–8.
82. Marklund M, Stenlund H, Franklin KA. Mandibular advancement devices in 630 men and women with obstructive sleep apnea and snoring: tolerability and predictors of treatment success. Chest. 2004;125(4):1270–8.
83. Liu Y, Lowe AA, Fleetham JA, Park YC. Cephalometric and physiologic predictors of the efficacy of an adjustable oral appliance for treating obstructive sleep apnea. Am J Orthod Dentofacial Orthop Off Publ Am Assoc Orthod Its Const Soc Am Board Orthod. 2001;120(6):639–47.

84. Sutherland K, Vanderveken OM, Tsuda H, Marklund M, Gagnadoux F, Kushida CA, et al. Oral appliance treatment for obstructive sleep apnea: an update. J Clin Sleep Med JCSM Off Publ Am Acad Sleep Med. 2014;10(2):215–27.
85. Gotsopoulos H, Kelly JJ, Cistulli PA. Oral appliance therapy reduces blood pressure in obstructive sleep apnea: a randomized, controlled trial. Sleep. 2004;27(5):934–41.
86. Barnes M, McEvoy RD, Banks S, Tarquinio N, Murray CG, Vowles N, et al. Efficacy of positive airway pressure and oral appliance in mild to moderate obstructive sleep apnea. Am J Respir Crit Care Med. 2004;170(6):656–64.
87. Andrén A, Sjöquist M, Tegelberg Å. Effects on blood pressure after treatment of obstructive sleep apnoea with a mandibular advancement appliance – a three-year follow-up. J Oral Rehabil. 2009;36(10):719–25.
88. Andrén A, Hedberg P, Walker-Engström M-L, Wahlén P, Tegelberg A. Effects of treatment with oral appliance on 24-h blood pressure in patients with obstructive sleep apnea and hypertension: a randomized clinical trial. Sleep Breath Schlaf Atm. 2013;17(2):705–12.
89. Iftikhar IH, Hays ER, Iverson M-A, Magalang UJ, Maas AK. Effect of oral appliances on blood pressure in obstructive sleep apnea: a systematic review and meta-analysis. J Clin Sleep Med JCSM Off Publ Am Acad Sleep Med. 2013;9(2):165–74.
90. Phillips CL, Grunstein RR, Darendeliler MA, Mihailidou AS, Srinivasan VK, Yee BJ, et al. Health outcomes of continuous positive airway pressure versus oral appliance treatment for obstructive sleep apnea. Am J Respir Crit Care Med. 2013;187(8):879–87.
91. Doff MHJ, Hoekema A, Wijkstra PJ, van der Hoeven JH, Huddleston Slater JJR, de Bont LGM, et al. Oral appliance versus continuous positive airway pressure in obstructive sleep apnea syndrome: a 2-year follow-up. Sleep. 2013;36(9):1289–96.
92. Anandam A, Patil M, Akinnusi M, Jaoude P, El-Solh AA. Cardiovascular mortality in obstructive sleep apnoea treated with continuous positive airway pressure or oral appliance: an observational study. Respirology. 2013;18(8):1184–90.
93. Marklund M. Long-term efficacy of an oral appliance in early treated patients with obstructive sleep apnea. Sleep Breath. 2015;20(2):689–94.
94. Gottlieb DJ, Punjabi NM, Mehra R, Patel SR, Quan SF, Babineau DC, et al. CPAP versus oxygen in obstructive sleep apnea. N Engl J Med. 2014;370(24):2276–85.
95. Caples SM, Rowley JA, Prinsell JR, Pallanch JF, Elamin MB, Katz SG, et al. Surgical modifications of the upper airway for obstructive sleep apnea in adults: a systematic review and meta-analysis. Sleep. 2010;33(10):1396–407.
96. Sundaram S, Bridgman SA, Lim J, Lasserson TJ. Surgery for obstructive sleep apnoea. Cochrane Database Syst Rev. 2005;(4):CD001004.

Chapter 14
Interference with Pharmacological Agents to Resistant Hypertension in Chronic Kidney Disease

Mikail Yarlioglues

Introduction

The accepted definition of resistant hypertension is a seated office systolic blood pressure (SBP) ≥140 mmHg or diastolic blood pressure (DBP) ≥90 mmHg on maximally tolerated doses of three or more antihypertensive agents, one of which must be a diuretic appropriate for the level of kidney function. The National Institute for Health and Care Excellence (NICE) guidelines recommend the use of triple combination therapy that includes a thiazide or a thiazide-like diuretic, a renin-angiotensin system (RAS) blocker including angiotensin converting enzyme inhibitors (ACEi) or angiotensin receptor blockers (ARB), and a calcium channel blocker [1]. White coat hypertension should be excluded using daytime ambulatory blood pressure measurement (ABPM) (readings of SBP ≥135 mmHg or DBP ≥85 mmHg on the same regimen) to confirm resistant hypertension.

True resistant hypertension is a diagnosis of exclusion of pseudo-resistance which refers the situation associated with poor drug adherence, secondary hypertension including endocrine and vascular causes, casual factors, and white coat hypertension. Inadequate blood pressure (BP) control is often related with poor drug adherence. It is very important to deal with barriers for optimum drug therapy including adverse effects of ongoing treatment, insufficient treatment, interfering vasopressor substance or medication, and excessive salt or alcohol intake. Therefore, the first step is to provide appropriate antihypertensive drug combinations with optimal dosage and good patient compliance [2].

M. Yarlioglues (✉)
Department of Cardiology, Ankara Education and Research Hospital, Ankara, Turkey
e-mail: drmikailyar@gmail.com

© Springer International Publishing AG 2017
A. Covic et al. (eds.), *Resistant Hypertension in Chronic Kidney Disease*,
DOI 10.1007/978-3-319-56827-0_14

The approach to treatment of resistant hypertension in patients with chronic kidney disease (CKD) should target several factors that contribute to the pathogenesis of hypertension including impaired handling of sodium and volume expansion, increased activity of the renin-angiotensin-aldosterone system, enhanced sympathetic activity, and reduced endothelium-dependent vasodilation [3]. In addition, particular attention should be given to non-dipping BP pattern which leads to increase the risk of target organ damage. In this chapter, we focus on the pharmacological agents to deal with resistant hypertension in CKD.

Treatment Options

Deal with Volume Overload and Salt Retention

Modifying Treatment According to Volume Status

Subclinical volume overload is present in more than one fifth of patients with CKD. It is an important contributor to resistant hypertension. The value of guiding resistant hypertension treatment based on subclinical extracellular fluid excess can be useful to arrange the appropriate type and dose of antihypertensive agents. Thoracic bioimpedance allows to get actual hemodynamic information about alterations in thoracic fluid volume, cardiac output, and systemic vascular resistance by the use of skin electrodes using together with BP measurement. It was tested in an interesting prospected study comparing hemodynamic management using thoracic bioimpedance to hypertension specialist care based on clinical evaluation during 3 months [4]. One hundred and four patients with resistant hypertension were randomized to group of drug selection based on thoracic bioimpedance findings and drug selection by a hypertension specialist. At the end of the study, target of ≤140/90 was gained in 56% of patient in hemodynamic measurement group while 33% of patients in specialist group. The number of patients taking diuretics did not differ between groups, but final diuretic dosage was higher in the hemodynamic group. Thus, impedance measurements can provide useful data about actual volume expansion resulting resistant hypertension in CKD patients (particularly in patients with subclinical volume overload) and may guide to determine appropriate diuretic dose.

Dietary Sodium Intake Leads to Resistant to RAS Blockage Agents

Dietary sodium intake is closely related with action of antihypertensive agents particularly those with RAS blockage. Both animal and human studies have indicated that it is closely interacting with RAS, particularly aldosterone, and mediates hypertension, vascular and tissue damage, and kidney disease [3, 5]. Most of patients with CKD are salt sensitive, increasing sodium intake causing BP elevation and failure in action of RAS blockers and diuretics. In a randomized study, 34 patients were prospectively enrolled to compare high and low-sodium diet according to antihypertensive and antiproteinuric effects of ARB and thiazide-type diuretic [6]. At the end of the study, investigators found that sodium restriction provides similar effects with diuretic in reducing proteinuria and BP when added to ARB. And, strongest effects on proteinuria and BP were obtained with combining of ARB, diuretic, and low sodium, together. They mentioned that sodium status is an effective method to maximize the antiproteinuric and antihypertensive efficacy of RAS blockade. Thus, approaches to reduce salt intake can be beneficial because of synergism with the actions of thiazides, ACEi, or ARB, resulting in improved BP control and less proteinuria. The Kidney Disease: Improving Global Outcomes (KDIGO) guideline on hypertension in patients with CKD recommends limiting sodium intake to 2–4 g per day in patients not on dialysis [7]. However, most of no added salt diets contain nearly 4 g sodium which already overdoes the limit that the kidney can excrete without diuretic administration in CKD patients. It should be noted that selection of low-sodium foods contributes to improving effectiveness of antihypertensive agents.

Appropriate Diuretic Therapy

Most commonly accepted hypothesis for resistant hypertension is excessive sodium retention due to impaired sodium excretion during the day. Usage of diuretics sufficiently to deal with sodium retention is one of the most effective treatments to achieve BP target. But diuretics remain underutilized and underdosed in many patients. Particularly, CKD patients are more predisposed to sodium retention and volume overload because of impaired renal function. Thus, the use of appropriate diuretics is principal therapy in patients with CKD and resistant hypertension.

Switching Thiazide-Like Diuretic to a More Potent Diuretic

Hydrochlorothiazide (HCTZ) is the most commonly prescribed antihypertensive drug worldwide. More than 97% of all HCTZ prescriptions are for 12.5–25 mg per day. But, in a meta-analysis of 14 studies of HCTZ dose 12.5–25 mg with 1234 patients and 5 studies of HCTZ dose 50 mg with 229 patients, it was reported that decrease in ABPM with HCTZ dose 12.5–25 mg (SBP:6.5 mmHg and DBP:4.5 mmHg) was inferior compared to the ABPM reduction of ACEi (mean BP reduction 12.9/7.7), ARB (mean BP reduction 13.3/7.8 mmHg), beta-blockers (mean BP reduction 11.2/8.5 mmHg), and calcium antagonists (mean BP reduction 11.0/8.1 mmHg) [8]. Another remarkable result was that there was no significant difference in both SBP and DBP in ABPM reduction between HCTZ 12.5 mg and HCTZ 25 mg, but HCTZ 50 mg provided significant higher reduction in ABPM which was comparable to that of other agents. Thus, first step using should be using HCTZ in appropriate dose before switching to other diuretics.

Chlorthalidone is approximately twice as potent as HCTZ with a much longer duration of action (8–15 h for HCTZ compared with >40 h for chlorthalidone) [9]. In a randomized study, investigators compared the effect of chlorthalidone 12.5 mg/day (force-titrated to 25 mg/day) and HCTZ 25 mg/day (force-titrated to 50 mg/day) on ABPM in untreated hypertensive patients after 8 weeks [10]. As compared to HCTZ, chlorthalidone indicated a greater reduction in SBP primarily due to its effect on reducing nighttime mean SBP (-13.5 ± 1.9 mmHg versus -6.4 ± 1.8 mmHg). Therefore, strong consideration should be given to using chlorthalidone over HCTZ, especially in patients with CKD. Thiazide diuretics are most effective in patients with an eGFR >50 mL/min/1.73 m^2, although chlorthalidone can be effective to a GFR of 30–40 mL/min/1.73 m^2 in the absence of severe hypoalbuminemia. Consequently, BP control can also be improved by increasing diuretic dosage or by switching to a more potent, thiazide-like diuretic with a longer duration of action than the existing drug such as chlorthalidone and indapamide instead of hydrochlorothiazide when GFR is 30 mL/min or over.

The Use of Loop Diuretics

A loop diuretic is preferred for patients with advanced CKD. It has suggested that loop diuretics should be prescribed when eGFR is less than 30 mL/min [11]. It is indicated in the presence of edema or volume overload due to nephrotic syndrome or heart failure. Furosemide and bumetanide should be administered twice daily (preferentially concurrent with sodium ingestion) because of their short duration of action, whereas longer-acting torasemide can be administered once daily. Higher loop diuretic doses might be needed in patients with severe chronic kidney disease with or without albuminuria. However, counter-regulatory rebound sodium retention could abolish the efficacy of loop diuretics in patients with chronic kidney disease in both the short and long term. To overcome this phenomenon, the diuretic dose or dosing frequency could be increased, or sequential nephron blockade using a combination of loop diuretics and thiazides might be needed for patients with resistant hypertension, especially in the presence of edema or heart failure [12]. But, careful monitoring of renal function, serum electrolytes, and fluid status is needed to detect dehydration, hypokalemia, hyponatremia, hypovolemia, or progressive renal dysfunction.

Aldosterone Blockage

Mineralocorticoid Receptor Antagonists as a Fourth-Line Therapy

The suggested fourth-line therapy is to add mineralocorticoid receptor antagonists (MRA, 12.5–25 mg per day spironolactone or 25–50 mg per day eplerenone, to be adapted according to eGFR level) in patients with GFR of 30 mL/min or over and plasma potassium concentrations 4.5 mmol/L or lower or in patients with other indications, such as heart failure with left ventricular dysfunction [13]. MRA reduces BP and left ventricular hypertrophy in patients with resistant hypertension and an eGFR 50–60 mL/min, but it doubles the risk of hyperkalemia when added to ACEi or ARB in patients with moderate chronic kidney disease (eGFR 30–90 mL/min per 1.73 m²) [14]. The long-term effects of MRA on renal and cardiovascular outcomes, mortality, and safety in patients with CKD still remain to be established. ESH guidelines do not recommend the routine use of MRA in patients with CKD, especially in combination with RAS blockers, because of the risk of further renal impairment and hyperkalemia [13].

Spironolactone Versus α-Blocker and/or Beta-Blocker

As mentioned previously, most commonly accepted hypothesis for resistant hypertension is excessive sodium retention due to impaired sodium excretion during the day. Usage of diuretics sufficiently to deal with sodium retention is also one of the most effective additional treatments. Thus, spironolactone would be superior to non-diuretic add-on drugs at lowering BP in resistant hypertension.

In this perspective, in PATHWAY study, investigators compared the effectiveness of spironolactone (25–50 mg) as add-on drugs to bisoprolol (5–10 mg), doxazosin modified release (4–8 mg), and placebo according to BP control during 12 months [15]. They enrolled 314 patients with resistant hypertension who were receiving at least three antihypertensive agents, including a diuretic, at full or maximum tolerated doses in the study. The primary endpoints consisted of the difference in home SBP between spironolactone versus placebo, average of doxazosin and bisoprolol, and each of doxazosin and bisoprolol. The average reduction in home SBP by spironolactone was superior to placebo (−8.70 mmHg), superior to the mean of the other two active treatments (doxazosin and bisoprolol; −4.26 mmHg), and superior when compared with the individual treatments, versus doxazosin (−4.03 mmHg) and versus bisoprolol (−4.48 mmHg). Spironolactone was the most effective treatment for almost 60% of all patients, and they concluded that it was at least three times the proportion in whom doxazosin or bisoprolol was the most effective. Spironolactone was well tolerated and did not increase drug discontinuation owing to renal impairment, hyperkalemia, or gynecomastia compared with placebo and the other active treatments. Serum potassium exceeded 6.0 mmol/L in only six of the 285 patients, who received spironolactone. Consequently, they suggested that spironolactone was the most effective add-on drug for the treatment of resistant hypertension. As indicated above, ESH guideline does not recommend the routine use of MRA in patients with CKD, especially in combination with RAS blockers, but 12.5–25 mg per day spironolactone can be given safely to patients as add-on drugs with eGFR of 30 mL/min or over and plasma potassium concentrations 4.5 mmol/L or lower, and close monitoring should be done when using higher dose of spironolactone.

Deal with Enhanced Sympathetic Activation: Beta-Blockers

The sympathetic nervous system is activated in CKD which acts an important role in the progression of renal dysfunction and contributes to the onset and progression of cardiovascular disease including resistant hypertension. It has demonstrated that patients treated with metoprolol had similar clinical composite outcomes (renal function decline, onset of end-stage renal disease, and/or death) with patients treated with amlodipine [16]. β-blockers are the drug of choice and can be used at any stage in CKD, especially in patients with coexisting coronary artery disease, heart failure, or arrhythmias. If BP remains uncontrolled, a β-blocker (preferably with a hepatic elimination route including metoprolol, carvedilol, nebivolol, and propranolol to avoid drug accumulation which could lead to an increased risk of bradyarrhythmias) could be appropriate agent to deal with resistant hypertension [2].

A New Approach: Endothelin Receptor Antagonists

Endothelin is a potent vasoconstrictor peptide derived from the endothelium. Increased circulating endothelin concentrations are determined in patients with hypertension indicating the potential therapeutic value of the endothelin receptor blockade. Especially, it might meet a significant need in patients with resistant hypertension. Because none of the standard antihypertensive therapies including renin-angiotensin system blockers, diuretics, and calcium-channel blockers do not inhibit vasoconstrictor effects of endothelin type A receptor, effectively. To date, several clinical studies have investigated whether endothelin receptor antagonists (ERAs), both selective and nonselective, might be a promising treatment option in hypertensive patients.

Bosentan is a nonselective, sulfonamide-type ERA which is often used in pulmonary hypertension. Its antihypertensive effect was studied in 93 patients with mild-to-moderate essential hypertension [17]. Patients were randomly assigned to receive one of four oral doses of bosentan (100, 500, or 1000 mg once daily or 1000 mg twice daily), placebo, or the enalapril (20 mg once daily) for 4 weeks. As compared with placebo, bosentan provided further decline in both DPB and SBP with a daily dose of 500 or 2000 mg (an absolute reduction of 5.7 mmHg at each dose in DBP) which was similar to the reduction with enalapril (5.8 mmHg) without activation of the sympathetic nervous system. In addition, the reductions in mean 24-h, daytime, and nighttime DP in the bosentan groups (greatest with 2000 mg) were significantly larger than those in the placebo group.

Darusentan is a selective, propionic acid-based ERA with higher affinity for the type A receptor. In a multicenter randomized, dose-response study, 392 patients with stage 1 or 2 hypertension were randomized to darusentan (10 mg, 30 mg, and 100 mg) and placebo [18]. As compared with placebo, darusentan at a dose of 100 mg once daily significantly decreased both DBP (8.3 mmHg) and SBP

(11.3 mmHg) after 6 weeks of treatment. Later studies have focused on the impact of ERAs in the setting of resistant hypertension. In a randomized trial, 379 patients (96 of them were CKD patients) with resistant hypertension who were receiving at least three antihypertensive agent, including a diuretic, at full or maximum tolerated doses were randomly assigned to 14 weeks treatment with placebo or darusentan 50 mg, 100 mg, or 300 mg taken once daily [19]. The primary endpoints were changes in office SBP and DBP. As compared to placebo, darusentan provided further reduction in both SBP (9 mmHg) and DBP (5 mmHg) in patients with resistant hypertension who already receiving standard antihypertensive treatment. In addition, darusentan produced sustained BP reductions across the 24-h dosing interval and obtained significant reduction in ABPM. Moreover, in subgroup analysis, similar decreases in SBP and DBP with darusentan were achieved in CKD patients with resistant hypertension. Generally, darusentan was well tolerated, the main adverse effects being related to fluid retention.

Despite clear evidence of a key role for the endothelin system in BP control and hypertension, the clinical use of ERAs to treat hypertension has not yet been approved. A major disadvantage has been the relatively high incidence of side effects, notably hepatotoxicity with the sulfonamide drugs bosentan, and fluid retention with all ERAs. Fluid retention fortunately seems amenable to management with diuretics, and to some degree, these side effects appear dose related, and certain studies have been criticized for excessive dosing. Probably ERAs will not have been destined to become first-line therapy for treating essential hypertension, but ERAs have excellent potential for providing benefit to select subgroups of patients especially with resistant hypertension accompanied by fluid management with effective diuretic therapy.

Dual ACE/ARB Inhibition

Proteinuria can be lowered by dual RAS blockade with ACEi and ARBs or with direct renin inhibitors to a greater extent than either RAS blocker alone. However, this combination has not been shown to improve BP control or improve cardiovascular outcomes compared with single RAS blockade in patients with resistant hypertension, although it might preserve renal function in patients with diabetes and chronic kidney disease to some extent, according to a recent network meta-analysis [20]. Additionally, this combination increases the risk of hyperkalemia, hypotension, and acute renal failure. Dual RAS blockade is discouraged by the guidelines [13]. Replacement of ACEi and ARB with other antihypertensive drugs in patients with advanced chronic kidney disease (stages 4–5) should be considered when there are no contraindications, such as heart failure or when discontinuation of the drug is expected to relieve side effects such as hyperkalemia, acute kidney injury, or symptomatic hypotension [2].

Deal with Non-dipping Status: Chronotherapy

The non-dipping pattern refers the situation of impaired circadian BP rhythm, and it is defined as decrement in SDP and/or DBP less than 10% during the night. Non-dipper has particular importance, and the prevalence of abnormally high sleep BP is very often in CKD patients. It was shown that the capacity of excreting sodium during daytime is a significant determinant of nocturnal BP and dipping pattern as reduced capacity leads to higher nocturnal BP and non-dipping pattern [21]. Non-dipping BP is associated with target organ damage including left ventricular hypertrophy, higher prevalence of proteinuria and higher risk of CKD progression, and poorer cardiovascular outcomes. In patients with true resistant hypertension, non-dipping pattern is associated with nearly twofold increased risk of cardiovascular morbidity and mortality. Thus, therapeutic restoration of normal physiologic BP reduction during nighttime sleep (dipping status) is the most significant independent predictor of decreased risk and the basis for the chronotherapy. Chronotherapy is a therapeutic strategy of taking at least one dose of antihypertensive medications at bedtime, instead of all in the morning time to provide dipping status (normal circadial variation) and ABMP control.

Chronotherapy Against to Non-dipping Pattern

Several studies have investigated the effect of chronotherapy on the ABPM control and the non-dipping pattern. The Monitorización Ambulatoria para Predicción de Eventos Cardiovasculares (MAPEC) is a prospective randomized study which examines the effect of chronotherapy on ABPM and clinical outcomes (primary endpoint including composite of all-cause mortality and cardiovascular events) in 2156 patients with untreated or resistant hypertension [22]. Study population divided into two groups consisting of control group, took all antihypertensive medications in the morning and the treatment group and took one or more antihypertensive at bedtime. Patients were followed during median of 5.6 years with a primary composite endpoint of all-cause mortality and total cardiovascular events. 48-h ABPM was performed to patients at least annually. Patients randomized to the treatment arm (bedtime administration) demonstrated lower sleep-time BP, a higher rate of controlled ABPM (62% vs. 53%, $p < 0.001$), and a much lower incidence of the non-dipper status (34% versus 62%, $p < 0.001$). As a clinical outcome, those in the bedtime administration group had a reduction in the primary endpoint of 11.95 versus 27.8 events per 1000 patient-years, NNT = 63 over 1 year. All-cause mortality alone was also reduced (2.11 versus 4.16 events per 1000 patient-years, NNT 488 over 1 year). It has been concluded that switching at least one medication to bedtime administration is cost-effective, simple intervention that contributes to improve BP control and reduce cardiovascular events. In another interesting study, 27 consecutive patients with resistant hypertension and non-dipper BP pattern on ABPM were enrolled to investigate whether shifting all non-diuretic antihypertensive drugs from morning to evening (maintaining the same drugs at the same doses) improves ABPM control after 6 weeks. At the end of the study, they determined significant decrement in ABPM (SBP: 140.5 ± 10.4 to 135.7 ± 12.5 mmHg and DBP: 80.5 ± 9.6 to 73.8 ± 9.3 mmHg), and 15% of the patients restored dipping pattern (normal circadian rhythm) after the drug shift, while no changes were observed in the control group [23]. Consequently, chronotherapy suggests a prospect to recover nocturnal BP control and the non-dipper pattern without changing the total number of medications.

Chronotherapy: A Promising Approach in Hypertensive Patients with CKD

Several studies suggest that chronotherapy is a promising approach in hypertensive patients with CKD. In one of them, 32 patients with CKD (eGFR of 46 ± 12 mL/min/$1.73m^2$) and night-day ratio of mean ABPM greater than 0.9 indicating non-dipper status but with normal daytime ABPM (<135/85 mmHg) were enrolled in the study [24]. They were treated with 2.4 ± 1.4 of antihypertensive drugs consisted of ACEi, ARB, thiazide diuretic, calcium channel blockers, and beta-blockers. It was investigated whether shifting 1 antihypertensive drug from morning to evening (except diuretics to avoid patient discomfort caused by nocturnal diuresis) after 8 weeks provides changing in the percentage of patients with night-day ratio of mean ABPM from greater than 0.9–0.9 or less. After the drug shift, normal circadian rhythm is restored in 87.5% of patients independently from number and class of shifted drug. In addition, significant decrement in office blood pressure in the morning (from SBP: 136 ± 16 to131 ± 13, DBP: 77 ± 10 to 75 ± 8 mmHg) and in proteinuria (especially in patients with >300 mg proteinuria) were obtained at the end of the study. It was concluded that changing the timing of antihypertensive therapy decreased nocturnal blood pressure and proteinuria in non-dipper patients with CKD with limitation of the absence of a control group and patients with severe proteinuria or uncontrolled daytime ABPM. Consequently, it has shown that time of ingestion of hypertension medications can affect circadian patterns of BP in this study, but whether this translates into an effect on clinical outcomes has been investigated in another prospective, randomized study. They enrolled 661 patients with CKD (eGFR <60 mL/min/$1.73m^2$ and/or albuminuria defined as albumin excretion ≥ 30 mg/24-h urine) to compare the effects of taking at least one of prescribed hypertension medications at bedtime to taking them all upon awakening according to cardiovascular outcomes (a composite of death, myocardial infarction, angina pectoris, revascularization, heart failure, arterial occlusion of lower extremities, occlusion of the retinal artery, and stroke) [25]. After a median follow-up period of 5.4 years, it was reported that patients who took at least one antihypertensive medication at bedtime had nearly one third risk of patients who took all medications upon awakening for total cardiovascular events. In addition, patients on bedtime treatment had a significantly lower mean sleep-time BP and a greater proportion demonstrated control of their ABPM (56% versus 45%, $P = 0.003$). Each 5-mmHg decrease in mean sleep-time systolic BP was related with a 14% reduction in the risk for cardiovascular events during follow-up. They concluded that patients with CKD and hypertension, taking at least one antihypertensive medication at bedtime, improve control of BP and reduce the risk for cardiovascular events. Therefore, changing at least one antihypertensive medication to bedtime dosing should be considered in CKD patients with resistant and/or non-dipping hypertension.

Other Drugs

If BP remains uncontrolled, an α-blocker or a centrally acting α-agonists, which preferably do not require dose adjustments (methyldopa or clonidine), could be used. Direct vasodilators such as hydralazine or minoxidil are sometimes used but could induce severe fluid retention and tachycardia, especially minoxidil which has other side effects (hirsutism, pericardial effusion).

Conclusion

Resistant hypertension is failure to achieve target blood pressure despite the use of three or more appropriately dosed antihypertensive drugs including a diuretic. It is still a common clinical problem, especially in patients with chronic kidney disease. First approach should be dealing with barriers for optimum drug therapy including adverse effects of ongoing treatment, insufficient treatment, interfering vasopressor substance or medication, and excessive salt or alcohol intake. Subsequently, next approach should target factors that contribute to the resistant hypertension including impaired handling of sodium and volume expansion, increased activity of the renin-angiotensin-aldosterone system, enhanced sympathetic activity, and reduced endothelium-dependent vasodilation. Pharmacological interferences should be applied including appropriate diuretic therapy, aldosterone blockage, beta-blocker, and chronotherapy to deal with resistant hypertension in chronic kidney disease. An algorithm for resistant hypertension treatment in CKD is shown in Fig. 14.1.

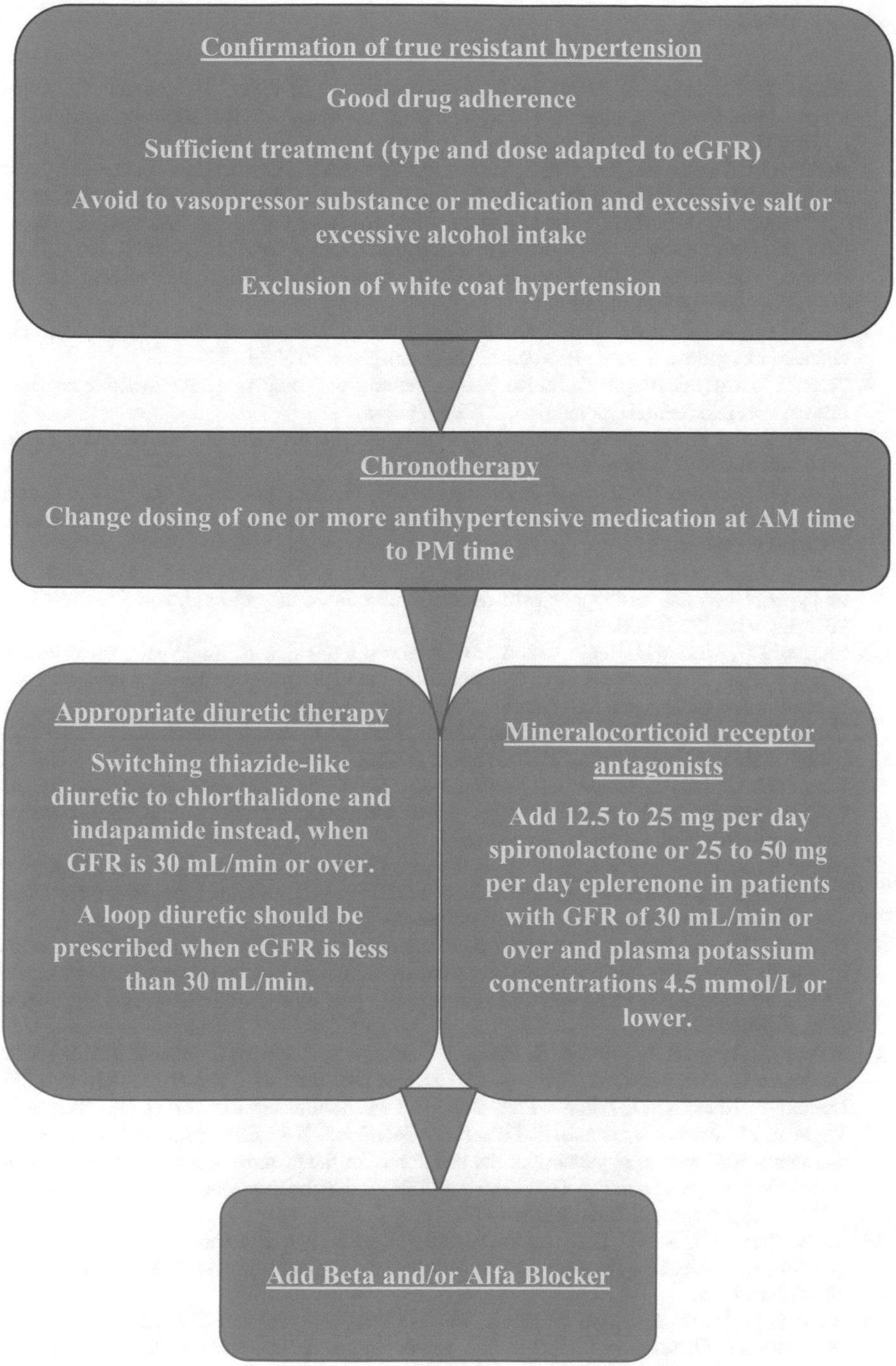

Confirmation of true resistant hypertension

Good drug adherence

Sufficient treatment (type and dose adapted to eGFR)

Avoid to vasopressor substance or medication and excessive salt or excessive alcohol intake

Exclusion of white coat hypertension

Chronotherapy

Change dosing of one or more antihypertensive medication at AM time to PM time

Appropriate diuretic therapy

Switching thiazide-like diuretic to chlorthalidone and indapamide instead, when GFR is 30 mL/min or over.

A loop diuretic should be prescribed when eGFR is less than 30 mL/min.

Mineralocorticoid receptor antagonists

Add 12.5 to 25 mg per day spironolactone or 25 to 50 mg per day eplerenone in patients with GFR of 30 mL/min or over and plasma potassium concentrations 4.5 mmol/L or lower.

Add Beta and/or Alfa Blocker

Fig. 14.1 An algorithm for resistant hypertension treatment in chronic kidney disease

References

1. Krause T, Lovibond K, Caulfield M, McCormack T, Williams B, and the Guideline Development Group. Management of hypertension: summary of NICE guidance. BMJ. 2011; 343:d4891.
2. Rossignol P, Massy ZA, Azizi M, Bakris G, Ritz E, Covic A, Goldsmith D, Heine GH, Jager KJ, Kanbay M, Mallamaci F, Ortiz A, Vanholder R, Wiecek A, Zoccali C, London GM, Stengel B, Fouque D; ERA-EDTA EURECA-m working group; Red de Investigación Renal (REDINREN) network; Cardiovascular and Renal Clinical Trialists (F-CRIN INI-CRCT) network. The double challenge of resistant hypertension and chronic kidney disease. Lancet. 2015;386(10003):1588–98. Review.
3. Drexler YR, Bomback AS. Definition, identification and treatment of resistant hypertension in chronic kidney disease patients. Nephrol Dial Transplant. 2014;29:1327–35.
4. Taler SJ, Textor SC, Augustine JE. Resistant hypertension: comparing hemodynamic management to specialist care. Hypertension. 2002;39:982–8.
5. Sato A, Saruta T. Aldosterone-induced organ damage: plasma aldosterone level and inappropriate salt status. Hypertens Res. 2004;27:303–10.
6. Vogt L, Waanders F, Boomsma F, de Zeeuw D, Navis G. Effects of dietary sodium and hydrochlorothiazide on the antiproteinuric efficacy of losartan. J Am Soc Nephrol. 2008;19(5):999–1007.
7. Kidney Disease Outcomes Quality Initiative (KDOQI). K/DOQI clinical practice guidelines on hypertension and antihypertensive agents in chronic kidney disease. Am J Kidney Dis. 2004;43(suppl 1):S1–290.
8. Messerli FH, Makani H, Benjo A, Romero J, Alviar C, Bangalore S. Antihypertensive efficacy of hydrochlorothiazide as evaluated by ambulatory blood pressure monitoring: a meta-analysis of randomized trials. J Am Coll Cardiol. 2011;57(5):590–600.
9. Carter BL, Ernst ME, Cohen JD. Hydrochlorothiazide versus chlorthalidone: evidence supporting their interchangeability. Hypertension. 2004;43:4–9.
10. Ernst ME, Carter BL, Goerdt CJ, Steffensmeier JJ, Phillips BB, Zimmerman MB, Bergus GR. Comparative antihypertensive effects of hydrochlorothiazide and chlorthalidone on ambulatory and office blood pressure. Hypertension. 2006 Mar;47(3):352–8.
11. Dussol B, Moussi-Frances J, Morange S, Somma-Delpero C, Mundler O, Berland Y. A pilot study comparing furosemide and hydrochlorothiazide in patients with hypertension and stage 4 or 5 chronic kidney disease. J Clin Hypertens. 2012;14:32–7.
12. Bobrie G, Frank M, Azizi M, Peyrard S, Boutouyrie P, Chatellier G, Laurent S, Menard J, Plouin PF. Sequential nephron blockade versus sequential renin-angiotensin system blockade in resistant hypertension: a prospective, randomized, open blinded endpoint study. J Hypertens. 2012;30(8):1656–64.
13. Mancia G, Fagard R, Narkiewicz K, Redón J, Zanchetti A, Böhm M, Christiaens T, Cifkova R, De Backer G, Dominiczak A, Galderisi M, Grobbee DE, Jaarsma T, Kirchhof P, Kjeldsen SE, Laurent S, Manolis AJ, Nilsson PM, Ruilope LM, Schmieder RE, Sirnes PA, Sleight P, Viigimaa M, Waeber B, Zannad F, Task Force Members. 2013 ESH/ESC guidelines for the management of arterial hypertension: the task force for the management of arterial hypertension of the European Society of Hypertension (ESH) and of the European Society of Cardiology (ESC). J Hypertens. 2013;31(7):1281–357.
14. Liu G, Zheng XX, Xu YL, Lu J, Hui RT, Huang XH. Effect of aldosterone antagonists on blood pressure in patients with resistant hypertension: a meta-analysis. J Hum Hypertens. 2015;29:159–66.
15. Williams B, MacDonald TM, Morant S, Webb DJ, Sever P, McInnes G, Ford I, Cruickshank JK, Caulfield MJ, Salsbury J, Mackenzie I, Padmanabhan S, Brown MJ; British Hypertension Society's PATHWAY Studies Group. Spironolactone versus placebo, bisoprolol, and doxazosin to determine the optimal treatment for drug-resistant hypertension (PATHWAY-2): a randomized, double-blind, crossover trial. Lancet. 2015;386(10008):2059–68.

16. Tomiyama H, Yamashina A. Beta-blockers in the management of hypertension and/or chronic kidney disease. Int J Hypertens. 2014;2014:919256.
17. Krum H, Viskoper RJ, Lacourciere Y, Budde M, Charlon V. The effect of an endothelin-receptor antagonist, bosentan, on blood pressure in patients with essential hypertension. Bosentan hypertension investigators. N Engl J Med. 1998;338(12):784–90.
18. Nakov R, Pfarr E, Eberle S, on behalf of the HEAT Investigators. Darusentan: an effective endothelin receptor antagonist for treatment of hypertension. Am J Hypertens. 2002;15:583–89.
19. Weber MA, Black H, Bakris G, Krum H, Linas S, Weiss R, Linseman JV, Wiens BL, Warren MS, Lindholm LH. A selective endothelin-receptor antagonist to reduce blood pressure in patients with treatment-resistant hypertension: a randomised, double-blind, placebo-controlled trial. Lancet. 2009;374(9699):1423–31.
20. Palmer SC, Mavridis D, Navarese E, Craig JC, Tonelli M, Salanti G, Wiebe N, Ruospo M, Wheeler DC, Strippoli GF. Comparative efficacy and safety of blood pressure-lowering agents in adults with diabetes and kidney disease: a network meta-analysis. Lancet. 2015;385(9982):2047–56.
21. Bankir L, Bochud M, Maillard M, Bovet P, Gabriel A, Burnier M. Nighttime blood pressure and nocturnal dipping are associated with daytime urinary sodium excretion in African subjects. Hypertension. 2008;51(4):891–8.
22. Hermida RC, Ayala DE, Mojón A, Fernández JR. Influence of circadian time of hypertension treatment on cardiovascular risk: results of the MAPEC study. Chronobiol Int. 2010;27(8):1629–51.
23. Almirall J, Comas L, Martinez-Ocana JC, et al. Effects of chronotherapy on blood pressure control in non-dipper patients with refractory hypertension. Nephrol Dial Transplant. 2012;27:1855–9.
24. Minutolo R, Gabbai FB, Borrelli S, Scigliano R, Trucillo P, Baldanza D, Laurino S, Mascia S, Conte G, De Nicola L. Changing the timing of antihypertensive therapy to reduce nocturnal blood pressure in CKD: an 8-week uncontrolled trial. Am J Kidney Dis. 2007;50(6):908–17.
25. Hermida RC, Ayala DE, Mojón A, Fernández JR. Bedtime dosing of antihypertensive medications reduces cardiovascular risk in CKD. J Am Soc Nephrol. 2011;22(12):2313–21.

Chapter 15
Public Health Efforts for Earlier Resistant Hypertension Diagnosis, Reduction of Salt Content in Food, Promotion of the Use of Polypills to Facilitate Better Adherence, and Reimbursement Policies

Nursen Keles, Yusuf Yilmaz, and Mustafa Caliskan

Introduction

In the developed and developing world, one in three adults suffers from hypertension, which is the most common chronic condition that primary care physicians and other health practitioners deal with.

There are many other risk factors seen in patients alongside hypertension; these include lipid abnormalities, glucose intolerance or diabetes, a history in the family of early cardiovascular events, obesity, as well as smoking.

Even though there are well-established approaches to the diagnosis and treatment of the disease, there has been limited success in treating hypertension, and in many communities less than half of all hypertensive patients have well-controlled blood pressure [1].

Resistant Hypertension Definition in Patients with High Cardiovascular Risk

The Eighth Joint National Committee (JNC 8) has released hypertension guidelines which recommend the goal of treatment of hypertension to be <140/90 mmHg for patients with CKD although the American Society of Hypertension (ASH) in

N. Keles, M.D. • Y. Yilmaz, M.D.
Department of Cardiology, Istanbul Medeniyet University, Goztepe
Training and Research Hospital, Istanbul, Turkey

M. Caliskan, Prof (✉)
Department of Cardiology, Medeniyet University, Goztepe Training
and Research Hospital, Istanbul, Turkey
e-mail: caliskandr@gmail.com; caliskandr46@yahoo.com

© Springer International Publishing AG 2017   233
A. Covic et al. (eds.), *Resistant Hypertension in Chronic Kidney Disease*,
DOI 10.1007/978-3-319-56827-0_15

Table 15.1 Causes of
"pseudo-resistant"
hypertension

Inaccurate measurement of BP
Inappropriate drug choices or doses
Nonadherence to prescribed therapy
White-coat effect

collaboration with the International Society of Hypertension suggests the goal of treatment of hypertension to be <140/90 mmHg for patients with CKD without albuminuria, and they have also acknowledged that it is recommended by some experts that the goal of hypertension treatment be <130/80 mmHg for patients with CKD with albuminuria [1].

Resistant hypertension (RHT) is a clinical situation in which, despite concomitant intake of at least three antihypertensive drugs, one of these preferably being a diuretic at full doses, blood pressure remains uncontrolled [2]. The American Heart Association (AHA) [3] defines patients who need four or more drugs to control their blood pressure as resistant.

Originally defined to identify a group of high-risk patients who may benefit from specialized care, resistant hypertension included the evaluation and treatment of the secondary causes of hypertension. JNC 7 defined resistant hypertension as the inability to achieve blood pressure that is lower than 140/90 mmHg even with optimal doses of three of more hypertensive drugs including one diuretic [4]. Resistant hypertension is defined by the 2008 AHA as uncontrolled hypertension despite treatment with at least three hypertensive drugs or controlled hypertension with at least four drugs [3]. This definition of resistant hypertension does not even attempt to make a distinction between resistant and pseudo-resistant hypertension. Patients suffering from pseudo-resistant hypertension are those individuals with elevated office BPs due to white-coat hypertension, improper BP measurement, or medication nonadherence, which is not true resistant hypertension [5, 6] (Table 15.1). To emphasize that pseudo-resistance hadn't been excluded, the term apparent resistant hypertension was adopted in epidemiological studies for those patients with an office BP of >140/90 mmHg while taking ≥3 antihypertensive medications [7]. After 24 h of ambulatory BP monitoring, pseudo-resistance is excluded; the true resistance can be made from the apparent resistance through the proper office BP measurement technique and confirmation of medication adherence. Due to this, true resistant hypertension is defined as a properly measured office BP >140/90 mmHg with a mean 24-h ambulatory BP >130/80 mmHg in a patient confirmed to be taking ≥3 antihypertensive medications. Excluding participants from the test population with pseudo-resistant hypertension is one of the challenges in establishing the prevalence of true resistant hypertension.

Public Health Efforts for Earlier Resistant Hypertension Diagnosis

From a public health sense, hypertension is the flagship contributor to the pioneering cause of premature death and disability worldwide – cardiovascular disease [8]. For these reasons, family physicians have been overpowered over the years by information and admonishments concerning hypertension. Such information comes from diverse sources. Industry representatives encourage physicians to prescribe drug A instead of drug B. Specialists and key influencers provide complicated messages on which drugs and diagnostic or therapeutic strategies to exercise. Clinical trials are conflicting or contradictory from time to time. Guidelines are comprehensive and often seem to differ between various medical institutions. It is no doubt that family physician has confused for that reason. The last disrespect is that published articles, specialists, and various organizations continuously tell family physician what a loose job they are doing in the management of hypertension, either straight-out or by implication. Articles in journals assert that "specialized" hypertension care is better than "ordinary" care. On the contrary, publications that actually furnish real-life, helpful advice in hypertension management are scarce, if any. Furthermore, in spite of the reprimand toward family physicians, almost no infrastructure or resources have been given to improve the level of "ordinary" care. Many of these issues have begun to be recognized by professional institutions, health authorities, and governments. The constructive problems with regard to the hypertension management in primary care have not gone overlooked. Consequently, a few initiatives are initiated to give better support to family physicians and to the health-care system in the management of hypertension in general. Therefore, chronic care model is established to improve the level of care for persons having chronic diseases [9]. In this model, the presentation of care is treated under various domains that include health system organization, community resources, information systems, decision support, patient self-management, and delivery system design. Until now, there has been rare organized effort for prevention, early detection, and ongoing management of chronic diseases. Furthermore, two systems of care appear to be developed: the specialist-based acute care system and family physician-based primary care system. These two systems have separated and appear to function independently from each other. The diseases like hypertension are now being mentioned system-wide in an integrated fashion. For instance, the presentation of hypertension care may begin with a central disease registry. This lets the system to know a submitted patient with a particular disease. Later, the level of disease complexity and severity may pave the way for triaging patients to the most suitable care. This may refer to that patients such as those with just diagnosed hypertension are treated by family physician, whereas patients with resistant or complex hypertension are treated by a specialized team. The association of family doctors creates primary care networks that is responsible for managing patients with chronic diseases and granted with extra funding for this purpose. To cater this care, these primary care networks are recruiting allied health professionals such as nurses, nurse practitioners, pharmacists, social workers, and other individuals. These health-care professionals work with doctors, usually benefiting from care maps or algorithms to give care to patients with hypertension. A significant element of this partnership is the upkeep of ordinary follow-up, assuring guidelines are tracked, promoting patient self-management, and founding defined linkages to specialist services and the health-care infrastructure. In practice, when the hypertension is diagnosed, a clinic nurse may take patient's blood pressure regularly, arrange medications within preset parameters, and assure that necessary testing is conducted. The family physician may observe the patient periodically or in the event of difficulties that arise. If the primary care team faces difficulties in patient management, a specialist or specialty team should be consulted. In this system, there is a change in the responsibility of the specialist. First of all, the specialist may serve with their own multidisciplinary team. Instead of seeing every patient, the specialists now observe only the more complicated patients. While this may give way to more suitable use of specialist talents, it may also pave the way for financial fines for the specialist. Another responsibility of the specialist under the chronic care system is to help educate and coach the primary care-based physicians and teams. By this way, specialists may realize satellite clinics in primary care, communicate in academic detailing, ensue group education sessions, or be ready for several distant consultation. In this altered health-care system, extended evaluation and monitoring are predominant. Health-care teams and regions are responsible for results. Indicator's system is regularly expanded, with feedback being displayed to respective physicians and to the system in overall. For instance, a physician may submit an information on the number of hypertensive patients at blood pressure objectives in his or her practice. Definitely, the unnatural separation between diseases is eliminated, and the system endeavors to cure the patient as a whole rather than the disease.

Information systems are important for enabling the changes as specified above. An electronic central registry assures beneficial data to public health officers which enable preventative or screening measures for hypertension to be aimed at high-risk populations. A central registry also ensures information on disease load that supports in the planning and prediction of health-care services. Central registries are entwined to other data repositories to ensure patient and physician reminders and alerts. For instance, local disease management software may associate an accustomed lipid level with the fact that a patient is hypertensive, reminding the physician to start lipid-lowering therapy. Decision support installed in electronic schedules can cater for similar support at primary care. Care to patients with hypertension and other chronic diseases is generally compromised by the failure to share medical information about patients. By this way, the medication record of a patient with hypertension who alters physicians may not be fully recognized, potentially giving way to adverse drug effects. The Western Health Information Collaborative project is commonly financed by the federal government and four western regional governments. A significant aim of this project is to create data standards for chronic disease that will ensure the sharing of core data between jurisdictions and care providers [10]. Three main chronic diseases have been classified by the Western Health Information Collaborative project: diabetes, chronic kidney disease, and

Table 15.2 Lifestyle changes as adjunctive therapy for antihypertensive medication

Weight reduction
Increasing physical activity
Moderation of alcohol consumption
Adoption of the Dietary Approaches to Stop Hypertension (DASH) diet
Dietary salt reduction
Smoking cessation

hypertension. Thus, data sharing around hypertensive patients should be achievable in the four western provinces soon.

The self-management of hypertension is significant of its treatment. The patient can manage their conditions. For instance, blood pressure monitoring at home has been gradually underscored over the years, with available 2006 recommendations bringing forward that all patients with hypertension monitor themselves [11] and the results of the recent studies support that own blood pressure monitoring is useful prognostic predictor and succeed better in blood pressure control [12, 13]. In the similar way, adherence to lifestyle advice can also mostly enhance blood pressure levels and decline other cardiovascular risk factors (Table 15.2). The primary care physician is important for both introducing and continually reassuring patient self-management. In the same way, primary care groups or the health system itself can ease self-management by courtesy of the arrangement of educational and motivational programs, patient portals, and engagement of other community resources.

Pseudo-Resistant Hypertension due to Poor Medication Adherence

In the beginning, a large number of the patients were considered to have resistant hypertension; in clinical trials in which the participants were aggressively titrated to reach a target BP, the prevalence of RHT was estimated to be 20–30% [14]. Although a large amount of the studies determine RHT based on the medical adherence and optimal levels of drug prescriptions and blood pressure first, it should be confirmed that the patients with resistant hypertension do have true RHT; this can be done by ruling out or correcting factors associated with pseudo-resistance which include an inaccurate measurement of BP, inappropriate drug choices or doses, and the nonadherence to prescribed therapy or the white-coat effect [15, 16]. The prevalence of RHT has been re-estimated to be below 15% as a significant group of patients with RHT were actually considered to have "pseudo-resistant" hypertension [17].

A major methodological strength is the exclusion of patients with pseudo-resistance due to nonadherence with prescribed antihypertensive medications; this determination has been lacking in prior epidemiologic assessments of RHT [17]. It was observed that 152 (43.9%) of 359 patients did not adhere to antihypertensive therapy in an investigation to determine the association between adherence to anti-hypertensive treatment and BP control in hypertensive outpatients, and 40 patients (11.1%) met criteria for RHT. "Pseudo-resistance" is commonly misdiagnosed as resistant hypertension, so in that sample, 98 of the 157 (62.4%) patients who showed uncontrolled BP with the correct antihypertensive treatment were nonadherers and therefore could be diagnosed as patients with resistant hypertension. This data indicated that nonadherence is an important although lesser known problem with patients suffering from RHT. These data indicate that nonadherence is an important, yet lesser known, problem among patients with RHT. Prior studies on resistant hypertension are limited by the failure to apply a uniform definition of resistant hypertension, a lack of longitudinal blood pressure data, and an inability to identify "pseudo-resistant" hypertension due to poor medication adherence, according to Daugherty et al. [18]. Because of this, trained pairs of pharmacy students and health community agents used a standardized protocol to measure BP with the values of systolic (SBP) and diastolic (DBP) blood pressure being obtained by the mean of six blood pressure measurements, carried out by the research team during three visits over a 2 week period, using mercury sphygmomanometers calibrated with a minimum interval of 10 min between each double measurement. The measurements were taken at the patients' homes with the effect being the reduction of the influence of the white-coat effect [19]. A validated Portuguese version of the eight-item Morisky Medication Adherence Scale (MMAS-8) was used to assess adherence [20]. If the patients had a score greater or equal to 6 in the MMAS-8, they were considered to be adherent in this study [21]. Each patient supplied informed consent, and the study protocol and consent form was approved by the Federal University of Alagoas' institutional review board. As the self-reporting methods have a major limitation in underestimating the number of nonadherent individuals, the proportion of nonadherent patients could be even higher. The adherence behavior of patients and potential reasons for nonadherence can be gained from self-reporting scales as they are usually simple, rapid, noninvasive, and economical in their methods. An objective technique that is used to assess drug intake in these cases of apparent resistant hypertension is toxicological urine screenings. Since the 1980s, there has been a systematic development of the analytical procedures for a general toxicological screening in urine, first using gas chromatography–mass spectrometry (GC–MS) [22, 23]. The development of analytical procedures for the detection of various drug classes [24, 25] including antihypertensive drugs [26, 27] is thanks to the recent improvement of liquid chromatography–mass spectrometry (LC–MS) instrumentation. Individuals with a lower quality of life in terms of health are more likely to have lower adherence to antihypertensive medications, and therefore the diagnosis of resistant hypertension should fundamentally include investigation of nonadherence and its causes [28]. This may result in the successful treatment of hypertension as well as avoiding the expense and invasive therapeutic approaches that include excessive antihypertensive therapy (although polypharmacy is difficult to avoid because blood pressure can be controlled by using one drug in only about 50% of patients [17], electrical stimulation of carotid baroreceptors, catheter-based renal denervation, and recent drug therapies (e.g., selective endothelin type A compounds, such as darusentan)) [16]. To summarize, a relevant or possibly the main cause of pseudo-resistant hypertension appears to be nonadherence to prescribed anti-hypertensives. The identification and removing of this factor provides the normalization of BP levels and the ability of ruling out the resistant hypertension diagnosis that prevents overtreatment and expensive or excessive evaluation.

How the Public Health Policies Promote Lifestyle Interventions to Prevent Development of RHT

As the popularity of RHT is supposed to increase [3], effective treatments to enhance results among individuals with RHT are required. Treatment methods being researched for the management of RHT contain invasive, irreversible procedures or implantable devices such as renal denervation and carotid baroreceptor stimulation. Nonetheless, it is significant to specify the efficacy of less invasive approaches to spare individuals the inconvenience and possible complications that come from these procedures. Hypertension guidelines generally advise lifestyle changes, including weight reduction, increasing physical activity, moderation of alcohol consumption, adoption of the Dietary Approaches to Stop Hypertension (DASH) diet, dietary salt reduction, and smoking cessation, as adjunctive therapy to antihypertensive medication [2, 4]. Partly, these advices rise from studies that have shown a relation between lifestyle factors and morbidity/mortality among hypertensive individuals [29, 30].

   All patients with resistant hypertension should be advised on lifestyle changes to lower blood pressure. Sodium intake is a great factor contributing to resistant hypertension. Meta-analyses of clinical trials showed that sodium restriction to approximately 1.7 g/day was related with a reduction in office blood pressure by 5/3 mmHg in patients with mild uncomplicated hypertension [31]. The antihypertensive effects of sodium restriction are even more addressed in patients with resistant hypertension. In one study, 24-h ambulatory blood pressure was decreased by 23/9 mmHg when sodium intake was shortened to 1.1 g/day in patients with unchecked blood pressure on a 3-drug regimen that built a diuretic [32]. However, the average sodium consumption in the USA is higher than the level recommended (8.5 g of salt per day). Approximately 75% of the sodium consumed in the USA is acquired from processed foods or restaurant cuisine. Circa 25% of consumed sodium is added at meals [33]. Recommending the patients to read nutritional labels carefully is necessary to limit sodium intake and have a better blood pressure control. Physical inactivity has been specified in more than 40% of patients. Guidelines advised that patients with hypertension should engage in at least 30 min per day of aerobic physical activity most days of the week [2, 3]. A recent randomized trial containing patients with resistant hypertension indicated that a training program, making up of walking on a treadmill three times weekly for 8–12 weeks, significantly declined ambulatory blood pressure by 6/3 mmHg compared with a sedentary control group [34]. By this way, aerobic exercise should be suggested in most patients with resistant hypertension.

Although the value of lifestyle interventions in patients already taking antihypertensive drugs has not been widely examined, the current evidence, obtained firstly in patients treated with one or two drugs, seems promising. Regular exercise alone lowered DBP and led to regression of left ventricular hypertrophy (LVH) in a small study of medicated African-American men with uncontrolled hypertension [35], and the TONE study showed that in elderly patients receiving antihypertensive monotherapy, sodium restriction and weight loss paved the way for improved BP control [36]. Notably, there are limited data showing the effects of the DASH diet in medicated hypertensive patients. In a study of 55 hypertensive patients treated with an angiotensin receptor blocker (ARB), the DASH diet was related with a 5-mmHg greater reduction in ambulatory SBP compared to patients taking the ARB with their regular diet [37]. The ADAPT trial [38] was an Australian study of hypertensive patients treated with one or two drugs in which an intervention designed to promote consumption of a modified DASH diet gives way to a modest (4/2 mmHg), but statistically important, decline in ambulatory BP and declined dependence on antihypertensive medications. In the DEW-IT study [39], a 9-week "feeding" study of 44 overweight adults on a single BP-lowering agent and the DASH diet coupled with weight loss also resulted in significant BP reductions. Notably, lifestyle change has not been correctly evaluated in patients with RHT.

Several small studies, however, put forward that modifications in diet and physical activity have the potential to lower BP substantially in these persons. For instance, in a study of 12 subjects with RHT, 24-hour ambulatory BP was 23/9 mmHg lower on a 50 mmol/day (1150 mg/day) sodium diet compared to a 250 mmol/day (5750 mg/day) sodium diet [32]. In this study, however, the periods of treatment were short (7 days), and all food was prepared in a clinical research center. In the longer term and the absence of specially prepared meals, the similar results may not be accomplished. In another small study, Dimeo et al. [34] checked the value of physical activity in 50 patients with RHT who were randomized to thrice every week treadmill exercise or a control condition; exercise decreased ambulatory daytime BP by 6/3 mmHg. For that reason, preliminary evidence puts forward that lifestyle changes may be effective in diminishing BP in RHT patients, but these efforts required to be examined in more rigorous randomized clinical trials (RCTs.)

Public Policies for Prevention and Treatment of RHT in Europe and the USA

A thorough consideration of public policy is vital to efforts to both prevent and treat hypertension (Table 15.3). This is true not only in Europe, where the public sector is largely responsible for financing health care; it is also the case in the USA, home to an ever-increasing public tranche of costs since the 1960s' implementation of Medicare and Medicaid, growing to 45.6% by 2003, 48.1% in 2006, and predictions of close to 50% [40]. Unfortunately, public funds for prevention do not account for a large share of expenditure. Health data compiled by the Organisation for Economic

Table 15.3 Public policies for prevention and treatment of RHT in Europe and the USA

Patients' organizations
Pharmaceutical reimbursement
Prevention and financial incentives for physicians

Co-operation and Development (OECD) show a range of public spending on "prevention and public health" over 2003/2004 as varying from 7.6% of public sector expenditure in the USA and 8.3% Canada, down to 4.0% in Germany and just 0.8% in Italy [41]. Much of the spread of these figures can be explained by how the private sector is proportionately more important to North American health spending than it is in Europe; this leaves preventative spending greater room within the overall scope of public expenditure. The extent of public spending in Europe is also very likely underreported by the OECD due to official statistics describing state-sponsored prevention "programs" as health-care "treatments." A 2002 study conducted in France which incorporated statistics concerning both approaches concluded that, while spending formally dedicated to prevention was 2.9% of total health expenditure, a further 3.5% termed as "soins et biens médicaux" [medical care and goods] was preventative in nature, leading to a more robust total of 6.4%. This analysis explicitly adds hypertension to the latter group during its discussion of risk factors and the difficulty of distinguishing between care and prevention: "We have in effect considered that uncomplicated forms of diabetes, arterial hypertension and hyperlipidemia are not treated for themselves but rather in order to avoid the advent of serious cardiovascular illness, which justifies their inclusion in the area of prevention" [author's translation of the French original] [42]. And yet there is a large imbalance between preventative expenditures and those on treatment even after this expansion to the scope of prevention, due to the political and economic pressures on public budgets. Strong and immediate demands for medical treatment have effectively discouraged investments in prevention which would pay out in the longer term. In addition to direct public expenditure, policy stakeholders in the public sector can take steps either to advance or to retard private sector actions and spending in the fields of primary and secondary prevention.

Public Policy and Patients' Organizations

If we are to recognize "prehypertension" as being prognostic of possible illness, patients' organizations are natural and committed conduits to reach those people who could benefit from information and advice regarding lifestyle, medication, and risk factors as a means of realizing the challenging personal process of behavioral change. It was for this reason that patient groups organized around cardiovascular disease and hypertension were advised to expand their focus to encompass "pre-patient" education and assistance at the special session in St Gallen. To do so requires a certain, not large, outlay, but patient groups typically rely on outside funding, and some consumer activists suggest they may be vulnerable to financial or informational manipulation by pharmaceutical industry. Gaps in communication between medical professionals and patients could be bridged by a system offering accreditation from the public sector and/or opening the door to reimbursement or eligibility for funds from public coffers to organizations seeking effectively to prevent hypertension. The behavior-altering benefits for (pre-)patients of public funding for patients' organizations could be substantially cheaper and potentially more effective than the "top-down" model of most public sector programs.

Public Policy and Pharmaceutical Reimbursement

Throughout Europe, government intervention in pharmaceutical markets, including pricing and access to reimbursement, has a pronounced effect upon the access of patients to medication, whether this effect be one of denial, delay, rationing, or promotion. This governmental footprint is especially prominent for innovative products, costly as they often are. An overview of a series of Finnish studies of hypertension from 1982–2002 noted that the European emphasis has changed from detecting to treating high blood pressure. The report highlighted reimbursement as an important challenge above and beyond the doctor/patient issues discussed above: "In Finland, the strict reimbursement criteria for antihypertensive drug treatment presented by the national social insurance institution may also play some role in unsatisfactory BP control. In these criteria, the BP levels justifying the reimbursement of antihypertensive drug costs are clearly higher than those recommended by the hypertension guidelines," leading to the conclusion that "in particular, effective antihypertensive drug treatment should have been prescribed for individuals with a moderate or high absolute CVD risk more frequently than at present" [43]. To prescribe medications after the optimum moment, in insufficient amounts, or ones which are cheaper but less effective is hardly a phenomenon unique to Finland, but sadly merely one more instance of the public sector overvaluing short-term budgets over long-term prevention of cardiovascular disease. Governmental policies can stop their own hearts in this way.

Prevention and Financial Incentives for Physicians in the USA

The USA has been the site of a long-running debate on the merits of creating incentives for caregivers to emphasize preventive care. This debate is one more indication of the widely acknowledged need of the US system to provide significantly better care.

Compared with the monolithic nature of European national services, the pluralism characteristic of health-care finances in the USA is simultaneously advantageous and not toward providing incentives to hospitals and individual doctors. This pluralism promotes experimentation and the creation of multiple mechanisms, while systems based upon a "single-payer" principle are often inefficient and slow to change, albeit with exceptions such as the incentive system recently introduced by the NHS in the UK. Unfortunately, single payers have a tendency to hew to single models, often regardless of whether they work well or not.

The opposing weakness of the US system is the multiplicity of health-care insurers and purchasers, which greatly complicates efforts to create incentives effective with group practices and hospitals that may deal with patients insured by a plethora of health-care plans. This situation makes administrative costs high relative to financial incentives. One possible solution to motivate hospitals and physicians would be the creation of collaborative programs between large insurers, supported by CMS (Centers for Medicare and Medicaid Services) [44], the biggest public sector purchaser. One thousand interviews with 35 health plans across 12 major US metro areas indicated that 77% of the plans "...had hospital- or physician-based pay-for-performance strategies that were being actively developed or had pilot or full programs that had already been implemented. Most of the health plan efforts were new, with about one-third of all reported efforts being in the planning or developmental stages...(They) uniformly reported that their goal is to reduce costs through improved quality and provider efficiency." [45].

The same cannot be said of QOF – "Quality and Outcomes Framework" of the UK NHS.

Public Policy Developments in the UK: Financial Incentives for Physicians

QOF was introduced to general practitioners (GPs) in April 2004 by the NHS as a voluntary contractual component. In terms of cardiovascular disease and hypertension, the quality objectives of QOF are preventative to a strong degree, emphasizing improved outcomes by ensuring patients are on the right medication to meet their needs and through early and continued monitoring of risk factors, including cholesterol and BP. The incentives use a "point" system and are rewarded to practices, not single doctors. Good record keeping and diagnosis are reasons for points, as are management both initially and ongoing. The most points are awarded for such improvements of outcomes as meeting or surpassing clinical guidelines across a broad span of patients [46]. QOF is widely seen as a leap forward for preventative care. When it was introduced, an American observer called QOF "...the boldest such proposal attempted anywhere in the world...With one mighty leap, the NHS has vaulted over anything being attempted in the United States, the previous leader in quality improvement studies" [47].

Striking differences between QOF and initiatives forwarded in America include:

• Systemic and national extent
• The near unanimity over its goals and methods

- Its primary care scope, excluding hospitals
- Disinclusion of cost containment among its objectives
- Ample financial incentives to practices to amassing points
- The following steep increase in the NHS's costs, making cutting or ending the program risky for future governments.

Reports about P4P initiatives from America talk about "gaming the system" – a sport that the administrative bureaucracy even of schemes lean on great concepts and requests will often be a loser.

Regardless, although it will take time to see if the outcomes of QOF related to hypertension match the pronouncements of its advocates, it represents a noteworthy attempt to create a new incentive structure for preventative care.

Public Policies for Prevention and Treatment of RHT in Developing Countries Compared to Developed Countries

The low level of awareness of hypertension in developing countries is alarming, and outcomes relating to its treatment and control are no better. Most studies about perceptions of hypertension in these countries show that a mere third or so of their hypertensive population were aware of their condition at the beginning of the study [48–50], a rate which is as low as 18% in some areas [51]. Yet, for whatever reason, this form of self-knowledge is a challenge even in parts of developed countries, for example, Australia, where even with improved rates of screening, some poorer areas still report an awareness of their status among only approximately one-third of hypertensive patients [52]. Complicating the situation, in the developing world, the proportion of known hypertensive patients who have controlled the situation is still low [53]; a study of six middle-income nations reported that control rates were especially low among adult men. In Africa, few countries have a rate of control among hypertensive patients higher than 5% – Gabon reaches 5.6% [54], while one study from Tanzania reported that fewer than 1% of patients with hypertension had BP readings beneath 140/90 mmHg [55]. One way to account for these low rates of awareness and control is that national policy-makers across the developing world may underestimate or misunderstand the threat from noncommunicable diseases, which may be new threats in rapidly changing societies. Undeniably caused at least in part by a shortage of resources for health care, the bigger problem may sometimes be poor prioritization or a lack of medium- to long-term planning, leading to a lack of such basic elements of primary care detection and monitoring as a basic sphygmomanometer. Unfortunately, even when a sphygmomanometer is available, in large parts of the developing world, blood pressure is not measured routinely at primary care checkups. One explanation could be that practitioners are more alert to dramatic complaints such as trauma, infectious disease, or complications of pregnancy. Nonetheless, the threshold among primary care practitioners in middle- and low-income countries is known to be quite low [56]. Innovative new data compiled from collaborative and comparative studies in Southeast Asia and Africa [57] show that much or most of the poor detection and treatment may rise from lack of understanding of hypertension's chronicity made worse by the asymptomatic presentation of the disease, as well as underdeveloped societal conditions including the high cost of often poor-quality health care, the difficulty of finding proper treatment expertise and materials, and unequal access to often inefficient health services.

However, some of the risk factors for the development and for worse outcomes of hypertension appear to be both overnutrition and undernutrition. The complexities of many developing societies undergoing urban transitions are that both of these two forms of malnutrition will coexist within the same population.

One result of the convoluted nature of rapidly urbanizing societies in the developing world is that both forms of malnutrition can be found side-by-side in a population.

An ineluctable first step in the treatment of hypertension anywhere is to understand its epidemiology as well as its natural history; these are often underdescribed in poorer nations, especially in sub-Saharan Africa. Where systematic monitoring of hypertension is in its initial stages, it must be remembered that alongside greater incidence, early estimates may be exaggerated due to greater awareness among the population, facilitating detection, as well as better methods of control, allowing a greater number of people to survive with high BP [58]. A lessened intake of salt directly decreases hypertension [52] and, like obesity, is a rare reversible cause of high blood pressure. As such, it is key in the struggle with hypertension [59]. Additionally, salt intake may be restricted at the individual level through counseling as well as among the population at large through policies limiting the salt found in processed foods like bread [59, 60]. These policies work in the long run because an individual's taste buds can grow accustomed to differing levels of salt content in food. Unfortunately, it is much harder to grow accustomed to a lower salt content than to a higher one, so reducing salt intake will remain a serious challenge for health-care providers and officials [52]. Reducing salt taste thresholds can be done, however, as we know that high salt-content food typically loses its appeal within 4–6 weeks of switching to a diet low in salt [52]. This is why salt reduction at the population level has proved, to date, more cost-effective than clinical interventions [52]. The Global Burden of Disease Study from the World Health Organization (WHO) indicates that lowering the amount of salt in processed foods through action at the level of societies could preserve 21 million or more disability-adjusted life years worldwide – every year [61]. Beneficial effects on blood pressure have been shown to derive from fruit and vegetable fiber, magnesium, and potassium, as well as calcium from low-fat dairy [52, 62]. Obesity is a major cause of hypertension and the efforts increasing physical activity among the population beginning at young ages and decreasing caloric intake may lessen the prevelance of the obesity in the general population.

There have been many success stories in developed countries regarding decreased CVD risk stemming from reduced consumption at the population level of energy-dense and high-fat diets but few parallel examples in developing ones. One exception is Iran, which introduced a program based on the high-risk factor and population strategies to implement positive lifestyle choices in communities and notably brought down the prevalence of hypertriglyceridemia, hypercholesterolemia, abdominal obesity, and hypertension [63]. For individuals, it has been suggested to be beneficial for hypertension to walk a minimum of 10 min a day [49], which should be possible even in urban areas of developing countries.

It will remain difficult to implement clinical approaches to hypertension in poorer countries for a variety of reasons. Many countries in the developing world maintain no precise guidelines regarding hypertension management in their individual setting, and as much as practitioners will be able to look to international guidelines for guidance in their daily practice, the investigations, materials, and medications indicated there may not be available locally. Moreover, in following guidelines not adapted to local needs, considerable variation exists in which international guidelines are adhered to and at what point the practitioners begin to improvise. Adherence to orderly norms in the successful treatment of hypertension is required not just of practitioners, who must follow protocols regarding early detection, but also of patients, especially in taking their medication. Both practitioner awareness of and adherence to protocol were found to be low even where national guidelines had been introduced and broadly promoted among the clinical community [56]. Despite the inevitability of encountering patients with a greater or lesser degree of hypertensive resistance to treatment, the most common cause for poor control of BP remains patient noncompliance with his or her medication regimen.

Stroke is a relatively immediate complication of hypertension under poor control, and reports from South Africa indicate that, among hypertensive patients, those of African descent die at twice the rate of their European-descended counterparts [53]. This likely stems from the fraught interplay of poor education, unequal access to quality health care, and lack of patient compliance. The best way to encourage compliance from a patient's perspective is through education and making the medication regimens simpler. There was a treatment-adherence trial of 500-plus patients for hypertension in Nigeria, both urban and rural but all new to treatment [64]. The treatment program was led by nurses with a doctor for backup and involved the administration of simple treatment of a b-blocker and thiazide diuretic to patients at no charge. The patients were followed up once a month for 6 months. Impressively, after 6 months, 81% of the patients were adhering to treatment, and 66% have controlled hypertension. These excellent results likely come from high-quality patient education, a simple regimen for medication, and the free service they received at the hospital. In Africa, studies have shown that regular attendance at the clinic, avoidance of prescription medication of non-Western origin, and social support were among the factors positively affecting self-reported compliance [65]. Oddly or not, compliance was not associated with beliefs as to the cause thereof. Furthermore, similarly to the rest of the world, and regardless of the method of treatment (traditional or modern), many patients mistakenly believe that they can discontinue their medication when they feel better [66]. Yet data from other countries in the underdeveloped word demonstrates the avidity with which patients with hypertension, a fairly unobtrusive, silent disease, seek out informal care providers for answers and alleviation. Authorities in Bangladesh have acknowledged the importance in the public sector's struggle with an epidemic chronic disease of fostering relationships with informal allopathic practitioners and have acknowledged efforts to standardize information and practice among them [66].

On the whole, the key to increasing medication compliance and to sponsoring healthier lifestyles seems to be education, whether personalized or of a population overall. In both Pakistan and across several different Asian communities, the combined effects of health education at home and a trained GP in controlling blood pressure have been shown to have better cost-effectiveness than standard strategies or either intervention alone, at the same time as being affordable.

Portable kiosks to distribute health information outside either the home or the clinic have proven themselves as an effective means of health education in settings both rural and urban [67]. An alliance of traditional and conventional means of health care was sought in Tanzania by means of the founding of an institute of traditional medicine. These efforts and similar ones in varied developing countries discussed by Joshi et al. [67] are widely perceived as beneficial. Closer to the formal health-care system, pharmacists are often providers of instant BP monitoring and advice about medication. Reports on the impact of pharmacist-provided services suggest improvements to hypertension control and overall quality of life but only in countries with middle-income profiles [68], potentially because of greater use of superior guidelines concerning hypertension management in such countries and more effective regulation and monitoring of pharmacist practice in those countries. A high-tech intervention that takes into account the reliance upon mobile technologies in countries where many have never had home Internet or land-based phone service is the use of cell phones to remind patients when to take their tablets. In combination with BP monitoring performed at home according to clear step-by-step guidance, automated management of this sort has been shown as beneficial for hypertension outcomes [69]. A telephone-based management system, using an automated caller to remind the patient when to take their medication and which gives self-care management tips to each patient based on their own BP measurements and diet, has been shown as beneficial in two middle-to-low-income countries in South America. These systems can even travel over the head of the patients to contact health workers when a patient might be having excessively many high BP readings or if they have self-reported a suboptimal level of compliance [69]. Finally, the lack of social support shown to contribute to poor levels of compliance [70] is addressed with weekly updates sent to a close friend or family member [69]. Unsurprisingly, the greatest reductions in blood pressure were seen among those with lower levels of literacy and those requiring frequent communications regarding the blood pressure – the most vulnerable groups in conventional practice in terms of worse outcomes. This intervention seems in these ways to have hurdled the provider-to-patient barrier in the management of hypertension. Still, like any other intervention, there are gaps concerning our knowledge of the risks, acceptability, effects, and costs over the long term [71].

Treatment of Resistant Hypertension

Medical Treatment

The approach to treatment of resistant hypertension in patients with CKD should have objective to address the multitude of factors that contribute to the pathogenesis of hypertension in this population, including disturbed handling of sodium and volume expansion, increased activity of the renin–angiotensin–aldosterone system (RAAS), improved sympathetic activity, and declined endothelium-dependent vasodilatation. Specific focus should be on the patterns of elevated blood pressure that have been discovered to be more prevalent in this population and to enhance the risk of target organ damage, including elevated nighttime BP and the presence of non-dipping.

Volume

Salt restriction has been indicated to lower blood pressure in patients with and without hypertension. In the Dietary Approaches to Stop Hypertension (DASH)-Sodium trial, sodium reduction from 100 to 50 mmol per day generally had twice the effect on blood pressure as reduction from 150 to 100 mmol per day [72]. The effect of dietary sodium restriction on the degree of BP reduction seems to be particularly powerful in patients with resistant hypertension. In a small, randomized crossover trial of patients with resistant hypertension, a low (50 mmol/day) compared with high (250 mmol/day) sodium diet diminished mean office SBP by 22.7 mmHg and initiated significant declines in daytime, nighttime, and 24-h ambulatory blood pressure [32]. For that reason, patients with resistant hypertension, as well as those with CKD, show salt-sensitive hypertension. Patients with CKD have an impaired skill to effectively excrete sodium and will reply to a sodium load by increasing blood pressure for reconstructing salt balance; this "pressure natriuresis" arrives at the expense of hypertension-related target organ damage [73]. Besides, dietary sodium intake has been indicated to interact with the RAAS, especially aldosterone, in both animal models and human studies, to mediate hypertension, vascular and tissue damage, and kidney disease [74]. In a study of patients with resistant hypertension and high 24-h urinary aldosterone, urinary protein excretion increased considerably with progressively greater salt intake, putting forward that aldosterone excess and high dietary sodium intake interact to increase proteinuria [75]. In fact, in a randomized, double-blind, placebo-controlled crossover study in proteinuric patients without diabetes, salt restriction itself exerted an antihypertensive and antiproteinuric effect and further enhanced the antiproteinuric effects of RAAS blockade to almost the same magnitude as, and in an additive manner with, diuretics [76]. While this study and others have showed the beneficial impact of sodium restriction on intermediate renal outcomes in CKD, it is significant to address that no large cohort studies have indicated sodium restriction to decline BP or long-term cardiovascular and general mortality specifically in CKD patients [77]. For that reason, the recommendation for sodium restriction in the treatment of hypertension in CKD and in the decline of cardiovascular and general mortality in CKD patients is largely opinion-based. The salt-excreting handicap of CKD and resulting extracellular volume expansion also ensures the basis for treating hypertensive CKD patients with diuretics. Studies of resistant hypertension bring forward that, even in the absence of CKD, this group of patients manifest enhanced extracellular volume, as measured by brain-type natriuretic peptide (BNP) and atrial natriuretic peptide (ANP) [78]. For that reason, the use of appropriate diuretics is a milestone of therapy in patients with CKD and resistant hypertension [4]. Nevertheless, diuretics remain underutilized and underdosed, and a modification in diuretic therapy may help a significant proportion of patients with resistant hypertension to achieve BP goals [79]. For instance, while the major trials supporting the use of diuretic therapy used chlorthalidone at 25 mg/day, the weaker hydrochlorothiazide (HCTZ) at doses of 12.5–25 mg/day remains the most commonly prescribed antihypertensive medication worldwide [80]. However, when evaluated with 24-h ambulatory BP monitoring (ABPM), the antihypertensive efficacy of HCTZ at doses of 12.5–25 mg/day has been indicated to be inferior to that of other commonly prescribed drug classes [80]. Chlorthalidone is approximately twice as potent as HCTZ with a much longer duration of action (8–15 h for HCTZ compared with >40 h for chlorthalidone) [81]. In clinical studies using 24-h ABPM, chlorthalidone 25 mg/day results in greater reductions in 24-h mean SBP compared with HCTZ 50 mg/day, primarily due to its effect on reducing nighttime mean SBP [82]. For that reason, strong consideration should be given to using chlorthalidone over HCTZ, especially given the growing importance of nocturnal blood pressure on cardiovascular results and kidney disease progression in patients with CKD. Thiazide diuretics are most effective in patients with a GFR >50 mL/min/1.73 m², although chlorthalidone can be effective to a GFR of 30–40 mL/min/1.73 m² in the absence of severe hypoalbuminemia [79]. A loop diuretic is preferred for patients with advanced CKD. Typically, loop diuretics such as furosemide and bumetanide should be dosed at least twice daily given their short duration of action and the potential for intermittent natriuresis leading to a reactive increase in the RAAS (with ensuing sodium retention) if dosed once daily [83]. The longer-acting torsemide can be dosed once or twice daily. Consideration should also be granted to combining the loop diuretic with a diuretic that acts more distally in the nephron, such as a thiazide or a low-dose potassium-sparing diuretic [84].

Cost-Effectiveness and Public Health Benefit of Primary and Secondary Cardiovascular Disease Prevention from Improved Adherence Using a Polypill

The complexity of the treatment regimen, socioeconomic status, lifestyle, and psychological influences affect adherence to medication [85]. With regard to the factors that can be modified, reducing dosage demands is defined as the most effective single approach to improve adherence by the European Society of Cardiology [86]. Reducing dosing can be provided by the use of a fixed-dose combination (FDC) polypill consisting of the recommended treatments in a single daily capsule. This approach has improved adherence and reduced costs [87–90]. For this purpose, Wald and Law have originally suggested a polypill that contains aspirin, thiazide, β-blocker, ACE inhibitors, statin, and folic acid, in 2003 for primary prevention. A simpler and more evidence-based formulation consisting of an aspirin, a statin, and ACE inhibitors for the secondary prevention of cardiovascular (CV) events was developed in Spain by a private–public partnership between the Centro Nacional de Investigaciones Cardiovasculares (CNIC) and Ferrer Internacional [88]. This latter polypill contains 100 mg aspirin, 20 mg atorvastatin, and 2.5, 5, or 10 mg ramipril.

Several studies have been reported on the efficacy, safety, tolerability, and affordability of FDC polypills for the primary and secondary prevention of cardiovascular diseases (CVD).

Several pilot studies have showed the feasibility of the primary prevention strategy [91–94]. These are TIPS-1 (Indian Polycap Study) [91], PolyIran (Phase II Study of Heart Polypill Safety and Efficacy in Primary Prevention of CV Disease) [92], Combination Therapy Trial [93], and IMPACT (Improving Adherence Using Combination Therapy) [94]. The large one TIPS-1 was a phase II randomized trial that included 2053 participants aged 40–80 years without CVD and with at least one CV risk factor in India [91]. The polypills used in those studies contained aspirin, statin, ACE inhibitors, and thiazide diuretics at various doses. The outcomes of those trials were feasibility, effect on risk factor levels, safety, and tolerability of polypills.

The IMPACT (Improving Adherence Using Combination Therapy) trial included 513 adults at high risk of CVD (with established CVD or 5-year risk of ≥15%). They were suggested for treatment with antiplatelet, statin, and ≥2 BP-lowering drugs, and were randomized to continued usual care or to FDC treatment. The investigators discovered that, parallel to other studies, adherence to all 4 suggested drugs was greater among FDC than usual care participants at 12 months (81% vs. 46%; relative risk, 1.75 [95% confidence interval, 1.52 to 2.03]; $p < 0.001$) [94].

For secondary prevention, TIPS-2 (Second Indian Polycap Study) [95] reported significant declines in BP and low density lipoprotein (LDL-C) in patients with stable CVD or diabetes with the use of the combination drugs used in TIPS-1.

The UMPIRE (Use of a Multidrug Pill in Reducing Cardiovascular Events) study that was the first randomized trial designed to detect the long-term effect of a FDC strategy in improving patients' adherence to medication in CV prevention has recently announced [96]. Adherence to medication in the polypill group was 85%, compared with 60% in the standard-care group ($p < 0.001$). BP and LDL-C levels were decreased with the FDC strategy to a greater extent than with standard care. No significant differences were noted in the incidence of serious adverse effects between the groups [96].

The latest trial to investigate the effect on adherence of the polypill in secondary prevention has just been noticed, and 623 patients with CVD or an estimated 5-year CVD risk ≥15% were enrolled in this study. After a median of 18 months, patients randomized to the polypill exposed a significantly higher adherence than those receiving usual care (70% vs. 47%; $p < 0.001$). The study showed no significant differences in BP or LDL-C levels between groups, possibly due to the limited power of the study.

Available clinical data aid the viability of the polypill in CVD prevention and management but with a limited area. The role of the polypill in CV prevention has been gradually described. Further research of the polypill is necessary, with the collective results to have the potential power changing the face of health care across the world.

Chronotherapy

Investigators have assessed whether chronotherapy – the strategy of bedtime, rather than morning, dosing of antihypertensive medications – can have an influence on the circadian rhythm of BP, including 24-h ambulatory BP control and the prevalence of non-dipping. In the study of 250 patients with resistant hypertension, patients who were randomly selected to the strategy of modifying one drug but administering the new drug at bedtime showed a statistically important ambulatory blood pressure reduction (9.4/6.0 mmHg for systolic/diastolic BP, $p < 0.001$) compared with the strategy of modifying one drug but continuing all medications in a single morning dose [97]. The effect was greater on the nocturnal than on the diurnal mean BP, and the prevalence of non-dipping diminished from 84 to 43% over the 12-week study period. The benefit of chronotherapy has also been showed in resistant hypertension by moving all non-diuretic antihypertensive drugs from morning to bedtime dosing without altering any medications or doses [98]. By this way, chronotherapy gives an opportunity to enhance nocturnal BP control and the non-dipper pattern without changing the total number of medications with CKD are encouraging.

Device Therapy for Resistant Hypertension

Devices to treat resistant hypertension significantly aim the sympathetic nervous system, which is recognized to contribute to the pathogenesis of necessary hypertension and many forms of secondary hypertension [99] (Table 15.4). However, these devices are not uniformly fruitful in treating resistant hypertension. Chronic electrical stimulation of the carotid sinus nerves with a surgically implantable device, which was designated to trigger baroreflex-mediated inhibition of sympathetic nerve activity, has been indicated to decline blood pressure in 54% of patients with resistant hypertension in a randomized, double-blind, parallel-designed clinical trial ($n = 181$) [100]. However, enhanced blood pressure con control was also examined in 46%of control group patients ($n = 81$) in whom the devices were

Table 15.4 Device therapy
for resistant hypertension

Chronic electrical stimulation of the carotid sinus nerves with a surgically implantable device
Catheter-based renal sympathetic denervation

deactivated for unknown reasons ($p = 0.97$) [100]. Catheter-based renal sympathetic denervation is another potential therapeutic strategy for resistant hypertension. This technique exercises radiofrequency energy to ablate renal nerves alongside renal arteries in the adventitial layers [101]. Although the initial unblended trial using this technology showed fruitful results [101], a subsequent randomized sham-controlled trial (SYMPLICITY-HTN3) [102] indicated no difference in the office blood pressure or 24-h ambulatory blood pressure in a denervation group compared with a sham-procedure group treated with medical therapy alone. It is unclear whether renal denervation may benefit a subset of patients with resistant hypertension.

Conclusions

One of the major causes of pseudo-resistant hypertension appears to be nonadherence to prescribed anti-hypertensives, and modifications in diet and physical activity have the potential to lower BP substantially in patients with RHT. On the other hand, it is not obvious whether renal denervation benefits a subset of patients with RHT. Therefore; the best choice for treatment of RHT appears to be providing well adherence to medication and lifestyle change of patients with RHT. The public policy is vital to efforts to both prevent and treat RHT.

References

1. Weber MA, Schiffrin EL, William B, White WB, et al. Clinical practice guidelines for the management of hypertension in the community a statement by the American Society of Hypertension and the International Society of Hypertension. J Clin Hypertens. 2014;16(1):14–26.
2. Mancia G, Fagard R, Narkiewicz K, et al. ESH/ESC guidelines for the management of arterial hypertension: the task force for the management of arterial hypertension of the European Society of Hypertension (ESH) and of the European Society of Cardiology (ESC). J Hypertens. 2013;31:1281–357.
3. Calhoun DA, Jones D, Textor S, et al. Resistant hypertension: diagnosis, evaluation, and treatment. Circulation. 2008;117:e510–26.
4. Chobanian AV, Bakris GL, Black HR, National Heart, Lung, and Blood Institute Joint National Committee on Prevention, Detection, Evaluation, and Treatment of High Blood Pressure; National High Blood Pressure Education Program Coordinating Committee, et al. The seventh report of the Joint National Committee on prevention, detection, evaluation, and treatment of high blood pressure: the JNC 7 report. JAMA. 2003;289(19):2560–72.

5. Sarafidis PA. Epidemiology of resistant hypertension. J Clin Hypertens (Greenwich). 2011;13:523–8.
6. Sarafidis PA, Georgianos P, Bakris GL, et al. Resistant hypertension—its identification and epidemiology. Nat Rev Nephrol. 2013;9:51–8.
7. Calhoun DA. Apparent and true resistant hypertension: why not the same? J Am Soc Hypertens. 2013;7(6):509–11.
8. World Health Organization. The world health report – reducing risks, promoting healthy life. (2002). www.who.int/whr/2002/en (Version current at April 26, 2006).
9. Wagner EH, Davis C, Schaefer J, et al. A survey of leading chronic disease management programs: are they consistent with the literature? Manag Care Q. 1999;7:56–66.
10. The WHIC Chronic Disease Management (CDM) Infostructure Initiative. 2006. www.whic. org/public/profiles/cdm.html (Version current at April 26, 2006).
11. Canadian Hypertension Education Program. 2006. www.hypertension.ca/CHEP2006/ CHEP_2006_complete.pdf (Version current at May 9, 2006).
12. Haynes RB, Sackett DL, Gibson ES, et al. Improvement of medication compliance in uncontrolled hypertension. Lancet. 1976;1:1265–8.
13. Ashida T, Yokoyama S, Ebihara A, et al. Profiles of patients who control the doses of their antihypertensive drugs by self-monitoring of home blood pressure. Hypertens Res. 2001;24:203–7.
14. Moser M, Setaro JF. Clinical practice. Resistant or difficult-to-control hypertension. N Engl J Med. 2006;355(4):385–92.
15. Pimenta E, Calhoun DA, Oparil S. Mechanisms and treatment of resistant hypertension.Arq. Bras Cardiol. 2007;88(6):683–92.
16. Makris A, Seferou M, Papadopoulos DP. Resistant hypertension workup and approach to treatment. Int J Hypertens. 2010;2011:598694.
17. Pimenta E, Calhoun DA. Resistant hypertension: incidence, prevalence, and prognosis. Circulation. 2012;125(13):1594–6.
18. Daugherty SL, Powers JD, Magid DJ, et al. Incidence and prognosis of resistant hypertension in hypertensive patients. Circulation. 2012;125(13):1635–42.
19. Khan TV, Khan SS, Akhondi A, et al. White coat hypertension: relevance to clinical and emergency medical services personnel. Med Gen Med. 2007;9(1):52.
20. Oliveira-Filho AD, Barreto-Filho JA, Neves SJ, et al. Association between the 8-item Morisky medication adherence scale (MMAS-8) and blood pressure control. Arq Bras Cardiol. 2012;99(1):649–58.
21. Morisky DE, Ang A, Krousel-Wood M, et al. Predictive validity of a medication adherence measure in an outpatient setting. J ClinHypertens (Greenwich). 2008;10(5):348–54.
22. Maurer H, Pfleger K. Identification and differentiation of beta-blockers and their metabolites in urine by computerized gas chromatography mass spectrometry. J Chromatogr. 1986;382:147–65.
23. Maurer HH. Systematic toxicological analysis procedures for acidic drugs and/or metabolites relevant to clinical and forensic toxicology and/or doping control. J Chromatogr B Biomed Sci Appl. 1999;733:3–25.
24. Maurer HH. Perspectives of liquid chromatography coupled to lowand high-resolution mass spectrometry for screening, identification, and quantification of drugs in clinical and forensic toxicology. Ther Drug Monit. 2010;32:324–7.
25. Ojanpera L, Pelander A, Laks S, et al. Application of accurate mass measurement to urine drug screening. J Anal Toxicol. 2005;29:34–40.
26. Maurer HH, Tenberken O, Kratzsch C, et al. Screening for library-assisted identification and fully validated quantification of 22 beta-blockers in blood plasma by liquid chromatographymass spectrometry with atmospheric pressure chemical ionization. J Chromatogr A. 2004;1058:169–81.
27. Kristoffersen L, Øiestad EL, Opdal MS, et al. Simultaneous determination of 6 beta-blockers, 3 calcium-channel antagonists, 4 angiotensin-II antagonists and 1 antiarrhythmic drug in

postmortem whole blood by automated solid phase extraction and liquid chromatography mass spectrometry-method development and robustness testing by experimental design. J Chromatogr B Analyt Technol Biomed Life Sci. 2007;850:147–60.

28. Zyoud SH, Al-Jabi SW, Sweileh WM, et al. Health-related quality of life associated with treatment adherence in patients with hypertension: a cross-sectional study. Int J Cardiol. 2013;168(3):2981–3.

29. Parikh A, Lipsitz SR, Natarajan S, et al. Association between a DASH-like diet and mortality in adults with hypertension: findings from a populationbased follow-up study. Am J Hypertens. 2009;22:409–16.

30. Rossi A, Dikareva A, Bacon SL, et al. The impact of physical activity on mortality in patients with high blood pressure: a systematic review. J Hypertens. 2012;30:1277–88.

31. He FJ, Li J, Macgregor GA. Effect of longer term modest salt reduction on blood pressure. BMJ. 2013;346:f1325.

32. Pimenta E, Gaddam KK, Oparil S, et al. Effects of dietary sodium reduction on blood pressure in subjects with resistant hypertension. Hypertension. 2009;54(3):475–81.

33. Centers for Disease Control and Prevention (CDC). Usual sodium intakes compared with current dietary guidelines—United States, 2005-2008. MMWR Morb Mortal WklyRep. 2011;60(41):1413–7.

34. Dimeo F, Pagonas N, Seibert F, et al. Aerobic exercise reduces blood pressure in resistant hypertension. Hypertension. 2012;60(3):653–8.

35. Kokkinos PF, Narayan P, Colleran JA, et al. Effects of regular exercise on blood pressure and left ventricular hypertrophy in African-American men with severe hypertension. N Engl J Med. 1995;333(22):1462–7.

36. Whelton PK, Appel LJ, Espeland MA, et al. Sodium reduction and weight loss in the treatment of hypertension in older persons: a randomized controlled trial of nonpharmacologic interventions in the elderly (TONE). JAMA J Am Med Assoc. 1998;279(11):839–46.

37. Conlin PR, Erlinger TP, Bohannon A, et al. The DASH diet enhances the blood pressure response to losartan in hypertensive patients. Am J Hypertens. 2003;16(5 Pt 1):337–42.

38. Burke V, Beilin LJ, Cutt HE, et al. Effects of a lifestyle programme on ambulatory blood pressure and drug dosage in treated hypertensive patients: a randomized controlled trial. J Hypertens. 2005;23(6):1241–9.

39. Miller ER 3rd, Erlinger TP, Young DR, et al. Results of the diet, exercise, and weight loss intervention trial (DEW-IT). Hypertension. 2002;40(5):612–8.

40. Heffler S, Smith S, Keehan S, et al. US Health Spending Projections for 2004–2014, Health Affairs doi:10.1377/hlthaff.w5.74. (2005).

41. OECD Indicators. The OECD register. http://www.oecd.org/health/health-systems/44117530. pdf. Accessed Nov 2009. (2006).

42. Fe'nina A, Geffroy Y, Minc C, Renaud T, Sarlon E, Sermet C. Lesde'penses de pre'vention et lesde'penses de soins par pathologie en France. IRDES, Bulletind'information en e'conomie de la sante´ No.111, Juillet 2006.

43. Kastarinen MJ, Antikainen RL, Laatikainen TK, et al. Trends in hypertensioncare in eastern and south-western Finland during 1982–20. J Hypertens. 2006;24:829–35.

44. Thomas C. Fenter Sonya J. Lewis RPh. Pay-for-Performance Initiatives. J Manag Care Pharm. 2008;14(6)(suppl S-c):S12–5.

45. Trude S, Au M, Christianson JB, et al. Health plan pay-for-performance strategies. Am J Manag Care. 2006;12:537–42.

46. National Health Service 2006/2007 The NHS register. www.nhsemployers.org/primary/primary-890.cfm. Accessed April 2006.

47. Roland M. Linkingphysicians' pay tothequality of care--a majorexperiment in the United kingdom. N Engl J Med. 2004;351:1448–54.

48. Dzudie A, Kengne AP, Muna WF, et al. Prevalence, awareness, treatment and control of hypertension in a self-selectedsub-SaharanAfrican urban population: a cross-sectionalstudy. BMJ. 2012;2:e001217.

49. Awoke A, Awoke T, Alemu S, et al. Prevalence and associated factors of hypertension among adults in Gondar, Northwest Ethiopia: a community based cross-sectional study. BMC Cardiovasc Disord. 2012;12:113.
50. Chow CK, Teo KK, Rangarajan S, et al. Prevalence, awareness, treatment, and control of hypertension in rural and urban communities in high-, middle-, and low-income countries. JAMA. 2013;310:959–68.
51. Damasceno A, Azevedo A, Silva-Matos C, et al. Hypertension prevalence, awareness, treatment, and control in Mozambique: urban/rural gap during epidemiological transition. Hypertension. 2009;54:77–83.
52. Food and SafetyAuthority of Ireland (FSAI). The FSAI register. https://www.fsai.ie/upload-edFiles/Science_and_Health/salt_report-1.pdf. Accessed 2005. (2005).
53. Opie L, Seedat YK. Hypertension in sub-Saharan African populations. Circulation. 2005;112:3562–8.
54. Ngoungou EB, Aboyans V, Kouna P, et al. Prevalence of cardiovascular disease in Gabon: a population study. Arch Cardiovasc Dis. 2012;105:77–83.
55. Bovet P, Gervasoni JP, Mkamba M, et al. Low utilization of health care services following screening for hypertension in Dar es salaam (Tanzania): a prospective population-basedstudy. BMC Public Health. 2008;8:407.
56. Rayner B, Blockman M, Baines D, et al. A survey of hypertensive practices at two community health centres in Cape Town. S Afr Med J. 2007;97:280–4.
57. Mohan V, Seedat YK, Pradeepa R, et al. The rising burden of diabetes and hypertension in south east Asian and African regions: need for effective strategies for prevention and control in primary health care settings. Int J Hypertens. 2013;2013:409083.
58. Tu K, Chen Z, Lipscombe LL, et al. Canadian hypertension education program outcomes research taskforce. Prevalence and incidence of hypertension from 1995 to 2005: a population-basedstudy. CMAJ. 2008;178:1429–35.
59. Forte JG, Miguel JM, Miguel MJ, et al. Salt and blood pressure: a community trial. J Hum Hypertens. 1989;3:179–84.
60. Bertram MY, Steyn K, Wentzel-Viljoen E, et al. Reducing the sodium content of high-salt foods: effect on cardiovascular disease in South Africa. S AfrMed J. 2012;102:743–5.
61. Murray CJ, Lauer JA, Hutubessy RC, et al. Effectiveness and costs of interventions to reduce systolic blood pressure and cholesterol: a global and regional analysis on reduction of cardiovascular-disease risk. Lancet. 2003;361:717–25.
62. Danaei G, Singh GM, Paciorek CJ, et al. The global cardiovascular risk transition: associations of four metabolic risk factors with national income, urbanization, and western diet in 1980 and 2008. Circulation. 2013;127:1493–502.
63. Sarrafzadegan N, Kelishadi R, Sadri G, et al. Outcomes of a comprehensive healthy lifestyle program on cardiometabolic risk factors in a developing country: the Isfahan healthyheart program. Arch Iran Med. 2013;16:4–11.
64. Adeyemo A, Tayo BO, Luke A, et al. The Nigerian antihypertensive adherence trial: a community-basedrandomizedtrial. J Hypertens. 2013;31:201–7.
65. Osamor PE, Owumi BE. Factors associated with treatment compliance in hypertension in southwest Nigeria. J Health Popul Nutr. 2011;29:619–28.
66. Parr J, Lindeboom W, Khanam M, et al. Informal allopathic provider knowledge and practice regarding hypertension in urban and rural Bangladesh. PLoSOne. 2012;7:e48056.
67. Joshi A, Puricelli Perin DM, Arora M, et al. Using portable health information kiosk to assess chronic disease burden in remote settings. Rural Remote Health. 2013;13:2279.
68. Pande S, Hiller JE, Nkansah N, et al. The effect of pharmacist provided non-dispensing services on patient outcomes, health service utilisation and costs in low- and middle-income countries. Cochrane Database SystRev. 2013;2:CD010398.
69. Piette JD, Datwani H, Gaudioso S, et al. Hypertension management using mobile technology and home blood pressure monitoring: results of a randomized trial in two low/middle-income countries. Telemed J E Health. 2012;18:613–20.

70. Malaza A, Mossong J, Bärnighausen T, et al. Hypertension and obesity in adults living in a high HIV prevalence rural area in South Africa. PLoS One. 2012;7:e47761.
71. de Jongh T, Gurol-Urganci I, Vodopivec-Jamsek V, et al. Mobile phone messaging for facilitating self-management of long-term illnesses. Cochrane Database Syst Rev. 2012;12:CD007459.
72. Bray GA, Vollmer WM, Sacks FM, et al. A further subgroup analysis of the effects of the DASH diet and three dietary sodium levels on blood pressure: results of the DASH-sodium trial. Am J Cardiol. 2004;94:222–7.
73. Hall JE, Mizelle HL, Hildebrandt DA, et al. Abnormal pressure natriuresis. A cause or a consequence of hypertension? Hypertension. 1990;15(6 Pt 1):547–59.
74. Sato A, Saruta T. Aldosterone-induced organ damage: plasma aldosterone level and inappropriate salt status. Hypertens Res. 2004;27:303–10.
75. Pimenta E, Gaddam KK, Pratt-Ubunama MN, et al. Relation of dietary salt and aldosterone to urinary protein excretion in subjects with resistant hypertension. Hypertension. 2008;51:339–44.
76. Vogt L, Waanders F, Boomsma F, et al. Effects of dietary sodium and hydrochlorothiazide on the antiproteinuric efficacy of losartan. J Am Soc Nephrol. 2008;19:999–1007.
77. Krikken JA, Laverman GD, Navis G, et al. Benefits of dietary sodium restriction in the management of chronic kidney disease. Curr Opin Nephrol Hypertens. 2009;18:531–8.
78. Gaddam KK, Nishizaka MK, Pratt-Ubunama MN, et al. Characterization of resistant hypertension: association between resistant hypertension, aldosterone, and persistent intravascular volume expansion. Arch Intern Med. 2008;168:1159–64.
79. Sarafidis PA, Bakris GL. Resistant hypertension: an overview of evaluation and treatment. J Am Coll Cardiol. 2008;52:1749–57.
80. Messerli FH, Makani H, Benjo A, et al. Antihypertensive efficacy of hydrochlorothiazide as evaluated by ambulatory blood pressure monitoring: a meta-analysis of randomized trials. J Am Coll Cardiol. 2011;57:590–600.
81. Carter BL, Ernst ME, Cohen JD, et al. Hydrochlorothiazide versus chlorthalidone: evidence supporting their interchangeability. Hypertension. 2004;43:4–9.
82. Ernst ME, Carter BL, Goerdt CJ, et al. Comparative antihypertensive effects of hydrochlorothiazide and chlorthalidone on ambulatory and office blood pressure. Hypertension. 2006;47:352–8.
83. Moser M, Cushman W, Handler J. Resistant or difficult-to-treat hypertension. J ClinHypertens (Greenwich). 2006;8:434–40.
84. Ernst ME, Gordon JA. Diuretic therapy: key aspects in hypertension and renal disease. J Nephrol. 2010;23:487–93.
85. Jin J, Sklar GE, Min Sen Oh V, et al. Factors affecting therapeutic compliance: a review from the patient's perspective. Ther Clin Risk Manag. 2008;4:269–86.
86. Perk J, De Backer G, Gohlke H, et al. European guidelines on cardiovascular disease prevention in clinical practice (version 2012). The fifth Joint task force of the European Society of Cardiology and Other Societies on cardiovascular disease prevention in clinical practice (constituted by representatives of nine societies and by invited experts). Eur Heart J. 2012;33:1635–701.
87. Muntner P, Mann D, Wildman RP, et al. Projected impact of polypill use among US adults: medication use, cardiovascular risk reduction, and side effects. Am Heart J. 2011;161:719–25.
88. Sanz G, Fuster V. Fixed-dose combination therapy and secondary cardiovascular prevention: rationale, selection of drugs and target population. Nat Clin Pract Cardiovasc Med. 2009;6:101–10.
89. Wald NJ, Law MR. A strategy to reduce cardiovascular disease by more than 80%. BMJ. 2003;326:1419–23.
90. Zeymer U, Junger C, Zahn R, et al. Effects of a secondary prevention combination therapy with an aspirin, an ACE inhibitor and a statin on 1-year mortality of patients with acute myo-

cardial infarction treated with a beta-blocker. Support for a polypill approach. Curr Med Res Opin. 2011;27:1563–70.

91. Indian Polycap S, Yusuf S, Pais P, et al. Effects of a polypill (Polycap) on risk factors in middle aged individuals without cardiovascular disease (TIPS): a phase II, double-blind, randomised trial. Lancet. 2009;373:1341–51.

92. Malekzadeh F, Marshall T, Pourshams A, et al. A pilot double-blind randomised placebo controlled trial of the effects of fixed-dose combination therapy ('polypill') on cardiovascular risk factors. Int J Clin Pract. 2010;64:1220–7.

93. Soliman EZ, Mendis S, Dissanayake WP, et al. A polypill for primary prevention of cardiovascular disease: a feasibility study of the World Health Organization. Trials. 2011;12:3.

94. Rodgers A, Patel A, Berwanger O, et al. An international randomised placebo-controlled trial of a four-component combination pill ("polypill") in people with raised cardiovascular risk. PloS One. 2011;6:e19857.

95. Yusuf S, Pais P, Sigamani A, et al. Comparison of risk factor reduction and tolerability of a fulldosepolypill (with potassium) versus low-dose polypill (Polycap) in individuals at high risk of cardiovascular diseases: the second Indian Polycap study (TIPS-2) investigators. Circ Cardiovasc Qual Outcomes. 2012;5:463–71.

96. Thom S, Poulter N, Field J, et al. Effects of a fixed-dose combination strategy on adherence and risk factors in patients with or at high risk of CVD: the UMPIRE randomized clinical trial. JAMA. 2013;310:918–29.

97. Hermida RC, Ayala DE, Fernandez JR, et al. Chronotherapy improves blood pressure control and reverts the nondipper pattern in patients with resistant hypertension. Hypertension. 2008;51:69–76 .

98. Almirall J, Comas L, Martinez-Ocana JC, et al. Effects of chronotherapy on blood pressure control in non-dipper patients with refractory hypertension. Nephrol Dial Transplant. 2012;27:1855–9.

99. KontakAC WZ, Arbique D, et al. Reversible sympathetic overactivity in hypertensive patients with primary aldosteronism. J Clin Endocrinol Metab. 2010;95(10):4756–61.

100. Bisognano JD, Bakris G, Nadim MK, et al. Baroreflex activation therapy lowers blood pressure in patients with resistant hypertension: results from the double-blind, randomized, placebo-controlled rheos pivotal trial. J Am Coll Cardiol. 2011;58(7):765–73.

101. Esler MD, Krum H, Sobotka PA, SYMPLICITY HTN-2 Investigators, et al. Renal sympathetic denervation in patients with treatment-resistant hypertension (the SYMPLICITY HTN-2 trial): a randomised controlled trial. Lancet. 2010;376(9756):1903–9.

102. Bhatt DL, Kandzari DE, WW O'N, SYMPLICITY HTN-3 Investigators, et al. A controlled trial of renal denervation for resistant hypertension. N Engl J Med. 2014;370:1393–401.

Chapter 16
Treatment of Hypertension in Light of the New Guidelines: Salt Intake

Baris Afsar and Alper Kirkpantur

Introduction

Presence of hypertension (HT) is commonly seen in patients with chronic kidney disease (CKD). Additionally, as kidney function declines, blood pressure (BP) elevation occurs and as BP rises, kidney function deteriorates [1]. This reciprocal interaction between kidney function and BP was observed both in experimental and clinical conditions. Besides, with advancing CKD, control of BP becomes more difficult [2]. Indeed, it can be stated that there is resistance to BP lowering effects of lifestyle modifications and antihypertensive drugs in CKD patients. The mechanisms of BP elevation and resistance to BP lowering in CKD are many but the exact causes are still unknown. However, one of the most important factors for resistant HT in CKD is salt intake. Indeed, nearly 2000 years ago, in ancient China, there is a statement of suspicion that there is link between renal disease, salt, and hypertension stated as: "when the pulse is full and hard ... the illness dominates the kidneys and has its seat therein." "If large amounts of salt are taken, the pulse will stiffen or harden" [3].

A part from increased HT prevalence, resistant hypertension (RHT) is also highly prevalent in CKD patients. Indeed, overt or incipient CKD has long been considered one of the most frequent medical causes of RHT [4–6].

In this chapter, we tried to summarize the definition, incidence, pathophysiologic mechanisms, and studies especially focusing on salt intake and resistant HT in CKD.

B. Afsar (✉)
Department of Internal Medicine, Division of Nephrology Çünür, Suleyman Demirel University, Doğu yerleşkesi, Isparta Merkez/Isparta, 32260, Turkey
e-mail: afsarbrs@yahoo.com; afsarbrs@gmail.com

A. Kirkpantur
Department of Nephrology, Acıbadem University Hospital, Ankara, Turkey

© Springer International Publishing AG 2017
A. Covic et al. (eds.), *Resistant Hypertension in Chronic Kidney Disease*,
DOI 10.1007/978-3-319-56827-0_16

Definition of Resistant Hypertension and Incidence in CKD

Resistant hypertension is a condition when BP is not controlled despite maximal effective dosing of ≥3 medications of different classes; one is being a diuretic [7]. Resistant hypertension should not be confused with pseudoresistance. Pseudoresistance implies uncontrolled office BP while receiving ≥3 medications in the setting of medication nonadherence, improper BP measurement technique, and/ or white coat HT. It is suggested that pseudoresistance is suggested to contribute to as much as 50% of RHT [8]. Factors associated with pseudoresistance include use of cuffs in an inappropriate size, recent smoking, improper BP measurement technique, inappropriate drug combinations and doses, poor compliance by patients to the prescribed antihypertensive regimen, poor doctor-patient relationship, and poor education of patients to the significance of achieving goal BP [9]. Thus it is important to differentiate true RHT or pseudoresistance while evaluating the patients and performing investigations.

Resistant hypertension is either not to be confused with refractory HT. Refractory HT is a condition which meet the definition of RHT but BP is not controlled despite maximal medical therapy (i.e., ≥4 antihypertensive medications at maximal effective dosing and of different class) [10, 11]. This means that patients with RHT may achieve target BP, patients with refractory HT cannot achieve optimal BP [12]. A part from RHT, one of the important concepts is masked hypertension (MHT) in CKD. This is important since as many as 40–70% of patients with CKD present MHT and MHT is related also with RHT [4, 13]. Masked hypertension was defined as controlled office BP (<140/90 mm Hg) with an elevated overall average BP by 24-h ABPM (>130/80 mm Hg) or home BP > 135/85 mm Hg [14].

Despite all these confirmed data, there is only scarce data regarding epidemiology of RHT both in general and CKD population. This is due to fact that until a few years ago, information regarding the epidemiology of RHT was obtained from indirect sources, such as cross-sectional studies on hypertension control in large cohorts from tertiary hypertension centers and outcome trials in hypertension. However, during recent years, large population- based studies have provided direct epidemiologic data on RHT and estimated its prevalence at 8–12% of adult patients with hypertension. Chronic kidney disease in particular has been long considered a frequent underlying cause of RHT; however, recently, direct epidemiologic data for this entity in patients with CKD were brought to light again, suggesting an even higher prevalence of resistant hypertension (approximately 20–35%) among such individuals. In one study which specifically focused on RHT in CKD, De Nicola et al. demonstrated that in 300 hypertensive CKD patients, 38% had RHT after 6 months of BP management, with a higher prevalence of diabetic nephropathy and higher levels of proteinuria with RHT [15]. Furthermore, recent prospective cohort studies have suggested incident RHT to be associated with increased cardiovascular and renal risk in both the general hypertensive population and patients with CKD [9].

Thus it is of no question that RHT is prevalent and has potential impact on cardiovascular outcomes in patients with HT including CKD.

Blood Pressure Targets in CKD

In recent years, there are a number of guidelines in medical literature providing recommendations for the management of high BP in HT including patients with CKD [16–20]. The potential danger in such guidelines resides in the fact that they focus on setting a BP threshold for treatment yet harm may exist with overtreatment of HTN in patients with CKD. In a cohort of over 650,000 Veteran Americans with CKD, extremes of both high and low BPs were associated with increased mortality, with the highest mortality for patients with high pulse pressures. The authors conclude that it may not be advantageous to achieve an ideal systolic BP (<130 mm Hg) in patients who have existing low diastolic BP (<70 mm Hg) [21].

Looking at this perspective, it is surprising to realize that there is still no sufficient evidence to recommend a lower BP goal less than 140/90 mm Hg in patients with CKD [8]. It is also a fact that, though some evidence informing the best treatment BP target in CKD is available, not all groups looking at the same data agree on exactly what the evidence shows.

The other important issue in CKD is the presence of albuminuria/proteinuria, and increased urine protein/albumin excretion needs extra level of consideration [22]. Thus the Kidney Disease Improving Global Outcomes BP work group advised a lower BP goal of less than 130/80 mm Hg for individuals with CKD and moderate-to-severe albuminuria (e.g., urine albumin-to-creatinine ratio > 30 mg/g) [23]. However, as suggested this recommendation was based on an evidence level equivalent to expert opinion.

Thus studies especially interventional ones are still needed to determine which BP values are optimal for better health outcomes in CKD patients.

Salt and Resistant Hypertension in CKD: Pathophysiologic View

The detailed pathophysiologic explanation for the RHT is beyond the scope of this chapter. However, a brief explanation will be useful. Before beginning, it is important to remember that the exact pathobiology of RHT is not known, although many factors are thought to play a role. These include increased reduced renal mass, age, arterial stiffness, vascular calcification and endothelial dysfunction, presence of diabetes, increased sympathetic nervous system activation renin angiotensin aldosterone system (RAAS) imbalance, and altered sodium chloride handling in the distal nephron or some combination of the earlier mentioned conditions [24] (Fig. 16.1).

It is also well recognized that high dietary salt intake not only exacerbates HT in patients with CKD but also has the potential to directly worsen kidney function. Rats receiving a high salt diet show sustained increases in kidney levels of transforming growth factor-β, polypeptides associated with kidney fibrosis [25]. Since this chapter is primarily focused on RHT in CKD, from now on we will explain this issue in more detail.

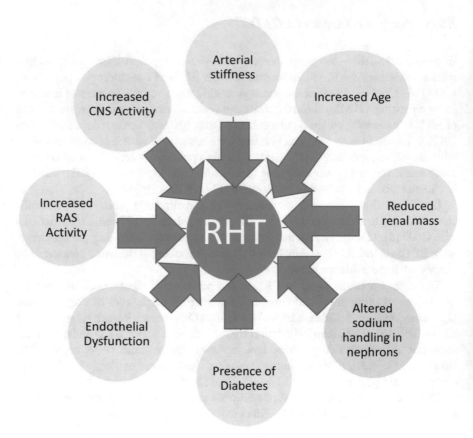

Fig. 16.1 Factors related with the development of resistant hypertension (*CNS* central nervous system, *RAS* renin angiotensin system)

The most important thing is to acknowledge that BP in CKD is very closely related with salt and salt intake in CKD patients. This relationship between salt and BP is also valid in patients with RHT in which salt is thought to play a major role in the development of RHT, a condition known as "salt sensitivity."

But how does salt induce RHT? To answer this question one must first know the normal physiology. Under normal physiologic conditions with healthy kidneys, there is autoregulation of BP after salt intake within certain limits. This means that under normal physiologic conditions, a high sodium intake drives sodium excretion by increasing blood volume, BP, cardiac output, and filtered sodium load [26]. This classical concept known as pressure-natriuresis describes the association between BP and sodium balance. As CKD develops and advances, this physiologic adaptation is lost gradually and kidney damage alters pressure-natriuresis curve and results in positive sodium balance with increased salt intake. This is due to fact that, as

CKD progresses, glomerular filtration rate (GFR) is reduced and, consequently, filtered sodium and fluid load is reduced. It is important to realize that this net fall in GFR is due to decreased GFR in some nephrons while hyperfiltration in other nephrons. This brings additional risk of glomerular damage and microalbuminuria in remaining nephrons and additional decrease of GFR in time [27].

There is also an opinion that high salt intake directly blunts kidney autoregulation, which exposes the glomerulus to higher filtration pressures [28]. Over time, the high glomerular filtration pressure leads to glomerular sclerosis and nephron loss. However, these compensatory mechanisms may be inadequate as CKD progresses and, hence, the resultant sodium retention and ECV expansion cause HT.

Second mechanism between salt intake and RHT may reside an amplification of the effects of constrictors including angiotensin II or norepinephrine [26, 29].

Third mechanism may be independent of BP; salt has unwanted effects on vessel wall structure and endothelial function. Ying et al. have shown the involvement of the fibrosis-promoting cytokine transforming growth factor-β (TGF-β) by salt. Dietary salt intake, working through shearing stress at the endothelial level, activates the proline-enriched tyrosine kinase-2 pathway. Proline-enriched tyrosine kinase-2, in turn, signals endothelial cells to produce TGF-β. By stimulating TGF-β production, salt contributes to accelerated aging and fibrosis in the vessel wall [30]. It was also concluded that an excess of total body salt likely also contributes to arterial stiffness, which is approximated by pulse pressure and known to be associated with worsened kidney function [31].

Johnson and colleagues hypothesized a fourth mechanism regarding CKD, hypertension, and salt. They have suggested that primary subclinical renal microvascular disease leading to afferent arteriolopathy and tubulointerstitial disease may be responsible for the development of HT [32]. Progressive tubulointerstitial disease will eventually result in microalbuminuria before the development of clinically apparent impairment of glomerular filtration. Concurrent microvascular damage is thought to result in renal vasoconstriction and subsequent local generation of angiotensin II. The resulting increased vascular resistance, reduced rate of ultrafiltration, and decreased sodium excretion cause sodium retention, volume expansion, and hypertension [33].

Thus by the light of aforementioned data one can say that BP in CKD patients is salt sensitive and with decreasing renal function, the salt sensitivity of BP increases [34]. The potential mechanisms related with increased salt and development of HT in CKD are summarized in Table 16.1.

Indeed clinical observations have also confirmed the specific role of salt in HT in CKD patients. For instance, salt-loading in CKD patients and healthy subjects over several days results in a predictable expansion of ECV and an increased fractional excretion of sodium; however, patients with CKD show an increase in arterial BP concomitant with the increase in ECV, whereas healthy subjects have no significant change in arterial BP [35]. It is also interesting to observe that the extent of ECV expansion correlates with the severity of renal impairment and contributes to approximately 5–10% of body weight even in the absence of peripheral edema [36].

Table 16.1 The potential mechanisms related with increased salt and development of HT in CKD

↑ in extracellular volume and glomerular hypertension
↑ effect of vasoconstrictor substances and ↓ the effect of vasodilator substances
↑ sympathetic activity
Potentially ↑ the structural and functional pathologies in the vessel wall (vascular sclerosis, endothelial dysfunction)
↑ oxidative stress
↑ urinary protein and albumin excretion
Blunts the effect of antihypertensive drugs (diuretics, ACE inhibitors, etc.)
↑ transforming growth factor-β production and kidney fibrosis

A recent systematic review also demonstrated that worsened kidney function, defined as a decline in creatinine clearance, doubling of serum creatinine, or progression to end-stage renal disease, is associated with high sodium intake compared to a low sodium intake [37].

Other proofs regarding salt and HT include reduced salt intake which is associated with an enhanced response to antihypertensive therapy [38] and high salt intake that diminishes nighttime dipping of BP in salt-sensitive HT [39].

Thus all these data suggest that salt has an extraordinary role in development, maintenance, and resistance of HT in CKD. Indeed, it was suggested that salt and water balance in the kidney plays a role as the central long-term regulator of BP and one can reasonably attribute a large portion of HTN in CKD to an impaired salt excretion that is exacerbated by excess salt intake [24].

In sum, all of these findings suggest that there is very close relationship between salt and RHT in CKD [29, 40].

In the next section we will summarize the performed studies regarding salt, RHT, and CKD.

Studies

Despite all these extensive research, it is very surprising to find that there are very few studies regarding salt intake, salt restriction, and BP in CKD patients [41]. The studies are mostly observational, have low patients numbers, and lack of control groups. Therefore, as suggested above, the recommendation for sodium restriction in the treatment of hypertension in CKD and in the reduction of cardiovascular and overall mortality in CKD patients remains largely opinion-based.

Yu et al. investigated the role of dietary sodium intake on BP control among non-dialysis Chinese CKD patients. They included 176 non-dialysis hypertensive CKD patients. Sodium intake was measured by 24-h urine sodium excretion (24-h UNa). Additionally, 20 patients with immunoglobulin A nephropathy (IgAN) participated in a 7-day sodium restriction study (100 mmol/day). The average 24-h UNa of the study cohort was 149.0 ± 66.4 mmol/day. The OR for each 17 mmol increment in

24-h UNa (salt 1 g/day) for BP > 130/80 mm Hg was 1.26 (95% CI 1.10–1.44, $P = 0.001$). The sodium restriction group achieved significantly more reduction in systolic BP (-11.1 mm Hg vs. -5.0 mmHg, $P = 0.022$), diastolic BP (-9.4 mm Hg vs. -2.1 mmHg, $P = 0.009$), and urine protein excretion [-465 (-855 to -340) mg/day vs. -150 (-570 to 40) mg/day, $P = 0.024$]. A positive correlation was observed between the change of 24-h UNa and the change of SBP ($r = 0.450$, $P = 0.047$) in the sodium restriction group. The change of 24-h UNa was also correlated with the 24-h TGF-β1 excretion ($r = 0.558$, $P = 0.011$) in these patient. The authors recommended that dietary sodium intake restriction should be monitored and intensified in the treatment of Chinese CKD patients [42].

In one recent observational study, Meng et al. investigated the relationship between salt intake and BPs in non-dialysis CKD patients. To determine salt intake, patients were given written instructions on how to collect the 24-h urine under normal eating habits. A urine aliquot (100 ml) from the 24-h urine collection was assayed. BP/dietary sodium intake was regarded as salt sensitivity index. The authors demonstrated that there was a linear positive relationship between the salt intake and the SBP but there was no relationship between salt intake and DBP. According to CKD stages, there was no correlation between the salt intake and the SBP in stage 1–2, but there was a linear regression relationship in stage 3, 4 and strongest in stage 5 [43].

Regarding the effect of salt intake on resistant HT, there is even scarce data. In an evaluation of subjects with severe hypertension (but not specifically mentioned as resistant HT), Fotherby et al. assessed the BP effects of low dietary salt ingestion in 17 untreated hypertensive subjects with a mean office BP of 176 ± 17 and 96 ± 11 mm Hg. After 5 weeks of low-salt diet (80–100 mmol/24 h), 24-h systolic and diastolic BP decreased by 5 and 2 mm Hg [44].

In a study by Gavras et al., a greater BP reduction was observed with extreme dietary salt restriction in combination with intense diuretic therapy in subjects with uncontrolled BP on maximal doses of at least two agents (a diuretic and a sympatholytic agent). In this study, BP decreased on average by 21/7 mm Hg during ingestion of a diet limited to 10 mmol of sodium with concurrent administration of either hydrochlorothiazide 100 mg or furosemide 80–200 mg daily. However, again there was no specific mention on RHT in this study [45].

The direct evidence between salt intake and RHT was shown in at least one clinical study. Pimenta et al. examined the effects of dietary salt restriction on office and 24-h ambulatory blood pressure in 12 subjects with resistant hypertension on an average of 3.4 ± 0.5 antihypertensive medications and a mean office BP of $145.8 \pm 10.8/83.9 \pm 11.2$ mm Hg. Patients entered into a randomized crossover evaluation of low (50 mmol/24 h × 7 days) and high sodium diets (250 mmol/24 h × 7 days) separated by a 2-week washout period. The mean urinary sodium excretion was 46.1 ± 26.8 versus 252.2 ± 64.6 mmol/24 h during low-salt versus high-salt intake. A low-salt compared with a high-salt diet decreased office systolic and diastolic BPs by 22.7 and 9.1 mm Hg, respectively. This was the first study, to assess the effects of low dietary salt ingestion in subjects with resistant hypertension. However, in this study patients with creatinine clearance <60 mL/min were excluded from the study [46].

In another trial, the effect of sodium restriction on BP and proteinuria was investigated in CKD patients. The study involved 20 hypertensive stage 3–4 CKD patients. Dietary education was individualized to the participant's food preferences and was provided by an accredited practicing dietitian. A double-blind placebo-controlled randomized crossover trial was performed to assess the effects of high versus low sodium intake on ambulatory BP, 24-h protein and albumin excretion, fluid status (body composition monitor), renin and aldosterone levels, and arterial stiffness (pulse wave velocity and augmentation index) in 20 adult patients with hypertensive stage 3–4 CKD as phase 1 of the LowSALT CKD study. Ambulatory BP showed a mean reduction of 9.7/3.9 mm Hg (systolic BP/ diastolic BP) which was achieved from the high salt period to the low salt period. Fluid volume, body weight, proteinuria, and albuminuria were also reduced in the low salt period. Plasma renin and plasma aldosterone increased. This is the first double-blind randomized controlled trial to assess the effect of sodium restriction on ambulatory BP and other cardiovascular risk factors in non-dialyzed, non-transplanted CKD patients. This study found that reducing dietary sodium intake by 100 mmol reduced extracellular volume by 0.8 L with concurrent BP reductions of approximately 10/4 mm Hg SBP/DBP, a considerable magnitude of change comparable with that expected from the addition of an antihypertensive medication [47].

In the post hoc analysis of LowSALT CKD study, peripheral systolic BP was reduced by mean 10 [95% CI 1–20] mm Hg from mean ±SD 159 ± 14 mm Hg at the high sodium period to 148 ± 21 mm Hg at the low sodium period ($p = 0.04$), while diastolic BP was reduced by 6 [95% CI 1–10] mm Hg from 87 ± 10 mm Hg at the high sodium to 82 ± 12 mm Hg at the low sodium period ($p = 0.03$). Central systolic BP was reduced by 13 [95% CI 2–24] mm Hg from 143 ± 20 mm Hg at the high sodium period to 130 ± 21 mm Hg at the low sodium period ($p = 0.03$) Central pulse pressure was significantly reduced by 9 [95% CI 2–17] mm Hg from 59 ± 16 mm Hg at the high sodium period to 50 ± 12 mm Hg at the low sodium period ($p = 0.02$). Fluid markers including extracellular/intracellular fluid ratio and NT–proBNP were decreased in low sodium group compared to high sodium group [48].

In hemodialysis (HD) patients, sodium mass balance is primarily dependent on dietary salt intake and sodium removal during dialysis. Thus simply reducing sodium intake is the most logical approach to prevent hypervolemia. However, salt restriction has not been performed in many dialysis centers [49] though the fact that plasma sodium is closely related with BP in hemodialysis patients [50, 51]. In hypertensive peritoneal dialysis patients, total sodium load, daily total sodium removal, extracellular water, and normalized extracellular water were all higher compared to normotensive group [52].

Kayikcioglu et al. investigated the effect of salt restriction in HD patients. They divided the patients into two groups. In first group (n: 190) salt restriction strategy (5 g/day) was performed. In second group (n: 204) antihypertensive-based strategy was applied. Salt restriction was defined as managing high BP via lowering dry weight by strict salt restriction and insistent ultrafiltration without using antihypertensive drugs. Antihypertensive drugs were used in 7% of the patients in first group and 42% in second group ($P < 0.01$); interdialytic weight gain was significantly lower in Centre A (2.29 ± 0.83 kg versus 3.31 ± 1.12 kg, $P < 0.001$). Mean systolic and diastolic BPs were similar in the two groups. However, first group had lower left ventricular (LV) mass index and cardiac hypertrophy [53].

In another prospective study, the effects of strict salt control on blood pressure and cardiac condition in end-stage renal disease were investigated. A total of 12 peritoneal dialysis (PD) and 15 prevalent hemodialysis (HD) patients were enrolled. All patients with either PD or HD were allocated to intervention of strict salt restriction according to basal hydration state of empty abdomen in PD and midweek pre-dialysis HD which were estimated by body composition monitor (BCM) and echocardiography. Systolic BP decreased in PD and HD from 133.1 ± 28 and 147.3 ± 28.5 to 114.8 ± 16.5 and 119.3 ± 12.1 mmHg, respectively ($P < 0.00$) [54].

Despite these studies showing the beneficial effect of sodium restriction, there are no large-scale, long-term prospective studies investigating the effect of strict sodium restriction on cardiovascular outcomes.

As seen, there are very few studies regarding sodium, CKD, and HT, especially resistant HT. It is obvious that more prospective, randomized studies are needed to define the role of salt restriction on BP and cardiovascular outcomes in CKD patients. The following chapter will focus on the management of RHT in CKD especially focusing on salt restriction.

Management of Salt Restriction

As suggested most patients with HT and CKD are salt sensitive. Sodium intake in CKD populations is generally high, and often above population average. Recent evidence suggests that independent of BP, high salt induces structural and functional deterioration in vessels. Additionally, moderately lower sodium intake in CKD patients is associated with substantially better long-term outcome of RAAS blockage, in diabetic and nondiabetic CKD, related to better effects of RAAS blockage on proteinuria independent of BP [55, 56].

Therefore, educating patients with CKD on a low salt diet is critical to achieving BP control while maintaining a simple BP medication regimen. However, it should be remembered that reducing salt intake is a hard task to achieve. Effectively reducing salt intake is not achieved even under supervision [57]. Due to low palatability of low sodium diets, convenience and lack of knowledge regarding the benefits of low sodium diet [58].

In 2005, the US Department of Health and Human Services recommended that adults consume no more than 2300 mg of sodium per day and those patients in specified subgroups (including persons with CKD) consume no more than 1500 mg/d. However, it was criticized that the evidence is not strong enough to indicate that these subgroups should be treated differently than the general US population [59].

In a double-blind placebo-controlled crossover trial, 20 hypertensive adults with stage 3–4 CKD were randomized to a low sodium diet by dietary education plus 120 mmol of sodium or a low sodium diet plus matched placebo capsules. Participants received each diet with capsules for 2 weeks with a 1-week washout period in between. Mean 24-h urinary sodium excretions were 168 mmol (95% confidence interval [CI], 146–219) and 75 mmol (95% CI, 58–112) for the high and low salt interventions, respectively. Mean BP by 24-h ambulatory monitoring was lower by 9.7/3.9 mm Hg (95% CI, 4.5–14.8/1.3–6.4) in the low salt intervention [47].

A modest dietary sodium restriction can enhance the effects of antihypertensive medications like angiotensin-converting enzyme inhibitors or angiotensin receptor blockers when treating HT in CKD. In a small randomized trial, 52 patients with nondiabetic nephropathy receiving lisinopril 40 mg daily were randomized to valsartan 320 mg daily or placebo combined with consecutively a low sodium (target 50 mmol/d) or a regular sodium (target 200 mmol/d) diet in a crossover design for four 6-week periods. Mean urinary sodium excretion was 106 and 184 mmol/d in the low and regular sodium interventions. This difference in dietary sodium intake resulted in a larger BP reduction (7% vs. 2% reduction, P: 0.003) compared with the addition of the angiotensin receptor blocker to lisinopril 40 mg daily. Besides, modest dietary sodium restriction inpatients receiving ACE medicines showed 11 mm Hg reduction in SBP in nondiabetic nephropathy [38].

Importantly, low dietary salt intake also augments the antiproteinuric effect of diuretics and RAAS blocking drugs. In 34 proteinuric patients with diabetes mellitus, reductions in mean baseline proteinuria were increased from 30% to 55% with the addition of a low salt diet to losartan monotherapy. The combination of a low salt diet and hydrochlorothiazide reduced proteinuria by 70% from baseline. Conversely, a high salt diet offsets the efficacy of diuretics and renin-angiotensin-aldosterone blockers to both reduce BP and proteinuria [60].

Thus these studies suggest that sodium restriction not only directly reduces BP but indirectly augments the natriuretic effects of antihypertensive drugs.

One of the important concern is the J-curve between sodium intake and renal and cardiovascular outcome during rigorous sodium restriction [61, 62]. However, these observational data should be interpreted with caution, as a habitual salt intake below 5 g daily is a rarity in the outpatient population, and quantification of sodium intake was questionable in some of the studies, by lack of 24-h urine data on sodium intake. This may have contributed to the substantial differences in the level of the nadir of the J-curve [55].

Future Directions

The most important issue is the need for prospective, placebo-controlled studies regarding reducing sodium intake and RHT. The interventional studies are also needed whether reducing salt intake will translate into health outcomes including cardiovascular diseases.

The second important concern is the education. Behavioral intervention studies have previously demonstrated that knowledge is a key contributing factor to adherence to low-salt diet [63] and that lack of knowledge is a key barrier in dietary modification and adherence [64]. Dietary advice to lower salt intake routinely given to patients with CKD in the form of an information sheet is ineffective. By contrast, the dietitian-led intervention may be of more value in decreasing sodium intake [65]. There is compelling evidence from behavioral sciences that sustained lifestyle changes require a dedicated, behavioral approach [66–68]. However, such approaches are not yet part of the clinical routine in renal care. Thus it is of paramount importance to educate patients actively to decrease sodium intake.

Cultural background and orientation are also important issues regarding salt intake. Efforts to understand their cultural mores interpret and convey health-promotion messages in culturally appropriate ways will probably result with a positive response in CKD patients [69].

A part from personalized care, national strategies regarding reducing salt intake is of paramount importance. The vitality of this action is already recognized and a review of salt reduction strategies undertaken in 2010 identified 32 national salt reduction strategies worldwide [70].

Although the limitation of salt intake as a national strategy seems a hard issue, salt reduction strategy has highlighted feasibility, demonstrating a 15% reduction in population salt intake between 2003 and 2011 in United Kingdom with average blood pressure in the adult population falling by 3/1.4 mm Hg over the same period [71].

It is important to remember that estimation of salt intake is a hard issue. The gold standard for the assessment of sodium intake is from well-collected 24-h urine, as dietary recall and food frequency questionnaires are notoriously unreliable due to fact that only 15% of the sodium ingested is added during cooking or during meals, whereas the remainder is present in the food in hidden form, as additives in processed foods [72]. For this reason, new, simple, and accurate methods should be performed to investigate sodium intake.

The potential strategies and suggested investigations regarding sodium restriction are summarized in Table 16.2.

Table 16.2 The potential strategies and suggested investigations regarding sodium restriction

Planning prospective, placebo-controlled studies regarding reducing sodium intake and RHT and exploring whether these studies will translate into better health outcomes
New, simple, and accurate methods should be performed to investigate sodium intake
Understand the cultural norms, beliefs, habits, and barriers regarding high sodium intake
Exploring strategies to reduce sodium intake nationally
Individual education to decrease sodium intake (better in the form of active education rather than passive dietary advice)
Explain the health gains regarding decreased sodium intake

Conclusions

Chronic kidney disease and RHT are closely related with each other and as CKD progresses, the proportion RHT increases. Although currently the cause and effect relationship cannot be suggested, studies confirm that there is reciprocal relationship between progression of CKD and development of RHT. The causes of RHT in CKD are thought to be many but the most important factor is the salt. Indeed the BP in CKD is salt sensitive. Although studies are rare, recent evidence suggests that salt intake is closely related with the development of RHT in CKD. Thus reduction of salt intake (both individually and nationally) is very important. To accomplish this issue, active education seems mandatory. Prospective, placebo-controlled studies are needed whether reducing salt intake will translate into heath outcomes including cardiovascular diseases.

References

1. Bakris GL, Williams M, Dworkin L, Elliott WJ, Epstein M, Toto R, Tuttle K, Douglas J, Hsueh W, Sowers J. Preserving renal function in adults with hypertension and diabetes: a consensus approach. National Kidney Foundation Hypertension and Diabetes Executive Committees Working Group. Am J Kidney Dis. 2000;36(3):646–61.
2. Cai G, Zheng Y, Sun X, Chen X. Survey of Prevalence, Awareness, and Treatment Rates in Chronic Kidney Disease Patients with Hypertension in China Collaborative Group. Prevalence, awareness, treatment, and control of hypertension in elderly adults with chronic kidney disease: results from the survey of Prevalence, Awareness, and Treatment Rates in Chronic Kidney Disease Patients with Hypertension in China. J Am Geriatr Soc. 2013;61(12):2160–7.
3. Michell AR. Salt, hypertension and renal disease: comparative medicine, models and real diseases. Postgrad Med J. 1994;70(828):686–94.
4. Drexler YR, Bomback AS. Definition, identification and treatment of resistant hypertension in chronic kidney disease patients. Nephrol Dial Transplant. 2014;29(7):1327–35.
5. Sarafidis PA. Epidemiology of resistant hypertension. J Clin Hypertens (Greenwich). 2011;13(7):523–8.
6. Borrelli S, De Nicola L, Stanzione G, Conte G, Minutolo R. Resistant hypertension in nondialysis chronic kidney disease. Int J Hypertens. 2013;2013:929183.
7. Calhoun DA, Jones D, Textor S, Goff DC, Murphy TP, Toto RD, White A, Cushman WC, White W, Sica D, Ferdinand K, Giles TD, Falkner B, Carey RM. Resistant hypertension: diagnosis, evaluation, and treatment. A scientific statement from the American Heart Association Professional Education Committee of the Council for High Blood Pressure Research. Hypertension. 2008;51(6):1403–19.
8. Judd E, Calhoun DA. Apparent and true resistant hypertension: definition, prevalence and outcomes. J Hum Hypertens. 2014;28(8):463–8.
9. Sarafidis PA, Georgianos PI, Zebekakis PE. Comparative epidemiology of resistant hypertension in chronic kidney disease and the general hypertensive population. Semin Nephrol. 2014;34(5):483–91.
10. Modolo R, de Faria AP, Sabbatini AR, Barbaro NR, Ritter AM, Moreno H. Refractory and resistant hypertension: characteristics and differences observed in a specialized clinic. J Am Soc Hypertens. 2015;9(5):397–402.
11. Sarafidis PA, Bakris GL. Resistant hypertension: an overview of evaluation and treatment. J Am Coll Cardiol. 2008;52(22):1749–57.

12. Acelajado MC, Pisoni R, Dudenbostel T, Dell'Italia LJ, Cartmill F, Zhang B, Cofield SS, Oparil S, Calhoun DA. Refractory hypertension: definition, prevalence, and patient characteristics. J Clin Hypertens (Greenwich). 2012;14(1):7–12.
13. Bangash F, Agarwal R. Masked hypertension and white-coat hypertension in chronic kidney disease: a meta-analysis. Clin J Am Soc Nephrol. 2009;4(3):656–64.
14. Parati G, Stergiou G, O'Brien E, Asmar R, Beilin L, Bilo G, Clement D, de laSierra A, de Leeuw P, Dolan E, Fagard R, Graves J, Head GA, Imai Y, Kario K, Lurbe E, Mallion JM, Mancia G, Mengden T, Myers M, Ogedegbe G, Ohkubo T, Omboni S, Palatini P, Redon J, Ruilope LM, Shennan A, Staessen JA, van Montfrans G, Verdecchia P, Waeber B, Wang J, Zanchetti A, Zhang Y. European Society of Hypertension Working Group on Blood Pressure Monitoring and Cardiovascular Variability. European Society of Hypertension practice guidelines for ambulatory blood pressure monitoring. J Hypertens. 2014;32(7):1359–66.
15. De Nicola L, Borrelli S, Gabbai FB, Chiodini P, Zamboli P, Iodice C, Vitiello S, Conte G, Minutolo R. Burden of resistant hypertension in hypertensive patients with non-dialysis chronic kidney disease. Kidney Blood Press Res. 2011;34(1):58–67.
16. James PA, Oparil S, Carter BL, Cushman WC, Dennison-Himmelfarb C, Handler J, Lackland DT, LeFevre ML, MacKenzie TD, Ogedegbe O, Smith SC Jr, Svetkey LP, Taler SJ, Townsend RR, Wright JT Jr, Narva AS, Ortiz E. 2014 evidence-based guideline for the management of high blood pressure in adults: report from the panel members appointed to the eighth joint National Committee (JNC 8). JAMA. 2014;311(5):507–20.
17. Dasgupta K, Quinn RR, Zarnke KB, Rabi DM, Ravani P, Daskalopoulou SS, Rabkin SW, Trudeau L, Feldman RD, Cloutier L, Prebtani A, Herman RJ, Bacon SL, Gilbert RE, Ruzicka M, McKay DW, Campbell TS, Grover S, Honos G, Schiffrin EL, Bolli P, Wilson TW, Lindsay P, Hill MD, Coutts SB, Gubitz G, Gelfer M, Vallée M, Prasad GV, Lebel M, McLean D, Arnold JM, Moe GW, Howlett JG, Boulanger JM, Larochelle P, Leiter LA, Jones C, Ogilvie RI, Woo V, Kaczorowski J, Burns KD, Petrella RJ, Hiremath S, Milot A, Stone JA, Drouin D, Lavoie KL, Lamarre-Cliche M, Tremblay G, Hamet P, Fodor G, Carruthers SG, Pylypchuk GB, Burgess E, Lewanczuk R, Dresser GK, Penner SB, Hegele RA, McFarlane PA, Khara M, Pipe A, Oh P, Selby P, Sharma M, Reid DJ, Tobe SW, Padwal RS, Poirier L. Canadian Hypertension Education Program. The 2014 Canadian Hypertension Education Program recommendations for blood pressure measurement, diagnosis, assessment of risk, prevention, and treatment of hypertension. Can J Cardiol. 2014;30(5):485–501.
18. Mancia G, Fagard R, Narkiewicz K, Redón J, Zanchetti A, Böhm M, Christiaens T, Cifkova R, De Backer G, Dominiczak A, Galderisi M, Grobbee DE, Jaarsma T, Kirchhof P, Kjeldsen SE, Laurent S, Manolis AJ, Nilsson PM, Ruilope LM, Schmieder RE, Sirnes PA, Sleight P, Viigimaa M, Waeber B, Zannad F, Members TF. 2013 ESH/ESC guidelines for the management of arterial hypertension: the task force for the management of arterial hypertension of the European Society of Hypertension (ESH) and of the European Society of Cardiology (ESC). J Hypertens. 2013;31(7):1281–357.
19. Taler SJ, Agarwal R, Bakris GL, Flynn JT, Nilsson PM, Rahman M, Sanders PW, Textor SC, Weir MR, Townsend RR. KDOQI US commentary on the 2012 KDIGO clinical practice guideline for management of blood pressure in CKD. Am J Kidney Dis. 2013;62(2):201–13.
20. Flack JM, Sica DA, Bakris G, Brown AL, Ferdinand KC, Grimm RH Jr, Hall WD, Jones WE, Kountz DS, Lea JP, Nasser S, Nesbitt SD, Saunders E, Scisney-Matlock M, Jamerson KA. International Society on Hypertension in Blacks. Management of high blood pressure in Blacks: an update of the International Society on Hypertension in Blacks consensus statement. Hypertension. 2010;56(5):780–800.
21. Kovesdy CP, Bleyer AJ, Molnar MZ, Ma JZ, Sim JJ, Cushman WC, Quarles LD, Kalantar-Zadeh K. Blood pressure and mortality in U.S. veterans with chronic kidney disease: a cohort study. Ann Intern Med. 2013;159(4):233–42.
22. Townsend RR. Blood pressure targets in CKD. Adv Chronic Kidney Dis. 2015;22(2):96–101.
23. KDIGO. Clinical practice guideline for the management of blood pressure in chronic kidney disease. Kidney Int Suppl. 2012;2(5):337–414.

24. Judd E, Calhoun DA. Management of Hypertension in CKD: beyond the guidelines. Adv Chronic Kidney Dis. 2015;22(2):116–22.
25. Ying WZ, Sanders PW. Dietary salt modulates renal production of transforming growth factor-beta in rats. Am J Phys. 1998;274(4 Pt 2):F635–41.
26. Sinnakirouchenan R, Kotchen TA. Role of sodium restriction and diuretic therapy for "resistant" hypertension in chronic kidney disease. Semin Nephrol. 2014;34(5):514–9.
27. Bigazzi R, Bianchi S, Baldari D, Sgherri G, Baldari G, Campese VM. Microalbuminuria in salt-sensitive patients. A marker for renal and cardio-vascular risk factors. Hypertension. 1994;23(2):195–9.
28. Fellner RC, Cook AK, O'Connor PM, Zhang S, Pollock DM, Inscho EW. High-salt diet blunts renal autoregulation by a reactive oxygen species-dependent mechanism. Am J Physiol Renal Physiol. 2014;307(1):F33–40.
29. Townsend RR. Pathogenesis of drug resistant hypertension. Semin Nephrol. 2014;34(5):506–13.
30. Ying WZ, Aaron K, Sanders PW. Mechanism of dietary salt mediated increase in intravascular production of TGF-beta1. Am J Physiol Renal Physiol. 2008;295(2):F406–14.
31. Townsend RR, Wimmer NJ, Chirinos JA, Parsa A, Weir M, Perumal K, Lash JP, Chen J, Steigerwalt SP, Flack J, Go AS, Rafey M, Rahman M, Sheridan A, Gadegbeku CA, Robinson NA, Joffe M. Aortic PWV in chronic kidney disease: a CRIC ancillary study. Am J Hypertens. 2010;23(3):282–9.
32. Johnson RJ, Herrera-Acosta J, Schreiner GF, Rodríguez-Iturbe B. Subtle acquired renal injury as a mechanism of salt-sensitive hypertension. N Engl J Med. 2002;346(12):913–23.
33. Oparil S, Zaman MA, Calhoun DA. Pathogenesis of hypertension. Ann Intern Med. 2003;139(9):761–76.
34. Koomans HA, Roos JC, Boer P, Geyskes GG, Mees EJ. Salt sensitivity of blood pressure in chronic renal failure. Evidence for renal control of body fluid distribution in man. Hypertension. 1982;4(2):190–7.
35. Blythe WB. Natural history of hypertension in renal parenchymal disease. Am J Kidney Dis. 1985;5(4):A50–6.
36. De Nicola L, Minutolo R, Bellizzi V, Zoccali C, Cianciaruso B, Andreucci VE, et al. investigators of the TArget Blood Pressure LEvels in Chronic Kidney Disease (TABLE in CKD) study group. Achievement of target blood pressure levels in chronic kidney disease: a salty question? Am J Kidney Dis. 2004;43(5):782–95.
37. Smyth A, O'Donnell MJ, Yusuf S, Clase CM, Teo KK, Canavan M, Reddan DN, Mann JF. Sodium intake and renal outcomes: a systematic review. Am J Hypertens. 2014;27(10):1277–84.
38. Slagman MC, Waanders F, Hemmelder MH, Woittiez AJ, Janssen WM, Lambers Heerspink HJ, Navis G, Laverman GD, HOlland NEphrology STudy Group. Moderate dietary sodium restriction added to angiotensin converting enzyme inhibition compared with dual blockade in lowering proteinuria and blood pressure: randomised controlled trial. BMJ. 2011;343:d4366.
39. Higashi Y, Oshima T, Ozono R, Nakano Y, Matsuura H, Kambe M, Kajiyama G. Nocturnal decline in blood pressure is attenuated by NaCl loading in salt-sensitive patients with essential hypertension: noninvasive 24-hour ambulatory blood pressure monitoring. Hypertension. 1997;30(2 Pt 1):163–7.
40. Egan BM, Basile JN, Rehman SU, Davis PB, Grob CH 3rd, Riehle JF, Walters CA, Lackland DT, Merali C, Sealey JE, Laragh JH. Plasma renin test-guided drug treatment algorithm for correcting patients with treated but uncontrolled hypertension: a randomized controlled trial. Am J Hypertens. 2009;22(7):792–801.
41. Krikken JA, Laverman GD, Navis G. Benefits of dietary sodium restriction in the management of chronic kidney disease. Curr Opin Nephrol Hypertens. 2009;18(6):531–8.
42. Yu W, Luying S, Haiyan W, Xiaomei L. Importance and benefits of dietary sodium restriction in the management of chronic kidney disease patients: experience from a single Chinese center. Int Urol Nephrol. 2012;44(2):549–56.
43. Meng L, Fu B, Zhang T, Han Z, Yang M. Salt sensitivity of blood pressure in non-dialysis patients with chronic kidney disease. Ren Fail. 2014;36(3):345–50.

44. Fotherby MD, Potter JF. Effects of moderate sodium restriction on clinic and twenty-four- hour ambulatory blood pressure in elderly hypertensive subjects. J Hypertens. 1993;11(6):657–63.
45. Gavras H, Waeber B, Kershaw GR, Liang CS, Textor SC, Brunner HR, Tifft CP, Gavras I. Role of reactive hyperreninemia in blood pressure changes induced by sodium depletion in patients with refractory hypertension. Hypertension. 1981;3:441–7.
46. Pimenta E, Gaddam KK, Oparil S, Aban I, Husain S, Dell'Italia LJ, Calhoun DA. Effects of dietary sodium reduction on blood pressure in subjects with resistant hypertension: results from a randomized trial. Hypertension. 2009;54(3):475–81.
47. McMahon EJ, Bauer JD, Hawley CM, Isbel NM, Stowasser M, Johnson DW, Campbell KL. A randomized trial of dietary sodium restriction in CKD. J Am Soc Nephrol. 2013;24(12):2096–103.
48. Campbell KL, Johnson DW, Bauer JD, Hawley CM, Isbel NM, Stowasser M, Whitehead JP, Dimeski G, McMahon E. A randomized trial of sodium-restriction on kidney function, fluid volume and adipokines in CKD patients. BMC Nephrol. 2014;15:57. doi:10.1186/1471-2369-15-57.
49. Ok E. How to successfully achieve salt restriction in dialysis patients? What are the outcomes? Blood Purif. 2010;29(2):102–4.
50. He FJ, Fan S, Macgregor GA, Yaqoob MM. Plasma sodium and blood pressure in individuals on haemodialysis. J Hum Hypertens. 2013;27(2):85–9.
51. Lindley EJ. Reducing sodium intake in hemodialysis patients. Semin Dial. 2009;22(3):260–3.
52. Inal S, Erten Y, Akbulu G, Oneç K, Tek NA, Sahin G, Okyay GU, Sanlier N. Salt intake and hypervolemia in the development of hypertension in peritoneal dialysis patients. Adv Perit Dial. 2012;28:10–5.
53. Kayikcioglu M, Tumuklu M, Ozkahya M, Ozdogan O, Asci G, Duman S, Toz H, Can LH, Basci A, Ok E. The benefit of salt restriction in the treatment of end-stage renal disease by haemodialysis. Nephrol Dial Transplant. 2009;24(3):956–62.
54. Magden K, Hur E, Yildiz G, Kose SB, Bicak S, Yildirim I, Sayin MR, Duman S. The effects of strict salt control on blood pressure and cardiac condition in end-stage renal disease: prospective-study. Ren Fail. 2013;35(10):1344–7.
55. Humalda JK, Navis G. Dietary sodium restriction: a neglected therapeutic opportunity in chronic kidney disease. Curr Opin Nephrol Hypertens. 2014;23(6):533–40.
56. Krikken JA, Lely AT, Bakker SJ, Navis G. The effect of a shift in sodium intake on renal hemodynamics is determined by body mass index in healthy youngmen. Kidney Int. 2007;71(3):260–5.
57. De Nicola L, Minutolo R, Gallo C, Zoccali C, Cianciaruso B, Conte M, Lupo A, Fuiano G, Gallucci M, Bonomini M, Chiodini P, Signoriello G, Bellizzi V, Mallamaci F, Nappi F, Conte G. Management of hypertension in chronic kidney disease: the Italian multicentric study. J Nephrol. 2005;18(4):397–404.
58. McMahon EJ, Campbell KL, Mudge DW, Bauer JD. Achieving salt restriction in chronic kidney disease. Int J Nephrol. 2012;2012:720429.
59. Institute of Medicine of the National Academies. Sodium intake in populations: assessment of evidence. Washington, D.C.: The National Academies Press; 2013.
60. Vogt L, Waanders F, Boomsma F, de Zeeuw D, Navis G. Effects of dietary sodium and hydrochlorothiazide on the anti-proteinuric efficacy of losartan. J Am Soc Nephrol. 2008;19(5):999–1007.
61. Thomas MC, Moran J, Forsblom C, Harjutsalo V, Thorn L, Ahola A, Wadén J, Tolonen N, Saraheimo M, Gordin D. Groop PH; Finn Diane Study Group. The association between dietary sodium intake, ESRD, and all-cause mortality in patients with type 1 diabetes. Diabetes Care. 2011;34(4):861–6.
62. O'Donnell MJ, Yusuf S, Mente A, Gao P, Mann JF, Teo K, McQueen M, Sleight P, Sharma AM, Dans A, Probstfield J, Schmieder RE. Urinary sodium and potassium excretion and risk of cardiovascular events. JAMA. 2011;306(20):2229–38.

63. Appel LJ, Champagne CM, Harsha DW, Cooper LS, Obarzanek E, Elmer PJ, Stevens VJ, Vollmer WM, Lin PH, Svetkey LP, Stedman SW, Young DR. Writing Group of the PREMIER Collaborative Research Group. Effects of comprehensive lifestylemodification on blood pressure control: main results of the PREMIER clinicaltrial. JAMA. 2003;289(16):2083–93.
64. Ni H, Nauman D, Burgess D, Wise K, Crispell K, Hershberger RE. Factors influencing knowledge of and adherence to self-care among patients with heart failure. Arch Intern Med. 1999;159(14):1613–9.
65. de Brito-Ashurst I, Perry L, Sanders TA, Thomas JE, Dobbie H, Varagunam M, Yaqoob MM. The role of salt intake and salt sensitivity in the management ofhypertension in South Asian people with chronic kidney disease: a randomised controlled trial. Heart. 2013;99(17):1256–60.
66. Cook NR, Cutler JA, Obarzanek E, Buring JE, Rexrode KM, Kumanyika SK, Appel LJ, Whelton PK. Long term effects of dietary sodium reduction on cardiovascular disease outcomes: observational follow-up of the trials of hypertension prevention (TOHP). BMJ. 2007;334(7599):885–8.
67. Robare JF, Bayles CM, Newman AB, Williams K, Milas C, Boudreau R, McTigue K, Albert SM, Taylor C, Kuller LH. The "10 keys" to healthy aging: 24-month follow-up results from an innovative community-based prevention program. Health Educ Behav. 2011;38(4):379–88.
68. Zhang SX, Guo HW, Wan WT, Xue K. Nutrition education guided by dietary guidelines for Chinese residents on metabolic syndrome characteristics, adipokines and inflammatory markers. Asia Pac J Clin Nutr. 2011;20(1):77–86.
69. de Brito-Ashurst I, Perry L, Sanders TA, Thomas JE, Yaqoob MM, Dobbie H. Barriers and facilitators of dietary sodium restriction amongst Bangladeshi chronic kidney disease patients. J Hum Nutr Diet. 2011;24(1):86–95.
70. Webster JL, Dunford EK, Hawkes C, Neal BC. Salt reduction initiatives around the world. J Hypertens. 2011;29(6):1043–50.
71. He FJ, Pombo-Rodrigues S, Mac Gregor GA. Salt reduction in England from 2003 to 2011: its relationship to blood pressure, stroke and ischaemic heart disease mortality. BMJ Open. 2014;4(4):e004549.
72. Carrigan A, Klinger A, Choquette SS, Luzuriaga-McPherson A, Bell EK, Darnell B, Gutiérrez OM. Contribution of food additives to sodium and phosphorus content of diets rich in processed foods. J Ren Nutr. 2014;24(1):13–9. 19e1

Chapter 17
Treatment of Hypertension in Light of the New Guidelines: Drug Adherence

Alper Kirkpantur and Baris Afsar

Introduction

Hypertension is frequently observed in patients with chronic kidney disease (CKD) [1] with an increasing prevalence as the glomerular filtration rate falls. Hypertension is an important issue in the care of CKD patients as it is an important determinant of the progression to end-stage renal disease and to protect against cardiovascular disease [2]. Therefore, an adequate control of blood pressure in these patients results in a slower decline in renal function [3] and is recommended in all patients with CKD. However, to achieve these goals, adherence to treatment plays a major role.

When we examine the blood pressure control rates in CKD patients, the story is different. It was shown that the BP control rate remains low in CKD patients with 13.2% of patients having <130/80 mmHg Kidney Early Evaluation Program (KEEP) [4]. Moreover, blood pressure targets were achieved only in 35% of CKD patients in a more recent work [5]. Furthermore, in the Reasons for Geographic and Racial Differences in Stroke (REGARDS) study, while 36.2% of CKD patients had a BP of >140/90 mmHg, 61.6% of patients had a BP of >130/80 mmHg [6].

A. Kirkpantur (✉)
Department of Nephrology, Acıbadem University Hospital, Ankara, Turkey
e-mail: alperkirkpantur@yahoo.com; alper.kirkpantur@acibadem.edu.tr

B. Afsar
Department of Internal Medicine, Division of Nephrology Çünür, Suleyman Demirel University, Doğu yerleşkesi, Isparta Merkez/Isparta, 32260, Turkey

© Springer International Publishing AG 2017
A. Covic et al. (eds.), *Resistant Hypertension in Chronic Kidney Disease*,
DOI 10.1007/978-3-319-56827-0_17

The Term "Adherence" in Patients with Chronic Kidney Disease: The Facts

When the patient reaches to end-stage renal disease, clinical comorbidities like renal anemia, secondary hyperparathyroidism, and infection are much morely added to hypertension that all are involved in the clinical course and survival of the CKD patient. Therefore, progression of CKD is generally associated with introduction of new drugs to be taken by the patient to minimize the effects of these disorders that might be difficult to be controlled only by dietary measures and dialysis therapy itself. Pre-dialysis patients have been shown to be treated with a mean of 6–12 medications [2, 7]. Moreover, a recent study on maintenance dialysis therapy revealed a median number of 19 pills with one-quarter of them taking >25 medications daily [2, 8]. In the light of these findings, the term "drug adherence" defined as patient's respect to taking his/her prescribed medication(s) is a significant issue in this patient population. Additionally, adherence in hypertension emphasizes the need for agreement between the physician and patient in the treatment of hypertension and consequently focuses on the patient's ability and willingness to accept an antihypertensive regimen. Moreover, the World Health Organization (WHO) says that, "adherence is a person's behavior concerning taking medication, following a diet, and making changes in lifestyle in accordance with a medical or non-medical health professional recommendations" [9].

Studies in Chronic Kidney Disease Population

Adherence might be lower in these patients due to such a high pill burden in patients with CKD. Supporting this idea, a low adherence to drug treatments (down to 3%) as well as a low adherence to nutritional recommendations has been reported in CKD and dialysis patients [2, 10]. Moreover, adherence to drug therapy in CKD was assessed via the medication possession ratio [5] and the Morisky questionnaire [6]. The findings of these abovementioned studies revealed that more than 30% of the study patients which is a quite significant number were poorly adherent to medical therapy. Interestingly, a study measuring drug adherence in CKD patients reported improving drug adherence (by self-report) while renal function further declines – indicating both doctors and patients have become more interested in blood pressure control with the progression of CKD [11]. A pre-dialysis study showed that medication nonadherence was lower (17.4%) at the baseline period of the study than after 1 year of the study (26.8%) [11]. Compared to the baseline period, the percentage of adherent patients who became nonadherent (22%) was lower than the percentage of nonadherent patients who became adherent (50%) [11]. Similar numbers were demostrated in CKD patients not on dialysis by Moreira et al. (18.5%) [12] – using the self-report method and a drug profile – and by Lee et al. (18%) [13], based on two methods, pill count and electronic monitoring. It is also a common finding that in several studies in pre-dialysis, CKD patients reveal that [11, 14, 15] the number of nonadherent patients increases throughout the observation period. This study also showed that nonadherent CKD patients had a higher mean age, were using a larger amount of pills per day at baseline and at the final period, did not self-administer medications, and had higher mean serum creatinine, lower GFR, and a lower frequency of coronary heart disease [11]. In this study, the logistic regression model, adjusted for statistically significant variables in univariate analysis, showed that intake of five or more tablets per day, as well as drug administration by caregivers, was significantly associated with patient's nonadherence [11]. However, problems in adherence to antihypertensive therapy are common in end-stage renal disease patients on dialysis. An Italian hemodialysis study reported that 53% of patients were inadherent to their prescribed drugs, and younger age, male gender, poor social support, increased comorbidities, health beliefs, and depression were the main factors associated with poor adherence [16]. Another European study identified factors associated with nonadherence in hemodialysis patients [10]. Associated parameters were as follows: demographic factors (age, gender, educational level, marital status/living arrangements, race/ethnicity, income/employment status, cost/payment/insurance/socioeconomic situation, smoking/drinking/drug abuse, religion/religiosity), clinical factors (length of time on hemodialysis, chronicity/chronic conditions, diabetic status, former transplant history, treatment regimen complexity/high tablet burden, tablet size and taste, treatment side effects), and psychosocial factors (health beliefs/knowledge/motivation, self-esteem cognitive behaviour/function, health locus of control, social support and family dynamics, psychiatric illness like anxiety/depression) [10].

How can we detect adherence in our patients in a reliable way? Well, the methods – including the widely used Morisky questionnaire, used to measure drug adherence – have disadvantages. They were generally inconsistent and are not very reliable [2]. Moreover, antihypertensive pill counts, questionnaires, patient diaries, and measurement of plasma drug concentrations have been shown to overestimate treatment adherence. Also, there is absence of a common taxonomy in this area. More interesting is that, when different methods are used in the same study, large variations in adherence are observed [2]. Therefore, the lack of effective methods to diagnose adherence problems yields to ineffective improvement in adherence problems. Methods that can be named to near ideal have been mentioned recently [2] as follows: retrospective analysis of prescription refill records [17], analysis of chemical markers of drug exposure [18], and automatic electronic time stamping and compilation of events more or less strongly linked to the act of taking medication (e.g., package opening, dosage form dissolution) [19].

It should always be kept in mind that patients with CKD are so-called a complex medical population that might exhibit significant medication-related problems and medication safety issues during their clinical follow-up [20]. These problems are classified as adverse drug reactions, drug interactions, inappropriate doses, and suboptimal laboratory monitoring [21, 22]. Several studies have examined the rates of adherence to prescribed drugs in patients with CKD involving maintenance renal replacement therapies. The common result of these studies was the frequent finding of poor adherence among these patients [2]. For example, in recent years, two large studies on hypertension management in CKD population showed that approximately 30% of patients were defined to have a poor antihypertensive drug adherence resulting in uncontrolled blood pressure [5, 6]. Reduced adherence does not only lead to uncontrolled blood pressure but also to poor CKD outcomes [8, 23–25] and to increased mortality in hemodialysis patients as well [26].

Causes of Problems in Drug Adherence in CKD Patients

Potential reasons for nonadherence to pharmacological therapy in both CKD and non-CKD populations can be grouped under three main titles:

Patient-Related Reasons

There are several patient-related reasons for nonadherence to antihypertensive medications. These are as follows:

(a) Forgetting to take medication perhaps because of a busy work or social life [27],
(b) A negative behaviour toward medication
(c) Cultural beliefs
(d) Lack of education
(e) Preconceived beliefs regarding medication
(f) Poor language proficiency

Moreover, patients can make a conscious decision, that is, deciding for themselves the dose and frequency of their antihypertensive regimen.

Physician-Related Reasons

Main thing in this heading is the poor communication between physician and patient as a significant problem that may influence the adherence of patients [28, 29]. The lack of information given by the physician regarding the reason of the initiation of therapy, the impact of hypertension on cardiovascular risk, and the clinical consequences of discontinuation of therapy is of critical importance.

Medication-Related Reasons

Treatment characteristics like complicated regimens (i.e., multiple daily doses of medications), long duration of medical therapy, medications with high cost, and adverse side effect of prescribed therapies (i.e., impotence and effects on mood and sedation) might lead to lower adherence to antihypertensive therapy.

Solutions to Improve Adherence

There are various strategies that can be employed to improve adherence to medication in CKD patients with hypertension:

1. To identify reasons like concerns about polypharmacy, drug interactions, pill size and frequency, cost of drugs, and doubts on the real efficacy of some of the prescribed drugs [30]
2. To educate and maintain significant contact with the CKD patient and the family [31]:

   (a) Information about medications, when written in simple language, is useful [32].
   (b) To avoid broken appointments to clinics by mail, telephone, and clinician reminders [33].

3. To focus on both the patient's and physician's motivations on the necessity of taking antihypertensive therapy [2]
4. To work on simplifying antihypertensive regimens, i.e., the use of fixed-dose combinations or drugs with longer duration of action to prevent the effect of missed doses [2, 34]
5. To work on a team-based strategy involving nephrologists, specialized nurses, and/or community pharmacists in order to enhance the control rates of the various risk factors [35, 36]

Conclusions

Adherence to antihypertensive therapy is a critical component to reduce complications associated with elevated BP in CKD. We should keep in mind that nonadherence is a very common observation in CKD. All the physicians need to understand the importance of improving adherence in their patients and should use or develop the tools to be able to measure it effectively in order to make decisions regarding medication intensification. This would be necessary to achieve optimal clinical outcomes for their patients in the future.

References

1. Whaley-Connell AT, Sowers JR, Stevens LA, McFarlane SI, Shlipak MG, Norris KC, Chen SC, Qiu Y, Wang C, Li S, Vassalotti JA, Collins AJ, Kidney Early Evaluation Program Investigators. CKD in the United States: Kidney Early Evaluation Program (KEEP) and National Health and Nutrition Examination Survey (NHANES) 1999-2004. Am J Kidney Dis. 2008;51(4 Suppl 2): S13–20.

2. Burnier M, Pruijm M, Wuerzner G, Santschi V. Drug adherence in chronic kidney diseases and dialysis. Nephrol Dial Transplant. 2015;30(1):39–44.
3. Kidney Disease Outcomes Quality Initiative (K/DOQI). K/DOQI clinical practice guidelines on hypertension and antihypertensive agents in chronic kidney disease. Am J Kidney Dis. 2004;43(5 suppl):1–290.
4. Sarafidis PA, Li S, Chen SC, Collins AJ, Brown WW, Klag MJ, Bakris GL. Hypertension awareness, treatment, and control in chronic kidney disease. Am J Med. 2008;121(4):332–40.
5. Schmitt KE, Edie CF, Laflam P, Simbartl LA, Thakar CV. Adherence to antihypertensive agents and blood pressure control in chronic kidney disease. Am J Nephrol. 2010;32(6):541–8.
6. Muntner P, Judd SE, Krousel-Wood M, McClellan WM, Safford MM. Low medication adherence and hypertension control among adults with CKD: data from the REGARDS (Reasons for Geographic and Racial Differences in Stroke) Study. Am J Kidney Dis. 2010;56(3):447–57.
7. Bailie GR, Eisele G, Liu L, Roys E, Kiser M, Finkelstein F, Wolfe R, Port F, Burrows-Hudson S, Saran R. Patterns of medication use in the RRICKD study: focus on medications with cardiovascular effects. Nephrol Dial Transplant. 2005;20:1110–5.
8. Chiu YW, Teitelbaum I, Misra M, de Leon EM, Adzize T, Mehrotra R. Pill burden, adherence, hyperphosphatemia, and quality of life in maintenance dialysis patients. Clin J Am Soc Nephrol. 2009;4(6):1089–96.
9. Sabate E. Adherence to long-term therapies: evidence for action. Geneva: World Health Organization; 2003.
10. Schmid H, Hartmann B, Schiffl H. Adherence to prescribed oral medication in adult patients undergoing chronic hemodialysis: a critical review of the literature. Eur J Med Res. 2009;14(5):185–90.
11. Magacho EJ, Ribeiro LC, Chaoubah A, Bastos MG. Adherence to drug therapy in kidney disease. Braz J Med Biol Res. 2011;44(3):258–62.
12. Moreira L, Fernandes P, Monte S, Martins A. Adesão ao tratamento farmacológico em pacientes com doença renal crônica. J Bras Nefrol. 2008;30:113–9.
13. Lee JY, Greene PG, Douglas M, Grim C, Kirk KA, Kusek JW, Milligan S, Smith DE, Whelton PK. Appointment attendance, pill counts, and achievement of goal blood pressure in the African American Study of Kidney Disease and Hypertension Pilot Study. Control Clin Trials. 1996;17(4 Suppl):34S–9S.
14. Vrijens B, Vincze G, Kristanto P, Urquhart J, Burnier M. Adherence to prescribed antihypertensive drug treatments: longitudinal study of electronically compiled dosing histories. BMJ. 2008;336(7653):1114–7.
15. Grymonpre RE, Didur CD, Montgomery PR, Sitar DS. Pill count, self-report, and pharmacy claims data to measure medication adherence in the elderly. Ann Pharmacother. 1998;32(7-8):749–54.
16. Neri L, Martini A, Andreucci VE, Gallieni M, Rey LA, Brancaccio D, MigliorDialisi Study Group. Regimen complexity and prescription adherence in dialysis patients. Am J Nephrol. 2011;34(1):71–6.
17. Go AS, Chertow GM, Fan D, McCulloch CE, Hsu CY. Chronic kidney disease and the risks of death, cardiovascular events, and hospitalization. N Engl J Med. 2004;351(13):1296–305.
18. U.S. Renal Data System, USRDS. 2013 Annual data report: atlas of chronic kidney disease and end-stage renal disease in the United States. Bethesda: National Institutes of Health, National Institute of Diabetes and Digestive and Kidney Diseases; 2013.
19. Stevens LA, Coresh J, Greene T, Levey AS. Assessing kidney function—measured and estimated glomerular filtration rate. N Engl J Med. 2006;354(23):2473–83.
20. Hepler CD, Strand LM. Opportunities and responsibilities in pharmaceutical care. Am J Hosp Pharm. 1990;47(3):533–43.
21. McFarland MS, Cross LB, Gross B, Gentry C, Tunney J, Patel UP. Drug use evaluation of sitagliptin dosing by pharmacist versus nonpharmacist clinicians in an internal medicine department of a private physician-owned multispecialty clinic. J Manag Care Pharm. 2009;15(7):563–7.

22. Zhang M, Holman CD, Price SD, Sanfilippo FM, Preen DB, Bulsara MK. Comorbidity and repeat admission to hospital for adverse drug reactions in older adults: retrospective cohort study. BMJ. 2009;338:a2752.
23. Chang TI, Desai M, Solomon DH, Winkelmayer WC. Kidney function and long-term medication adherence after myocardial infarction in the elderly. Clin J Am Soc Nephrol. 2011;6(4):864–9.
24. Raymond CB, Wazny LD, Sood AR. Medication adherence in patients with chronic kidney disease. CANNT J. 2011;21(2):47–50.
25. Ibrahim N, Wong IC, Patey S, Tomlin S, Sinha MD, Jani Y. Drug-related problem in children with chronic kidney disease. Pediatr Nephrol. 2013;28(1):25–31.
26. Rosenthal Asher D, Ver Halen N, Cukor D. Depression and nonadherence predict mortality in hemodialysis treated end-stage renal disease patients. Hemodial Int. 2012;16(3):387–93.
27. Kressin NR, Wang F, Long J, Bokhour BG, Orner MB, Rothendler J, Clark C, Reddy S, Kozak W, Kroupa LP, Berlowitz DR. Hypertensive patients' race, health beliefs, process of care, and medication adherence. J Gen Intern Med. 2007;22(6):768–74.
28. Yiannakopoulou EC, Papadopulos JS, Cokkinos DV, Mountokalakis TD. Adherence to anti-hypertensive treatment: a critical factor for blood pressure control. Eur J Cardiovasc Prev Rehabil. 2005;12(3):243–9.
29. Erhardt L, Hobbs FD. Public perceptions of cardiovascular risk in five European countries: The react survey. Int J Clin Pract. 2002;56(9):638–44.
30. Rifkin DE, Laws MB, Rao M, Balakrishnan VS, Sarnak MJ, Wilson IB. Medication adherence behavior and priorities among older adults with CKD: a semistructured interview study. Am J Kidney Dis. 2010;56(3):439–46.
31. Daniels PR, Kardia SL, Hanis CL, Brown CA, Hutchinson R, Boerwinkle E, Turner ST, Genetic Epidemiology Network of Arteriopathy Study. Familial aggregation of hypertension treatment and control in the Genetic Epidemiology Network of Arteriopathy (GENOA) study. Am J Med. 2004;116(10):676–81.
32. Baker D, Roberts DE, Newcombe RG, Fox KA. Evaluation of drug information for cardiology patients. Br J Clin Pharmacol. 1991;31(5):525–31.
33. Macharia WM, Leon G, Rowe BH, Stephenson BJ, Haynes RB. An overview of interventions to improve compliance with appointment keeping for medical services. JAMA. 1992;267(13):1813–7.
34. Burnier M, Brown RE, Ong SH, Keskinaslan A, Khan ZM. Issues in blood pressure control and the potential role of single-pill combination therapies. Int J Clin Pract. 2009;63(5):790–8.
35. Mendelssohn DC. Coping with the CKD epidemic: the promise of multidisciplinary team-based care. Nephrol Dial Transplant. 2005;20:10–2.
36. Barrett BJ, Garg AX, Goeree R, Levin A, Molzahn A, Rigatto C, Singer J, Soltys G, Soroka S, Ayers D, Parfrey PS. A nurse-coordinated model of care versus usual care for stage 3/4 chronic kidney disease in the community: a randomized controlled trial. Clin J Am Soc Nephrol. 2011;6(6):1241–7.

Chapter 18
Treatment of Hypertension in Light of the New Guidelines: Pharmacologic Approaches Using Combination Therapies

Liviu Segall

Introduction

Resistant hypertension (RH) is very common in patients with chronic kidney disease (CKD), with a prevalence of 20–35%, according to various studies [1].

Unfortunately, since individuals with advanced CKD and end-stage renal disease (ESRD) have usually been excluded from randomized controlled trials (RCTs), there is very little evidence to guide the pharmacological therapy of hypertension, and particularly RH, in these patients [2].

Nevertheless, it is widely thought that the multifactorial pathogenesis of RH in CKD requires multiple drug therapy, to simultaneously target factors like the intravascular volume expansion and the hyperactivity of the renin-angiotensin system (RAS) and the sympathetic nervous system [3]. Combined therapy, however, has to be individualized, depending on the patient's pathophysiologic profile, comorbidities, and contraindications. Moreover, the optimal combination should be well tolerated, to ensure long-term adherence [3]. Most antihypertensive agents available for the general population can also be used in CKD patients, after consideration of their metabolism and dosing adjustments according to the level of renal function [4]. The pharmacological armamentarium includes diuretics, angiotensin-converting enzyme inhibitors (ACEIs), angiotensin receptor blockers (ARBs), calcium channel blockers (CCBs), beta-blockers (BBs), alpha-blockers, centrally acting drugs, and other vasodilators [3] (Table 18.1).

L. Segall (✉)
Nefrocare MS Dialysis Centre, Iaşi, Romania
e-mail: l_segall@yahoo.com

© Springer International Publishing AG 2017
A. Covic et al. (eds.), *Resistant Hypertension in Chronic Kidney Disease*,
DOI 10.1007/978-3-319-56827-0_18

Table 18.1 Indications, additional benefits, caution, and combined use of the different antihypertensive drug groups in CKD patients [5]

Type of drug	Other indications besides hypertension	Additional benefits	Caution	Combined use
RAS blockers				
ACEIs and ARBs	Proteinuria Heart failure Post-AMI	Reduction of intraglomerular pressure, reduction of proteinuria, and CKD progression Reduction of fibrosis and cardiovascular remodeling	Hyperkalemia Monitor kidney function and K$^+$ after starting treatment Use of NSAIDs Use of COX-2 inhibitors Combined use with other RAS blockers Bilateral renal artery stenosis Volume depletion	Diuretics CCBs BBs
MR antagonists	Heart failure Post-AMI	Reduction of albuminuria or proteinuria	Hyperkalemia Monitor kidney function and K+ after starting treatment Use of NSAIDs Use of COX-2 inhibitors	ACEIs ARBs
DRIs		Reduction of albuminuria or proteinuria	As above Increased risk of complications in diabetic or CKD patients when combined with ACEIs or ARBs	Diuretics CCBs
Diuretics				
Thiazides		Reduced risk of hyperkalemia	May aggravate hyperglycemia Replace with or add loop diuretic if GFR <30 ml/min/1.73 m^2	ACEIs ARBs
Loop diuretics	Edema	Reduced risk of hyperkalemia		
CCBs				
DHP	Angina			ACEIs ARBs BBs Diuretics
Non-DHP	Angina Supraventricular tachycardia	Reduction of intraglomerular pressure Reduction of heart rate	They increase the levels of CNIs and mTOR inhibitors Do not associate with BBs	ACEIs ARBs Diuretics

(continued)

Table 18.1 (continued)

Type of drug	Other indications besides hypertension	Additional benefits	Caution	Combined use
BBs				
	Heart failure (bisoprolol, carvedilol, and metoprolol) Angina Post-AMI	Reduction of heart rate	Risk of bradycardia Do not use with non-DHP CCBs	ACEIs ARBs Diuretics DHP CCBs
Others				
Centrally acting alpha-agonists			Reduce moxonidine dose if GFR <30 ml/min/1.73 m^2	Diuretics
Alpha-blockers	Prostatic hypertrophy		Orthostatic hypotension	BBs Diuretics
Direct vasodilators			Salt and water retention Tachycardia	BBs Diuretics

NSAIDs nonsteroidal anti-inflammatory drugs, *ARBs* angiotensin receptor blockers, *COX2* cyclooxygenase 2, *DHP* dihydropyridines, *CKD* chronic kidney disease, *AMI* acute myocardial infarction, *ACEIs* angiotensin-converting enzyme inhibitors, *RAS* renin-angiotensin system

Treatment of Resistant Hypertension in the General Population

Triple Therapy

For hypertensive patients requiring a triple therapy, the European Society of Hypertension (ESH) and the European Society of Cardiology (ESC) recommendation of 2013 indicates that the choice should be made between four classes of antihypertensive drugs: RAS inhibitors (ACEIs and ARBs), BBs, CCBs, and thiazide diuretics [6]. However, in the past decade, BBs have been slightly "downgraded," after the publication of a meta-analysis [7] which revealed the association of these drugs with a 16% higher stroke rate, as compared to the other agents [8]. Therefore, other expert societies, including the British Hypertension Society [9], American Heart Association [10], and French Society of Arterial Hypertension [11], suggest that the triple combination should consist of ACEI/ARB + CCB + diuretic (the "ACD regimen"), although there are no RCTs to support this suggestion.

Definition of RH

Resistant hypertension is defined as uncontrolled hypertension (i.e., office BP $\geq$140/90 mmHg in a patient <80 years or systolic blood pressure [BP] $\geq$150 mmHg in a patient $\geq$80 years, confirmed by home self-measurement or ambulatory monitoring of BP), despite antihypertensive treatment consisting of appropriate lifestyle changes and triple drug therapy for at least 4 weeks, in optimal doses, including a diuretic [11]. However, before making the diagnosis of RH, adherence to prescribed therapy should be confirmed (e.g., by using specific questionnaires or serum drug-level measurements), and possible interference of pro-hypertensive factors, such as high salt intake, excess alcohol consumption, or use of vasopressor drugs (like cyclosporine, steroids, erythropoietin, or oral contraceptives), should be searched for [11]. If true RH is established, causes of secondary hypertension including primary aldosteronism, pheochromocytoma, hypercorticism, renal artery stenosis, or sleep apnea syndrome should also be considered and investigated [11].

Treatment of RH

In patients with RH for which no curable cause can be identified, the addition of a fourth antihypertensive agent is indicated. This should preferably be an MR antagonist (spironolactone or eplerenone), in the absence of contraindications [11].

MR antagonists are weak diuretics, but they play a special role in the management of RH, for several reasons. Patients with RH often have secondary hyperaldosteronism and may also exhibit the so-called aldosterone escape or breakthrough. This phenomenon is defined as an increase in aldosterone levels after initiation of ACEIs or ARBs, most likely by non-ACE pathways of angiotensin II activation [12]. However, MR antagonists were shown to improve BP control in patients with RH, regardless of circulating aldosterone levels [13]. The RCT Addition of Spironolactone in Patients with Resistant Arterial Hypertension (ASPIRANT) [14] evaluated the antihypertensive effects of spironolactone 25 mg/day in 117 patients with RH after treatment for 8 weeks. Existing antihypertensive treatment was continued during this period. The study showed that systolic BP was reduced significantly in treated patients, with no adverse effects. More recently, the Prevention and Treatment of resistant Hypertension With Algorithm-Guided Therapy (PATHWAY-2) study [15] demonstrated the superior BP-lowering effect (and similarly good tolerance) of spironolactone 25–50 mg/ day, as compared to each of bisoprolol, doxazosin, and placebo, in patients with RH already on ACD regimen.

In cases with contraindications, resistance, or intolerance to spironolactone, the use of a BB, an alpha-blocker, or a centrally acting agent is recommended [11].

Another important therapeutic measure, given the role of volume overload in the pathogenesis of RH, is to reinforce diuretic medication, together with the low-salt diet [11]. This involves a dose increase or a change in diuretic therapy.

Recently, there has been much debate about which diuretic is better: hydro-chlorothiazide (HCTZ), chlorthalidone, or indapamide? Chlorthalidone is often thought to be superior to HCTZ in terms of efficacy and reduction of cardiovas-cular events, as it has been shown by two meta-analyses [16, 17]; however, in these meta-analyses there was no head-to-head comparison, and also, in the Multiple Risk Factor Intervention Trial (MRFIT), chlorthalidone was used in higher doses than HCTZ [13]. Indapamide is considered a good alternative to chlorthalidone. If the BP target is still not reached, a sequential blockade of tubular sodium reabsorption, using both thiazides and loop diuretics, is sug-gested [8].

With thiazides and/or loop diuretics, the risk of hypokalemia should be con-sidered and avoided. In contrast, with aldosterone antagonists, hyperkalemia may occur, in particular in cases of CKD or if combined with a RAS inhibitor, a BB or a nonsteroidal anti-inflammatory drug (NSAID). Therefore, during treat-ment with any of these drugs, monitoring of serum potassium and creatinine is indicated [8].

Some authors have proposed the guidance of antihypertensive therapy in RH by plasma renin activity (the Cambridge αβΔ-guideline) [8]. This method can be applied in patients without concomitant diseases, taking into consideration the results of plasma renin testing. According to this strategy, inadequately controlled patients should receive (in addition to the ACD regimen) a BB in case of high renin levels, an alpha-blocker in case of normal renin levels, and diuretic reinforcement in case of low renin levels [8]. In the PATHWAY-2 study, the BP response to spirono-lactone was superior to bisoprolol and doxazosin across most of the plasma renin distribution; however, the magnitude of spironolactone superiority was much higher at the low-renin pole of the distribution [15].

Other drugs, including centrally acting antihypertensive agents (e.g., clonidine) and direct vasodilators (e.g., minoxidil, hydralazine), are often indicated as drugs of last resort, when previously recommended treatments have failed. However, their use is not supported by evidence from large interventional studies [8]. Clonidine is a potent antihypertensive drug, and patients with RH seem to respond well to this medication [8]. Minoxidil is a strong vasodilator and has been successfully used for many years, as well as clonidine, in patients with RH, including those with advanced CKD. Its use is limited, however, because of numerous side effects, like tachycar-dia, salt retention, pericardial effusion, and hirsutism [8]. Hydralazine is less effec-tive than minoxidil but may be used in cases with contraindications or intolerance to the latter. Due to its short duration of action, hydralazine has to be administered three or four times daily. It can also induce tachycardia, requiring the association of BBs [8].

Treatment of Resistant Hypertension in Pre-dialysis CKD Patients

Definition of RH and Target BP According to Guidelines

The general definition of RH is largely applicable to the CKD population. Most of the current guidelines, including those from the ESH/ESC 2013 [6], American Society of Hypertension/International Society of Hypertension (ASH/ISH) 2014 [18], Eighth Joint National Committee (JNC 8) 2014 [19], American Heart Association/American College of Cardiology/Centers for Disease Control and Prevention (AHA/ACC/CDC) 2014 [20], Caring for Australasians with Renal Impairment (CARI) 2013 [21], and Canadian Hypertension Education Program (CHEP) 2014 [22], recommend a BP goal for these patients <140/90 mmHg, but some suggest a lower target (<130/80 mmHg) for the subgroup with proteinuria [6, 18, 21].

Triple Therapy

The triple regimen ACD seems to be a reasonable choice for patients with CKD and difficult-to-treat hypertension.

The efficacy/safety of the ARB olmesartan (OM) 40 mg, the CCB amlodipine 10 mg (AML), and the diuretic hydrochlorothiazide 25 mg (HCTZ) versus the component dual combinations (OM/AML, OM/HCTZ, and AML/HCTZ) was evaluated in participants with diabetes, CKD, or cardiovascular diseases in the Triple Therapy with Olmesartan Medoxomil, Amlodipine, and Hydrochlorothiazide in Hypertensive Patients Study (TRINITY) [23]. At 12 weeks, OM/AML/HCTZ resulted in significantly greater systolic BP reductions in participants with CKD. The BP goal achievement was greater for participants receiving triple-combination treatment compared with the dual-combination treatments. At week 52, there was sustained BP lowering with the OM/AML/HCTZ regimen. Overall, the triple combination was well tolerated.

Although RCTs comparing it with other triple therapies have never been performed, the ACD combination is thought to be scientifically sound, effective, and well tolerated, and it is widely used in everyday clinical practice. It should be tried in optimum doses as the first therapeutic step in patients with CKD and RH, in the absence of contraindications and after all forms of pseudo-resistance have been excluded. This regimen might be applied in terms of switching previous therapy or of treatment intensification in patients already using this combination in lower doses [3].

Table 18.2 Strategies to minimize risk of hyperkalemia caused by RAS inhibitors in patients with CKD [25]

Wherever possible, discontinue drugs that can impair renal potassium excretion (e.g., NSAIDs, including selective COX-2 inhibitors)
Prescribe a low-potassium diet; advise patients to avoid use of salt substitutes that contain potassium
Prescribe thiazide diuretics (and/or loop diuretics if estimated GFR is <30 mL/min/1.73 m^2)
Prescribe sodium bicarbonate to correct metabolic acidosis; decrease dose of ACEI or ARB
Measure serum potassium level 1 week after initiating ACEI or ARB therapy or after increasing the dose
If patient is taking some combination of an ACEI, an ARB, and a MR antagonist, discontinue one and recheck serum potassium level
Do not exceed a 25-mg daily dose of spironolactone when used in combination with an ACEI or an ARB

ACEIs and ARBs

ACEIs and ARBs are RAS blockers, with both cardioprotective and renoprotective effects. They reduce cardiac and vascular remodeling and myocardial fibrosis, as well as intraglomerular pressure and proteinuria [4, 5]. Therefore, they are not only very effective antihypertensive agents, but they are also beneficial in patients with heart failure, post-myocardial infarction, and proteinuric CKD [5], in whom they can prevent cardiovascular mortality and CKD progression, respectively.

Adverse effects of ACEIs and ARBs include hypotension, acute kidney injury, and hyperkalemia. Caution is required when using these drugs in patients with bilateral renal artery stenosis, volume depletion, and concurrent use of NSAIDs or other RAS inhibitors. Monitoring of serum creatinine and potassium is indicated after starting treatment, especially in such high-risk cases [5]. The use of these drugs in women of child-bearing age should be balanced with the risk of pregnancy, since they are potentially teratogenic [24].

Most available ACEIs have active moieties that are largely excreted in the urine. Fosinopril and trandolapril are partially (approximately 50%) excreted by the liver, such that the blood levels are less influenced by kidney failure than levels of other ACEIs which are predominantly excreted by the kidneys. Since ACEIs are generally titrated to achieve optimal clinical effect, the mode of excretion is not regarded as a major factor in dosing. If hyperkalemia occurs in CKD patients taking a renal-excreted ACEI, possible interventions include dietary advice, reducing the dose, or adding a potassium-losing diuretic [24]. If strategies to minimize hyperkalemia (Table 18.2) fail to maintain serum potassium concentrations below 5.6 mEq/L, the RAS inhibitor should be discontinued, and another class of antihypertensive drugs should be used instead [25].

Virtually all guidelines recommend ACEIs/ARBs as first-line therapeutic agents in hypertensive CKD patients, regardless of proteinuria levels and diabetic status [5, 6, 18–21, 24]. However, some guidelines suggest that these drugs are particularly preferable in CKD patients with micro- or macroalbuminuria [24, 26], in which they are associated with better kidney and cardiovascular outcomes [24]. ACEIs and ARBs are probably equivalent with respect to renal outcomes [26]. They should be considered for use particularly in patients with CKD who also have heart failure, recent myocardial infarction, a history of stroke, or a high cardiovascular risk, although this KDIGO recommendation is largely based on data from studies in non-CKD patients [24].

The support for the recommendation of ACEIs/ARBs as first-line therapeutic agents in hypertensive CKD patients is provided by several studies. The KDIGO recommendations cite five relevant trials: reanalyses of the Heart Outcomes Prevention Evaluation (HOPE) trial [27], the Candesartan Antihypertensive Survival Evaluation in Japan (CASE-J) trial [28], the Telmisartan Randomised Assessment Study in ACE Intolerant Subjects with Cardiovascular Disease (TRANSCEND) [29], as well as the Investigation on Type 2 Diabetic Nephropathy (INNOVATION) study [30] and the Irbesartan in Development of Nephropathy in Patients with Type 2 Diabetes (IDNT) trial [31]. A meta-analysis of 11 RCTs [32] included studies of patients with nondiabetic CKD treated with BP-lowering regimens containing ACEIs to those not containing ACEIs. All trials included in the analysis targeted a BP <140/90 mmHg, and nearly all patients were hypertensive at baseline. In this analysis, the use of an ACEI was associated with a significant reduction in the risk of progression of kidney disease as defined by doubling of serum creatinine or the need for dialysis. This effect was independent of other important covariates, including baseline BP and urinary protein excretion. Of relevance, there was no significant interaction between current urinary protein excretion and treatment allocation. In other words, there was no evidence that the degree of protein excretion modified the relationship between the use of ACEIs and the progression of kidney disease. The results of the meta-analysis suggest that ACEIs should be the antihypertensive drugs of choice in individuals with CKD. However, another analysis of the same data set [33] suggested that baseline urinary protein excretion was an important effect modifier, in that those with baseline urine protein excretion ≥500 mg/day seemed to have greater benefits with ACEI therapy. Those with proteinuria <500 mg/day at baseline appeared to receive little if any benefit compared to other antihypertensive regimens. TRANSCEND [34] randomized patients at high vascular risk to telmisartan or placebo. No difference was observed between groups in the primary cardiovascular endpoint or the secondary renal endpoint of dialysis, doubling of serum creatinine, or death. In a reanalysis of TRANSCEND, individuals without microalbuminuria had an increased risk of the renal endpoint, while there was no significant difference in those with urinary albumin excretion ≥30 mg/day, although the trend favored telmisartan.

There are also some other significant controversies between guidelines regarding ACEIs and ARBs. First, according to the ERBP guideline [35], it is unclear if the renoprotective superiority of ACEIs and ARBs is truly a BP-independent effect or simply a reflection of better BP control. Second, in contrast with the KDIGO guidelines, the authors of ERBP recommend that, due to increased risk of side effects, consideration should be given to stopping ACEIs/ARBs in patients with advanced CKD (stages 4 and 5) when there are no other compelling indications for these agents (such as heart failure), especially in those with renovascular disease, or when discontinuation of the drug may enable the start of renal replacement therapy to be postponed or avoided [35].

Diuretics

Diuretics are the cornerstone of hypertension treatment in CKD and, by definition, a component of any antihypertensive drug combination for RH. Most patients with CKD should receive a diuretic as their first or second agent to manage volume and sodium retention, with the possible exception of those with autosomal dominant polycystic kidney disease, in which there is concern that diuretic therapy can stimulate the RAS and subsequent cyst growth [4]. However, the efficacy of diuretics is limited in CKD, because both the tubular secretion of these drugs and the fractional reabsorption of sodium are reduced. Therefore, CKD patients often require large doses of diuretics, which are achieved in practice by sequentially doubling the dose until a response is seen or a ceiling dose is reached [12].

Verdalles et al. [36] used bioimpedance spectroscopy (BIS) to assess fluid status and guide the use of diuretics to treat hypertension in CKD patients not on dialysis. They treated 30 patients with extracellular volume (ECV) expansion with a diuretic, which were compared to 20 patients without ECV expansion who instead received another additional antihypertensive medication. At 6 months of follow-up, systolic BP decreased by 21 mmHg in patients with ECV expansion versus 9 mmHg in patients without ECV expansion ($P < 0.01$). In addition, 9 of 30 patients with ECV expansion and 2 of 20 without ECV expansion achieved the target BP of <140/90 mmHg at 6 months. This novel approach to managing hypertensive CKD patients based on BIS assessment of volume status will need further study in larger cohorts before it can be considered for wider use.

Except for diuretics, most antihypertensive drugs induce sodium retention and ECV expansion. Diuretics counteract this by inhibiting sodium reabsorption. In addition, diuretics may also reduce the risk of hyperkalemia associated with RAS inhibitors. On the other hand, volume loss caused by diuretics activates neurohormonal pathways, particularly the RAS. Hence, the combination of diuretics with an ACEI or an ARB is synergistic and very effective [12].

Thiazide diuretics are less potent than loop diuretics when used alone in patients with moderate-to-severe CKD, because only 3% to 5% of filtered sodium is reabsorbed at the thiazide site of action and because the decrease in filtered sodium load in CKD causes a reduction in sodium reabsorption [12]. Most clinicians choose to switch to a loop diuretic in patients with CKD stage 4, particularly if hypertension is becoming resistant to therapy or if edema is an issue [24]. However, thiazides may still be useful for the treatment of high BP in CKD, as they have been shown to possess multiple nephron target sites and also to lower peripheral vascular resistance, by direct or indirect mechanisms [12]. By sequential tubular blockade, thiazide diuretics may augment the natriuretic effect of loop diuretics and improve BP control. However, when thiazides and loop diuretics are used together, the incidence of adverse effects is higher and requires close monitoring [12]. Knauf and Mutschler [37] showed that HCTZ alone or in combination with furosemide increased diuresis in patients with CKD even at a GFR <30 ml/min/1.73 m². Dussol et al. [38] conducted an RCT involving 23 patients with hypertension and stage 4 or 5 CKD, who received long-acting furosemide (60 mg) and HCTZ (25 mg) for 3 months, and then both diuretics for the next 3 months. The authors found no differences between furosemide and HCTZ with respect to natriuresis and BP control. Another trial [39] enrolled 60 CKD patients with a mean eGFR of 39 ml/min/1.73 m² and a systolic BP of 151 mmHg, under 1.8 antihypertensive drugs on average. After a run-in phase, all patients were treated with chlorthalidone, and at the end of the 8-week intervention, systolic BP was significantly reduced by 20 mmHg. Notably, the nine patients with eGFR <30 ml/min/1.73 m² had a similar reduction in BP.

Calcium Channel Blockers

The major subclasses of CCBs are the dihydropyridines (e.g., amlodipine, nifedipine, lercanidipine) and the non-dihydropyridines, including benzothiazepines (diltiazem) and phenylalkylamines (verapamil). Dihydropyridines tend to be more selective for the vascular smooth muscle (vasodilation) than for the myocardium. Accordingly, the side effects may include fluid retention and ankle edema, which can be problematic in patients with CKD. Dizziness, headache, and facial flush are also common. Non-dihydropyridines have direct effects on the myocardium, including the sinoatrial and atrioventricular nodes, causing reductions in heart rate and contractility [24].

CCBs are widely used in the treatment of hypertension, angina, and supraventricular tachycardia. Non-dihydropyridine CCBs have been shown to reduce proteinuria. In contrast, dihydropyridines completely abolish renal autoregulation, which is already impaired in CKD, and may thus aggravate proteinuria when used as monotherapy. Therefore, the use of dihydropyridines is not advisable without concomitant use of an ACEI or ARB [24, 35].

Most CCBs do not accumulate in patients with impaired kidney function, with the exception of nicardipine and nimodipine. Accumulation of these agents may also be due to reduced blood flow to the liver in the elderly. Caution is thus advised when using these two agents in elderly patients with CKD [24].

The combination of a RAS inhibitor with a dihydropyridine CCB attenuates the reflex vasoconstriction and tachycardia resulting from increased sympathetic nervous system activity in response to CCB-induced systemic vasodilation [25]. Fluid retention, seen particularly with dihydropyridines, can be problematic in patients with CKD, such that avoiding other vasodilators may be sensible. The combination of non-dihydropyridines such as verapamil and diltiazem with BBs can lead to severe bradycardia, particularly in patients with advanced CKD and if drugs like atenolol and bisoprolol (which accumulate in CKD) are used. CCBs, particularly non-dihydropyridines, also interfere with the metabolism and excretion of calcineurin inhibitors (CNIs), as well as with the mammalian target of rapamycin (mTOR) inhibitors. In patients taking such combinations, careful monitoring of CNIs and mTOR inhibitor blood levels is required if drugs or dosages are changed [24].

Dual Blockade of the RAS

Although dual blockade of the RAS with ACEI + ARB or ACEI/ARB + direct renin inhibitor (DRI) combinations may seem like a rational strategy for improving renal and cardiovascular outcomes, there is no conclusive evidence of the long-term renal and cardiovascular benefit of such combinations in hypertensive CKD patients [25].

In Ongoing Telmisartan Alone and in Combination With Ramipril Global Endpoint Trial (ONTARGET) [40], investigators randomized patients ≥55 years of age with cardiovascular disease or diabetes with end-organ damage to ramipril, telmisartan, or the combination of both drugs. The primary outcome of interest was the combined endpoint of dialysis, doubling of serum creatinine, or death. There was no significant difference in this outcome between ramipril and telmisartan alone, whereas combination therapy actually increased the risk. In addition, the ONTARGET trial found no benefit of combination therapy over ramipril mono-therapy in reducing the cardiovascular risk. The Veterans Affairs Nephropathy in Diabetes (VA NEPHRON-D) trial [41] enrolled 1448 patients with diabetic nephropathy, with or without hypertension. Subjects were randomized to losartan + lisinopril versus losartan + placebo for prevention of a primary composite endpoint of renal events or death. The trial was halted early because of lack of efficacy, as well as because of increased risk of hyperkalemia and acute kidney injury in the dual therapy group. Notably, BP was not different between groups.

The Aliskiren in the Evaluation of Proteinuria in Diabetes (AVOID) trial [42] studied the DRI aliskiren in combination with the ARB losartan versus losartan alone in 599 patients with type 2 diabetes and diabetic nephropathy. Combination therapy reduced the urinary albumin/creatinine ratio by 20%, as compared with losartan alone. There were only small differences in BP between the two groups and no differences between the rates of adverse events. In contrast, the Aliskiren Trial in Type 2 Diabetes Using Cardiovascular and Renal Disease Endpoints (ALTITUDE) [43], involving the same combination of aliskiren + losartan in patients with diabetes and CKD, has been terminated early due to an increased risk of adverse events and no evidence of benefit in the dual therapy group. Consequently, the US Food and Drug Administration (FDA) [44] and the ERBP guideline [35] have counseled against the use of this combination.

Mineralocorticoid Receptor Antagonists

Aldosterone may mediate CKD progression, independently of its BP-increasing effect. Animal studies suggest that MR antagonists reduce proteinuria in diabetic nephropathy. MR antagonists may also ameliorate early renal injury and prevent renal fibrosis, presumably via the inhibition of macrophage infiltration, reduction in local oxidative stress, and the decreased expression of fibronectin, plasminogen activator inhibitor-1, and transforming growth factor-β1 [12].

In CKD, MR antagonists have been tried for anti-proteinuric and renoprotective purposes, as well as for the treatment of RH. In the largest relevant RCT [45] involving CKD patients with proteinuria and type 2 diabetes, the addition of eplerenone to enalapril resulted in a significant decrease in albuminuria, as compared to placebo, without an increase in the risk of hyperkalemia. The PATHWAY-2 study [15] unfortunately excluded patients with eGFR <45 ml/min. Based on current data, the long-term effects of MR antagonists on renal and cardiovascular outcomes, mortality, and safety in patients with CKD are unknown [24].

Because of the risk of hyperkalemia and acute kidney injury, MR antagonists should be used with caution in CKD patients. Plasma potassium levels and kidney function should be monitored closely during the introduction of these agents and during intercurrent illnesses, such as dehydration. Great care should be taken when MR antagonists are combined with ACEIs, ARBs, or NSAIDs. Caution is also advised when used together with other cytochrome P450-metabolized agents, such as verapamil [24]. Predictors of hyperkalemia include baseline renal function, serum potassium levels, the dose of MR antagonists, and the use of other RAS blockers or drugs that interfere with renal potassium handling [12]. MR antagonists are usually combined with thiazide or loop diuretics, which enhance potassium loss in the urine.

The ESH/ESC guidelines [6] suggest the addition of a MR antagonist as fourth-line therapy for RH (12.5–25 mg/day spironolactone or 25–50 mg/day eplerenone, to be adapted according to eGFR level) in patients with GFR $\geq$30 ml/min and plasma potassium concentrations $\leq$4–5 mmol/L or in patients with other indications, such as heart failure. However, the ESH guidelines do not recommend the routine use of MR antagonists in patients with CKD, especially in combination with RAS blockers, because of the risk of further renal impairment and hyperkalemia. The KDIGO [24] and ERBP [35] guidelines only state that the place of MR antagonists as an add-on therapy in hypertensive patients with CKD needs to be explored in further studies.

Beta-Blockers

BBs are one of the most extensively investigated drug classes, having been used to treat hypertension, as well as coronary artery disease, heart failure, and cardiac arrhythmias, for over 40 years. Although all BBs are effective for reducing BP, other issues may influence their indication in a given patient and which specific drug is chosen, since BBs vary widely in their pharmacological profile [24]. A recent systematic review and meta-analysis [46] endorsed the use of BBs in CKD patients with heart failure, but did not provide any definitive specific advice on their efficacy in preventing mortality, cardiovascular outcomes, or renal disease progression in CKD patients without heart failure [24].

Notable adverse effects associated with BBs include bradycardia, erectile dysfunction, fatigue, and lipid and glucose abnormalities [47]. In patients with CKD, the accumulation of BBs or active metabolites could exacerbate side effects like bradycardia. Such accumulation occurs with atenolol and bisoprolol, but not with carvedilol, propranolol, or metoprolol [24].

BBs have often been combined with diuretics in RCTs and clinical practice. They can also be combined with ACEIs or ARBs. On the other hand, the combination of atenolol or bisoprolol with bradycardia-inducing drugs such as nondihydropyridine CCBs is not recommended. The association of lipophilic BBs (e.g., propranolol and metoprolol), which cross the blood-brain barrier, with other centrally acting drugs such as clonidine may lead to drowsiness or confusion, particularly in the elderly [24].

Centrally Acting Alpha-Adrenergic Agonists

Centrally acting alpha-agonists cause vasodilatation by reducing sympathetic outflow from the brain. The main agents in use are methyldopa, clonidine, and moxonidine. The use of centrally acting alpha-antagonists is limited by side effects, but since they interact minimally with other antihypertensives, they are valuable as adjunct therapy for RH in CKD patients [24].

Doses of methyldopa or clonidine are not generally reduced in patients with impaired kidney function. Moxonidine is largely excreted by the kidney, and accordingly it has been recommended that the dosage should be decreased in the presence of a low GFR [24].

Combination of alpha-agonists with thiazides may be particularly advantageous to reduce vasodilatation-induced fluid retention. Because of the side-effect profile, however, caution is advised when using alpha-agonists in the elderly, in patients with advanced CKD, and in those taking sedating drugs. Since clonidine can slow the heart rate, it should be avoided if bradycardia or heart block is present [24].

Alpha-Blockers

Alpha-adrenergic blockers (e.g., prazosin, doxazosin, and terazosin) selectively act to reduce BP by causing peripheral vasodilatation. In general, they are not considered a preferred choice, because of common side effects like postural hypotension, tachycardia, and headache. These drugs should be started at a low dosage to avoid a first-dose hypotensive reaction. They are useful in CKD patients with RH, as well as in those with symptoms of prostatic hypertrophy. Vasodilatation can lead to peripheral edema, so they are commonly combined with diuretics. Alpha-blockers do not require dose modification in CKD, since they are excreted via the liver [24].

Direct Vasodilators

Hydralazine and minoxidil both act by directly causing vascular smooth-muscle relaxation and vasodilatation. Hydralazine is rarely used in CKD. Minoxidil is sometimes indicated in patients with RH; however, its side effects limit its use to the most resistant cases. Because of fluid retention and tachycardia, these drugs (especially minoxidil) are usually combined with a BB and a loop diuretic. Hydralazine and minoxidil do not require dose adjustment in patients with impaired kidney function [24].

Treatment of RH in Dialysis-Dependent (CKD-5D) Patients

In patients who are receiving renal replacement therapy, specific BP targets derived from RCTs are lacking. The National Kidney Foundation Kidney Disease Outcomes Quality Initiative (KDOQI) guidelines suggest that pre-hemodialysis (HD) and post-HD BP should be 140/90 mmHg and 130/80 mmHg, respectively, but these targets are mainly based on the expert judgment of the working group, applying weak evidence [48, 49].

ACEIs and ARBs

The KDOQI guidelines suggest RAS inhibitors to be the preferred antihypertensive agents in dialysis patients, particularly in those with diabetes or a history of heart failure [49].

Several studies demonstrated a 5–12 mmHg reduction in systolic BP with ACEIs [50, 51]. Retrospective analyses and small clinical trials also suggest that ACEIs may help preserve residual renal function [52], decrease arterial stiffness [50] and left ventricular hypertrophy [53], reduce mortality after acute coronary syndromes [54], and improve overall survival [55, 56] in HD patients. In the Fosinopril in Dialysis (FOSIDIAL) trial [51], 397 HD patients with left ventricular (LV) hypertrophy were randomized to fosinopril or placebo and followed for 2 years. The primary outcome was a combined endpoint of cardiovascular death, nonfatal myocardial infarction, unstable angina, stroke, cardiovascular revascularization, hospitalization for heart failure, and resuscitated cardiac arrest. At the end of the study, there was a nonsignificant reduction in the primary endpoint with fosinopril.

Some studies found ACEIs to be relatively safe in dialysis patients, with no significant effect on serum potassium, while others suggested that ACEIs may increase the risk of hyperkalemia in these patients, potentially by inhibiting extrarenal potassium loss. Therefore, monitoring of serum potassium after initiation of RAS inhibitors is recommended [47]. ACEIs have also been associated with higher dose requirements for erythropoietin-stimulating agents in HD [47].

Most ACEIs (with the exception of fosinopril) are removed by HD. This is not problematic in most hypertensive patients and may help avoid intradialytic hypotension. However, in those who experience intradialytic hypertension, dialyzable ACEIs should be switched to either fosinopril or an ARB [47].

The effects of ARBs on BP were variable in different studies. Some trials have shown an association of ARBs with a reduction of cardiovascular events and mortality in dialysis patients [57, 58], while others did not confirm this benefit [59].

ARBs can be administered once daily, they are not removed by HD, and they are well tolerated in dialysis patients [47]. In two trials, the use of an ARB was not associated with hyperkalemia or with higher erythropoietin requirements [57, 58].

Diuretics

In 16,420 HD patients from the Dialysis Outcomes and Practice Patterns Study (DOPPS) diuretic use was associated with lower interdialytic weight gain, lower risk of hyperkalemia (>6.0 mmol/L), and higher odds of retaining residual renal function after 1 year, as compared to patients not on diuretic therapy. Patients on diuretics also had a 7% lower all-cause mortality risk ($P = 0.12$) and 14% lower cardiac mortality risk ($P = 0.03$) than patients without diuretics [60].

Calcium Channel Blockers

CCBs can effectively lower BP in dialysis patients. They are not removed by HD and, thus, do not require additional post-dialysis dosing [47]. A recent RCT found that amlodipine lowered systolic BP by 10 mmHg more than placebo, without an increased risk of intradialytic hypotension [61]. In an RCT comparing amlodipine to placebo in 251 hypertensive HD patients, Tepel et al. [62] found no difference in all-cause mortality at 30 months; however, amlodipine significantly reduced the secondary combined endpoint of all-cause mortality and cardiovascular events.

Dual Blockade of the RAS

A small study [63] randomized 33 incident diabetic HD patients to an ACEI versus ARB versus combination of ACEI + ARB and achieved good BP control and regression of LV mass index (LVMI) at 1 year in all groups. However, the patients treated with the ACEI + ARB combination exhibited an additional 28% reduction in LVMI when compared with those treated with monotherapy. Larger studies are required to determine whether this therapeutic combination can improve cardiovascular outcomes in HD patients.

A multicenter RCT [64] investigated the antihypertensive effect of the DRI aliskiren in comparison with the CCB amlodipine in 83 HD patients with difficult-to-treat or resistant hypertension. The baseline medications were dual therapy in 60% and therapy with ≥3 drugs in 40% of cases. Most patients (77%) were on ARBs or ACEIs. A significant decrease in BP was found only in the amlodipine group, but not in the aliskiren group.

Mineralocorticoid Receptor Antagonists

The use of these agents in HD patients has not been thoroughly investigated, but it may be limited because of fear of the risk of hyperkalemia, particularly in anuric patients [47]. In two small open-label studies of low-dose (25 mg) spironolactone [65, 66], there was no significant increase in serum potassium with thrice weekly administration, but 7% of patients with daily dosage of the drug were withdrawn because of severe hyperkalemia. In a larger study of spironolactone 25 mg/day in 61 oligoanuric HD patients, potassium levels increased overall (from 4.6 to 5.0 mEq/l) with treatment; however, no patients had a potassium >6.8 mEq/l or required ion exchange resin therapy [67]. While these studies suggest that MR antagonists may be relatively safe, further research is required prior to their use in dialysis patients.

Beta-Blockers

BBs are important antihypertensive agents for HD patients and are particularly indicated in those with coronary artery disease and heart failure [47]. In a secondary analysis of 11,142 prevalent HD patients from the United States Renal Database Systems (USRDS) Wave 3 and 4 Study, Foley et al. [68] found that the use of BBs was associated with a 16% lower adjusted risk of death. Two small RCTs by Cice et al. [69, 70] showed that carvedilol therapy, as compared to placebo, improved cardiac structure and function, as well as survival, in HD patients with heart failure.

Atenolol and metoprolol are dialyzable and require supplementation after dialysis, while combined α- and β-blockers (e.g., carvedilol) are not significantly cleared by HD. Metoprolol is mainly metabolized by the liver and therefore does not require dose adjustment, while atenolol is excreted mainly by the kidneys, and, thus, its half-life is prolonged in HD patients. Carvedilol is a nonselective inhibitor of β-adrenergic receptors and, theoretically, may increase the risk of hyperkalemia [47].

Other Agents

Alpha-blockers are seldom used in dialysis patients. However, in those requiring multiple antihypertensive agents, they can be safely prescribed and do not require additional dosing after HD. Nocturnal administration is preferred, in order to prevent postural hypotension. These agents should be avoided in patients with intradialytic hypotension [47].

Centrally acting alpha-adrenergic agonists are also rarely used, because of their high rate of adverse side effects. However, they may still be useful in dialysis patients, particularly those with RH [47].

Hydralazine and minoxidil are potent vasodilators and can be effective in dialysis patients with RH. These drugs are not removed by HD. Because of reflex stimulation of the sympathetic nervous system, they should be administered together with a BB. Fluid retention, including pleural and pericardial effusions, may occur during therapy and may require drug discontinuation [47].

New Antihypertensive Agents for CKD Patients

Phosphodiesterase Type 5 (PDE5) Inhibitors

In CKD, relative deficiency of circulating nitric oxide (NO) may contribute to hypertension and atherosclerosis, whereas NO deficiency within the kidneys may promote a sharper decline in renal function. Abundant PDE5 expression has been identified in the kidney, and, therefore, it has been proposed that, through its inhibition, the function of the renal NO-cGMP pathway in the kidney can be enhanced, improving the NO deficit associated with CKD. The benefits of PDE5 inhibitors may extend from BP-lowering effects to renoprotective properties [71]. Experimental studies have demonstrated favorable effects of PDE5 inhibition on mesangial cell proliferation, extracellular matrix expansion, tubulointerstitial injury, renal cell apoptosis, oxidative stress, inflammation, and proteinuria in CKD models [71].

To date, only one clinical trial of PDE5 inhibition in CKD has been published [72]. In this study, 40 men with type 2 diabetes mellitus were treated for 1 month with either 50 mg sildenafil daily or placebo. The sildenafil-treated group had a 50% reduction in albuminuria and the drug was well tolerated. A randomized, placebo-controlled trial is currently investigating the impact of a long-acting PDE5 inhibitor on patients with diabetes mellitus and overt nephropathy [71].

Endothelin Antagonists

Endothelin-1 (ET-1) upregulation plays a pathogenic role in endothelial dysfunction and atherosclerosis and may also contribute to cardiovascular complications of CKD [71]. Selective endothelin type A (ETA) receptor antagonist darusentan, but not ETA/ETB receptor antagonist bosentan, prevented the aggravation of hypertension in renal failure rats treated with erythropoietin-stimulating agents [73]. Administration of a selective ETA receptor antagonist to hypertensive patients with CKD produced a substantial reduction in BP (10 mmHg) and increased renal blood flow [74]. In addition, chronic treatment with the mixed ETA/ETB receptor antagonist, avosentan [75], and the selective ETA receptor antagonist, atrasentan [76], in addition to standard ACEI/ARB treatment, substantially decreased albumin excretion in patients with diabetic nephropathy.

While ET receptor antagonists are generally well tolerated in clinical trials, the major adverse effects are peripheral edema, a mild decrease in hemoglobin (thought to be related to hemodilution secondary to increased extracellular fluid), headache, and flushing. As these drugs are primarily metabolized and eliminated by the liver, one significant adverse effect is hepatic dysfunction, which is dose dependent and reversible upon discontinuation of the drug [47].

Conclusions and Recommendations

In patients requiring a triple therapy, this should consist of an ACEI or ARB + CCB + diuretic (ACD regimen) for most patients. This regimen is thought to be effective and well tolerated in CKD. It should be tried in optimum doses as the first therapeutic step in patients with CKD and RH, in the absence of contraindications.

ACEIs and ARBs are especially preferred in patients with CKD and heart failure, post-myocardial infarction, and proteinuria. Adverse effects include hypotension, acute kidney injury, and hyperkalemia. Monitoring of serum creatinine and potassium is indicated after starting treatment. If strategies to minimize hyperkalemia fail to maintain serum potassium concentrations <5.6 mEq/l, the RAS inhibitor should be discontinued, and another class of antihypertensive drugs should be used instead. In patients with advanced CKD (stages 4 and 5), consideration should be given to stopping ACEIs/ARBs when there are no other compelling indications for these agents and especially when there is high risk of hyperkalemia and/or acute kidney injury, which may precipitate dialysis initiation. Dual therapy ACEI + ARB or ACEI/ARB + DRI is not indicated, because of increased risk of adverse events and lack of proven benefits.

Diuretics are the cornerstone of hypertension treatment in CKD and, by definition, a component of any antihypertensive drug combination for RH. The combination of diuretics with RAS inhibitors, CCBs, and BBs is synergistic and very effective. In patients with CKD stage 4 (GFR <30 ml/min/1.73 m^2) or with significant edema, thiazide diuretics should be replaced or combined with loop diuretics.

CCBs are particularly useful in hypertensive patients who also have angina and/ or supraventricular tachycardia. Most CCBs do not accumulate in patients with impaired renal function. Dihydropyridines may induce fluid retention, which can be counteracted with diuretics. Non-dihydropyridines should not be associated with BBs, because of risks of bradycardia and depression of myocardial inotropism.

MR antagonists may be used as fourth-line therapy for RH in patients with GFR ≥30 ml/min and plasma potassium concentrations ≤4–5 mmol/L or in patients with other indications, such as heart failure. However, they should be used with caution in CKD patients, particularly in combination with ACEIs or ARBs, because of increased risk of hyperkalemia and acute kidney injury. Although, these drugs were shown to be very effective in patients with essential RH, the long-term effects of MR antagonists on renal and cardiovascular outcomes, mortality, and safety in patients with CKD are still to be determined.

BBs have been widely used for decades to treat hypertension, as well as coronary artery disease, heart failure, and cardiac arrhythmias. Adverse effects associated with BBs include bradycardia, erectile dysfunction, fatigue, and lipid and glucose abnormalities. Agents like metoprolol and carvedilol should be preferred over atenolol, which may accumulate in patients with CKD.

Other fourth- or fifth-line antihypertensive agents include centrally acting alpha-agonists, alpha-blockers, and direct vasodilators. They are potent BP-lowering drugs and do not require dose adjustments in CKD (except for moxonidine). However, their use is limited by numerous side effects; among these, fluid retention usually requires the association with diuretics.

References

1. Sarafidis PA, Georgianos PI, Zebekakis PE. Comparative epidemiology of resistant hypertension in chronic kidney disease and the general hypertensive population. Semin Nephrol. 2014;34(5):483–91.
2. Sinha AD, Agarwal R. Hypertension treatment for patients with advanced chronic kidney disease. Curr Cardiovasc Risk Rep. 2014;8(10):pii: 400.
3. Doumas M, Tsioufis C, Faselis C, Lazaridis A, Grassos H, Papademetriou V. Non-interventional management of resistant hypertension. World J Cardiol. 2014;6(10):1080–90.
4. Townsend RR, Taler SJ. Management of hypertension in chronic kidney disease. Nat Rev Nephrol. 2015;11(9):555–63.
5. Gorostidi M, Santamaría R, Alcázar R, Fernández-Fresnedo G, Galcerán JM, Goicoechea M, Oliveras A, Portolés J, Rubio E, Segura J, Aranda P, de Francisco AL, Del Pino MD, Fernández-Vega F, Górriz JL, Luño J, Marín R, Martínez I, Martínez-Castelao A, Orte LM, Quereda C, Rodríguez-Pérez JC, Rodríguez M, Ruilope LM. Spanish Society of Nephrology document on KDIGO guidelines for the assessment and treatment of chronic kidney disease. Neftekhimi. 2014;34(3):302–16.
6. Mancia G, Fagard R, Narkiewicz K, Redón J, Zanchetti A, Böhm M, Christiaens T, Cifkova R, De Backer G, Dominiczak A, Galderisi M, Grobbee DE, Jaarsma T, Kirchhof P, Kjeldsen SE, Laurent S, Manolis AJ, Nilsson PM, Ruilope LM, Schmieder RE, Sirnes PA, Sleight P, Viiigimaa M, Waeber B, Zannad F, Members TF. 2013 ESH/ESC guidelines for the management of arterial hypertension: the task force for the management of arterial hypertension of the European Society of Hypertension (ESH) and of the European Society of Cardiology (ESC). J Hypertens. 2013;31(7):1281–357.
7. Lindholm LH, Carlberg B, Samuelsson O. Should beta blockers remain first choice in the treatment of primary hypertension? A meta-analysis. Lancet. 2005;366(9496):1545–53.

8. Weber F, Anlauf M. Treatment resistant hypertension—investigation and conservative management. Dtsch Arztebl Int. 2014;111(25):425–31.
9. Brown MJ, Cruickshank JK, Dominiczak AF, MacGregor GA, Poulter NR, Russell GI, Thom S, Williams B, Executive Committee, British Hypertension Society. Better blood pressure control: how to combine drugs. J Hum Hypertens. 2003;17(2):81–6.
10. Calhoun DA, Jones D, Textor S, Goff DC, Murphy TP, Toto RD, White A, Cushman WC, White W, Sica D, Ferdinand K, Giles TD, Falkner B, Carey RM, American Heart Association Professional Education Committee. Resistant hypertension: diagnosis, evaluation, and treatment: a scientific statement from the American Heart Association professional Education Committee of the Council for high blood pressure research. Circulation. 2008;117(25):e510–26.
11. Denolle T, Chamontin B, Doll G, Fauvel JP, Girerd X, Herpin D, Vaïsse B, Villeneuve F, Halimi JM. Management of resistant hypertension. Expert consensus statement from the French Society of Hypertension, an affiliate of the French Society of Cardiology. Presse Med. 2014;43(12 Pt 1):1325–31.
12. Sinnakirouchenan R, Kotchen TA. Role of sodium restriction and diuretic therapy for "resistant" hypertension in chronic kidney disease. Semin Nephrol. 2014;34(5):514–9.
13. Manolis AJ, Kallistratos MS, Doumas M, Pagoni S, Poulimenos L. Recent advances in the management of resistant hypertension. F1000Prime Rep. 2015;7:03.
14. Václavík J, Sedlák R, Plachy M, Navrátil K, Plásek J, Jarkovsky J, Václavík T, Husár R, Kociánová E, Táborsky M. Addition of spironolactone in patients with resistant arterial hypertension (ASPIRANT): a randomized, double-blind, placebo-controlled trial. Hypertension. 2011;57(6):1069–75.
15. Williams B, MacDonald TM, Morant S, Webb DJ, Sever P, McInnes G, Ford I, Cruickshank JK, Caulfield MJ, Salsbury J, MacKenzie I, Padmanabhan S, Brown MJ, British Hypertension Society's PATHWAY Studies Group. Spironolactone versus placebo, bisoprolol, and doxazosin to determine the optimal treatment for drug-resistant hypertension (PATHWAY-2): a randomised, double-blind, crossover trial. Lancet. 2015;386(10008):2059–68.
16. Peterzan MA, Hardy R, Chaturvedi N, Hughes AD. Meta-analysis of dose-response relationships for hydrochlorothiazide, chlorthalidone, and bendroflumethiazide on blood pressure, serum potassium, and urate. Hypertension. 2012;59(6):1104–9.
17. Roush GC, Holford TR, Guddati AK. Chlorthalidone compared with hydrochlorothiazide in reducing cardiovascular events: systematic review and network meta-analyses. Hypertension. 2012;59(6):1110–7.
18. Weber MA, Schiffrin EL, White WB, Mann S, Lindholm LH, Kenerson JG, Flack JM, Carter BL, Materson BJ, Ram CV, Cohen DL, Cadet JC, Jean-Charles RR, Taler S, Kountz D, Townsend R, Chalmers J, Ramirez AJ, Bakris GL, Wang J, Schutte AE, Bisognano JD, Touyz RM, Sica D, Harrap SB. Clinical practice guidelines for the management of hypertension in the community a statement by the American Society of Hypertension and the International Society of Hypertension. J Hypertens. 2014;32(1):3–15.
19. James PA, Oparil S, Carter BL, Cushman WC, Dennison-Himmelfarb C, Handler J, Lackland DT, LeFevre ML, MacKenzie TD, Ogedegbe O, Smith SC Jr, Svetkey LP, Taler SJ, Townsend RR, Wright JT Jr, Narva AS, Ortiz E. 2014 evidence-based guideline for the management of high blood pressure in adults: report from the panel members appointed to the eighth joint National Committee (JNC 8). JAMA. 2014;311(5):507–20.
20. Go AS, Bauman MA, Coleman King SM, Fonarow GC, Lawrence W, Williams KA, Sanchez E, American Heart Association; American College of Cardiology; Centers for Disease Control and Prevention. An effective approach to high blood pressure control: a science advisory from the American Heart Association, the American College of Cardiology, and the Centers for Disease Control and Prevention. Hypertension. 2014;63(4):878–85.
21. Johnson DW, Atai E, Chan M, Phoon RK, Scott C, Toussaint ND, Turner GL, Usherwood T, Wiggins KJ, KHA-CARI. KHA-CARI guideline: early chronic kidney disease: detection, prevention and management. Nephrology (Carlton). 2013;18(5):340–50.

22. Houle SK, Padwal R, Poirier L, Tsuyuki RT. The 2014 Canadian hypertension Education program (CHEP) guidelines for pharmacists: an update. Can Pharm J (Ott). 2014;147(4):203–8.
23. Kereiakes DJ, Chrysant SG, Izzo JL Jr, Littlejohn T 3rd, Melino M, Lee J, Fernandez V, Heyrman R. Olmesartan/amlodipine/hydrochlorothiazide in participants with hypertension and diabetes, chronic kidney disease, or chronic cardiovascular disease: a subanalysis of the multicenter, randomized, double-blind, parallel-group TRINITY study. Cardiovasc Diabetol. 2012;11:134.
24. Kidney Disease: Improving Global Outcomes (KDIGO) Blood Pressure Work Group. KDIGO clinical practice guideline for the management of blood pressure in chronic kidney disease. Kidney Int Suppl. 2012;2:337–414.
25. Palmer BF, Fenves AZ. Optimizing blood pressure control in patients with chronic kidney disease. Proc (Baylor Univ Med Cent). 2010;23(3):239–45.
26. Ruzicka M, Quinn RR, McFarlane P, Hemmelgarn B, Ramesh Prasad GV, Feber J, Nesrallah G, MacKinnon M, Tangri N, McCormick B, Tobe S, Blydt-Hansen TD, Hiremath S. Canadian society of nephrology commentary on the 2012 KDIGO clinical practice guideline for the management of blood pressure in CKD. Am J Kidney Dis. 2014;63(6):869–87.
27. Mann JF, Gerstein HC, Yi QL, Lonn EM, Hoogwerf BJ, Rashkow A, Yusuf S. Development of renal disease in people at high cardiovascular risk: results of the HOPE randomized study. J Am Soc Nephrol. 2003;14(3):641–7.
28. Saruta T, Hayashi K, Ogihara T, Nakao K, Fukui T, Fukiyama K, CASE-J Study Group. Effects of candesartan and amlodipine on cardiovascular events in hypertensive patients with chronic kidney disease: subanalysis of the CASE-J study. Hypertens Res. 2009;32(6):505–12.
29. Mann JF, Schmieder RE, Dyal L, McQueen MJ, Schumacher H, Pogue J, Wang X, Probstfield JL, Avezum A, Cardona-Munoz E, Dagenais GR, Diaz R, Fodor G, Maillon JM, Rydén L, Yu CM, Teo KK, Yusuf S, TRANSCEND (Telmisartan Randomised Assessment Study in ACE Intolerant Subjects with Cardiovascular Disease) Investigators. Effect of telmisartan on renal outcomes: a randomized trial. Ann Intern Med. 2009;151(1):1–10. W1-2
30. Makino H, Haneda M, Babazono T, Moriya T, Ito S, Iwamoto Y, Kawamori R, Takeuchi M, Katayama S, INNOVATION Study Group. Prevention of transition from incipient to overt nephropathy with telmisartan in patients with type 2 diabetes. Diabetes Care. 2007;30(6):1577–8.
31. Parving HH, Lehnert H, Bröchner-Mortensen J, Gomis R, Andersen S, Arner P, Irbesartan in Patients with Type 2 Diabetes and Microalbuminuria Study Group. The effect of irbesartan on the development of diabetic nephropathy in patients with type 2 diabetes. N Engl J Med. 2001;345(12):870–8.
32. Jafar TH, Stark PC, Schmid CH, et al. Progression of chronic kidney disease: the role of blood pressure control, proteinuria, and angiotensin-converting enzyme inhibition: a patient-level meta-analysis. Ann Intern Med. 2003;139(4):244–52.
33. Kent DM, Jafar TH, Hayward RA, et al. Progression risk, urinary protein excretion, and treatment effects of angiotensin-converting enzyme inhibitors in nondiabetic kidney disease. J Am Soc Nephrol. 2007;18(6):1959–65.
34. Telmisartan Randomised AssessmeNt Study in ACE iNtolerant subjects with cardiovascular Disease (TRANSCEND) Investigators, Yusuf S, Teo K, Anderson C, Pogue J, Dyal L, Copland I, Schumacher H, Dagenais G, Sleight P. Effects of the angiotensin-receptor blocker telmisartan on cardiovascular events in high-risk patients intolerant to angiotensin-converting enzyme inhibitors: a randomised controlled trial. Lancet. 2008;372(9644):1174–83.
35. Verbeke F, Lindley E, Van Bortel L, Vanholder R, London G, Cochat P, Wiecek A, Fouque D, Van Biesen W. A European renal best practice (ERBP) position statement on the kidney disease: improving Global outcomes (KDIGO) clinical practice guideline for the management of blood pressure in non-dialysis-dependent chronic kidney disease: an endorsement with some caveats for real-life application. Nephrol Dial Transplant. 2014;29(3):490–6.
36. Verdalles U, de Vinuesa SG, Goicoechea M, et al. Utility of bioimpedance spectroscopy (BIS) in the management of refractory hypertension in patients with chronic kidney disease (CKD). Nephrol Dial Transplant. 2012;27(Suppl 4):iv31–5.

37. Knauf H, Mutschler E. Diuretic effectiveness of hydrochlorothiazide and furosemide alone and in combination in chronic renal failure. J Cardiovasc Pharmacol. 1995;26(3):394–400.
38. Dussol B, Moussi-Frances J, Morange S, Somma-Delpero C, Mundler O, Berland Y. A pilot study comparing furosemide and hydrochlorothiazide in patients with hypertension and stage 4 or 5 chronic kidney disease. J Clin Hypertens (Greenwich). 2012;14(1):32–7.
39. Cirillo M, Marcarelli F, Mele AA, Romano M, Lombardi C, Bilancio G. Parallel-group 8-week study on chlorthalidone effects in hypertensives with low kidney function. Hypertension. 2014;63(4):692–7.
40. Mann JF, Schmieder RE, McQueen M, Dyal L, Schumacher H, Pogue J, Wang X, Maggioni A, Budaj A, Chaithiraphan S, Dickstein K, Keltai M, Metsärinne K, Oto A, Parkhomenko A, Piegas LS, Svendsen TL, Teo KK, Yusuf S, ONTARGET investigators. Renal outcomes with telmisartan, ramipril, or both, in people at high vascular risk (the ONTARGET study): a multicentre, randomised, double-blind, controlled trial. Lancet. 2008;372(9638):547–53.
41. Fried LF, Emanuele N, Zhang JH, Brophy M, Conner TA, Duckworth W, Leehey DJ, McCullough PA, O'Connor T, Palevsky PM, Reilly RF, Seliger SL, Warren SR, Watnick S, Peduzzi P, Guarino P, VA NEPHRON-D Investigators. Combined angiotensin inhibition for the treatment of diabetic nephropathy. N Engl J Med. 2013;369(20):1892–903.
42. Parving HH, Persson F, Lewis JB, Lewis EJ, Hollenberg NK, AVOID Study Investigators. Aliskiren combined with losartan in type 2 diabetes and nephropathy. N Engl J Med. 2008;358(23):2433–46.
43. Parving HH, Brenner BM, McMurray JJ, de Zeeuw D, Haffner SM, Solomon SD, Chaturvedi N, Persson F, Desai AS, Nicolaides M, Richard A, Xiang Z, Brunel P, Pfeffer MA, ALTITUDE Investigators. Cardiorenal end points in a trial of aliskiren for type 2 diabetes. N Engl J Med. 2012;367(23):2204–13.
44. US Food and Drug Administration. FDA drug safety communication: new warning and contraindication for blood pressure medicines containing aliskiren (Tekturna). http://www.fda.gov/Drugs/DrugSafety/ucm300889.htm
45. Epstein M, Williams GH, Weinberger M, Lewin A, Krause S, Mukherjee R, Patni R, Beckerman B. Selective aldosterone blockade with eplerenone reduces albuminuria in patients with type 2 diabetes. Clin J Am Soc Nephrol. 2006;1(5):940–51.
46. Badve SV, Roberts MA, Hawley CM, Cass A, Garg AX, Krum H, Tonkin A, Perkovic V. Effects of beta-adrenergic antagonists in patients with chronic kidney disease: a systematic review and meta-analysis. J Am Coll Cardiol. 2011;58(11):1152–61.
47. Inrig JK. Antihypertensive agents in hemodialysis patients: a current perspective. Semin Dial. 2010;23(3):290–7.
48. Covic A, Goldsmith D, Donciu MD, Siriopol D, Popa R, Kanbay M, London G. From profusion to confusion: the saga of managing hypertension in chronic kidney disease! J Clin Hypertens (Greenwich). 2015;17(6):421–7.
49. K/DOQI Workgroup. K/DOQI clinical practice guidelines for cardiovascular disease in dialysis patients. Am J Kidney Dis. 2005;45(4 Suppl 3):S1–153.
50. Ichihara A, Hayashi M, Kaneshiro Y, Takemitsu T, Homma K, Kanno Y, Yoshizawa M, Furukawa T, Takenaka T, Saruta T. Low doses of losartan and trandolapril improve arterial stiffness in hemodialysis patients. Am J Kidney Dis. 2005;45(5):866–74.
51. Zannad F, Kessler M, Lehert P, Grünfeld JP, Thuilliez C, Leizorovicz A, Lechat P. Prevention of cardiovascular events in end-stage renal disease: results of a randomized trial of fosinopril and implications for future studies. Kidney Int. 2006;70(7):1318–24.
52. Moist LM, Port FK, Orzol SM, Young EW, Ostbye T, Wolfe RA, Hulbert-Shearon T, Jones CA, Bloembergen WE. Predictors of loss of residual renal function among new dialysis patients. J Am Soc Nephrol. 2000;11(3):556–64.
53. Matsumoto N, Ishimitsu T, Okamura A, Seta H, Takahashi M, Matsuoka H. Effects of imidapril on left ventricular mass in chronic hemodialysis patients. Hypertens Res. 2006;29(4):253–60.

54. Berger AK, Duval S, Krumholz HM. Aspirin, beta-blocker, and angiotensin-converting enzyme inhibitor therapy in patients with end-stage renal disease and an acute myocardial infarction. J Am Coll Cardiol. 2003;42(2):201–8.
55. Efrati S, Zaidenstein R, Dishy V, Beberashvili I, Sharist M, Averbukh Z, Golik A, Weissgarten J. ACE inhibitors and survival of hemodialysis patients. Am J Kidney Dis. 2002;40(5):1023–9.
56. McCullough PA, Sandberg KR, Yee J, Hudson MP. Mortality benefit of angiotensin-converting enzyme inhibitors after cardiac events in patients with end-stage renal disease. J Renin-Angiotensin-Aldosterone Syst. 2002;3(3):188–91.
57. Takahashi A, Takase H, Toriyama T, Sugiura T, Kurita Y, Ueda R, Dohi Y. Candesartan, an angiotensin II type-1 receptor blocker, reduces cardiovascular events in patients on chronic haemodialysis—a randomized study. Nephrol Dial Transplant. 2006;21(9):2507–12.
58. Suzuki H, Kanno Y, Sugahara S, Ikeda N, Shoda J, Takenaka T, Inoue T, Araki R. Effect of angiotensin receptor blockers on cardiovascular events in patients undergoing hemodialysis: an open-label randomized controlled trial. Am J Kidney Dis. 2008;52(3):501–6.
59. Iseki K, Arima H, Kohagura K, Komiya I, Ueda S, Tokuyama K, Shiohira Y, Uehara H, Toma S, Olmesartan Clinical Trial in Okinawan Patients Under OKIDS (OCTOPUS) Group. Effects of angiotensin receptor blockade (ARB) on mortality and cardiovascular outcomes in patients with long-term haemodialysis: a randomized controlled trial. Nephrol Dial Transplant. 2013;28(6):1579–89.
60. Bragg-Gresham JL, Fissell RB, Mason NA, Bailie GR, Gillespie BW, Wizemann V, Cruz JM, Akiba T, Kurokawa K, Ramirez S, Young EW. Diuretic use, residual renal function, and mortality among hemodialysis patients in the Dialysis Outcomes and Practice Pattern Study (DOPPS). Am J Kidney Dis. 2007;49(3):426–31.
61. Kestenbaum B, Gillen DL, Sherrard DJ, Seliger S, Ball A, Stehman-Breen C. Calcium channel blocker use and mortality among patients with end-stage renal disease. Kidney Int. 2002;61(6):2157–64.
62. Tepel M, Hopfenmueller W, Scholze A, Maier A, Zidek W. Effect of amlodipine on cardiovascular events in hypertensive haemodialysis patients. Nephrol Dial Transplant. 2008;23(11):3605–12.
63. Suzuki H, Kanno Y, Kaneko K, Kaneko M, Kotaki S, Mimura T, Takane H. Comparison of the effects of angiotensin receptor antagonist, angiotensin converting enzyme inhibitor, and their combination on regression of left ventricular hypertrophy of diabetes type 2 patients on recent onset hemodialysis therapy. Ther Apher Dial. 2004;8(4):320–7.
64. Kuriyama S, Yokoyama K, Hara Y, Sugano N, Yokoo T, Hosoya T. Effect of aliskiren in chronic kidney disease patients with refractory hypertension undergoing hemodialysis: a randomized controlled multicenter study. Clin Exp Nephrol. 2014;18(5):821–30.
65. Saudan P, Mach F, Perneger T, Schnetzler B, Stoermann C, Fumeaux Z, Rossier M, Martin PY. Safety of low-dose spironolactone administration in chronic haemodialysis patients. Nephrol Dial Transplant. 2003;18(11):2359–63.
66. Hussain S, Dreyfus DE, Marcus RJ, Biederman RW, McGill RL. Is spironolactone safe for dialysis patients? Nephrol Dial Transplant. 2003;18(11):2364–8.
67. Matsumoto Y, Kageyama S, Yakushigawa T, Arihara K, Sugiyama T, Mori Y, Sugiyama H, Ohmura H, Shio N. Long-term low-dose spironolactone therapy is safe in oligoanuric hemodialysis patients. Cardiology. 2009;114(1):32–8.
68. Foley RN, Herzog CA, Collins AJ, United States Renal Data System. Blood pressure and long-term mortality in United States hemodialysis patients: USRDS waves 3 and 4 study. Kidney Int. 2002;62(5):1784–90.
69. Cice G, Ferrara L, Di Benedetto A, Russo PE, Marinelli G, Pavese F, Iacono A. Dilated cardiomyopathy in dialysis patients—beneficial effects of carvedilol: a double-blind, placebo-controlled trial. J Am Coll Cardiol. 2001;37(2):407–11.

70. Cice G, Ferrara L, D'Andrea A, D'Isa S, Di Benedetto A, Cittadini A, Russo PE, Golino P, Calabrò R. Carvedilol increases two-year survival in dialysis patients with dilated cardiomy-opathy: a prospective, placebo-controlled trial. J Am Coll Cardiol. 2003;41(9):1438–44.
71. Brown KE, Dhaun N, Goddard J, Webb DJ. Potential therapeutic role of phosphodiesterase type 5 inhibition in hypertension and chronic kidney disease. Hypertension. 2014;63(1): 5–11.
72. Grover-Páez F, Villegas Rivera G, Guillén OR. Sildenafil citrate diminishes microalbuminuria and the percentage of A1c in male patients with type 2 diabetes. Diabetes Res Clin Pract. 2007;78(1):136–40.
73. Brochu E, Lacasse S, Larivière R, Kingma I, Grose JH, Lebel M. Differential effects of endo-thelin-1 antagonists on erythropoietin-induced hypertension in renal failure. J Am Soc Nephrol. 1999;10(7):1440–6.
74. Goddard J, Johnston NR, Hand MF, Cumming AD, Rabelink TJ, Rankin AJ, Webb DJ. Endothelin-a receptor antagonism reduces blood pressure and increases renal blood flow in hypertensive patients with chronic renal failure: a comparison of selective and combined endothelin receptor blockade. Circulation. 2004;109(9):1186–93.
75. Wenzel RR, Littke T, Kuranoff S, Jürgens C, Bruck H, Ritz E, Philipp T. Mitchell a; SPP301 (Avosentan) Endothelin antagonist evaluation in diabetic nephropathy study investigators. Avosentan reduces albumin excretion in diabetics with macroalbuminuria. J Am Soc Nephrol. 2009 Mar;20(3):655–64.
76. Kohan DE, Pritchett Y, Molitch M, Wen S, Garimella T, Audhya P, Andress DL. Addition of atrasentan to renin-angiotensin system blockade reduces albuminuria in diabetic nephropathy. J Am Soc Nephrol. 2011 Apr;22(4):763–72.

Chapter 19
Devices for Neural Modulation (Renal Denervation, Barostimulation)

Marcin Adamczak, Magdalena Bartmańska, and Andrzej Więcek

Introduction

One of the pathogenic factors of arterial hypertension in chronic kidney disease (CKD) patients besides others like hypervolemia, increased activity of renin angiotensin system (RAS), or endothelial dysfunction is increased activity of the sympathetic nervous system (SNS). In CKD patients, SNS overactivity may also contribute to the pathogenesis of cardiovascular morbidity, mortality, and progression toward end-stage kidney disease (ESKD). In this chapter, first the issue of SNS activity in CKD patients will be briefly discussed. Next, we will review the current status of interventional nonpharmacological methods of treatment which aim to reduce SNS activity = such as renal denervation (RDN) and baroreflex activation therapy (BAT) in resistant hypertension and experience with such therapies in patients with CKD.

Sympathetic Nervous System Overactivity in Chronic Kidney Disease

Early observations of the sympathetic nervous system overactivity in CKD were based on increased catecholamines plasma concentrations. More precisely, SNS activity can be estimated directly by the analysis of nerve discharge of the *nervus peronaeus*, i.e., by the muscle sympathetic nerve activity (MSNA) measurement. Converse et al. in 1992 were first to report that MSNA is increased in hemodialysis CKD patients. They showed about 2.5-fold MSNA increase in hemodialysis CKD patients when compared to healthy subjects. In this study, it was also shown that

M. Adamczak • M. Bartmańska • A. Więcek (✉)
Department of Nephrology, Transplantation and Internal Medicine,
Medical University of Silesia, Katowice, Poland
e-mail: awiecek@sum.edu.pl

© Springer International Publishing AG 2017
A. Covic et al. (eds.), *Resistant Hypertension in Chronic Kidney Disease*,
DOI 10.1007/978-3-319-56827-0_19

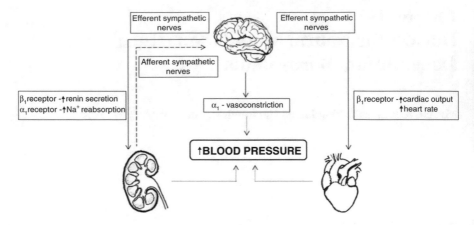

Fig. 19.1 The role of renal sympathetic nerves in blood pressure regulation

MSNA in CKD patients undergoing hemodialysis after bilateral nephrectomy did not differ from healthy subjects [1]. Hausberg et al. have proven that despite correction of uremia in patients after renal transplantation with adequate transplanted kidney function but preserved native kidneys, MSNA is increased as in CKD hemodialysis patients. MSNA in kidney transplant patients after bilateral nephrectomy was comparable to healthy volunteers [2]. Increased MSNA has been also reported in patients with autosomal dominant polycystic kidney disease (ADPKD) even in the presence of a normal glomerular filtration rate (GFR). In another study, Grassi et al. demonstrated that increased activation of SNS is present in the early stages of CKD (mean estimated glomerular filtration rate – eGFR – in the studied patients: 41 ml/min per 1.73 m^2) [3]. Results of the above-quoted clinical studies suggest that SNS overactivity in CKD is caused by diseased kidneys themselves.

Results of the animal experiments confirmed such a hypothesis. Ye et al. showed that applying a small lesion in one kidney by an intrarenal phenol injection, not affecting kidney function, increases SNS activity and leads to a long-term increase of noradrenaline secretion and arterial hypertension. These effects are abolished by afferent surgical denervation [4]. It has been showed in subtotally nephrectomized rats that blood pressure increase and elevation of norepinephrine (NE) turnover in sympathetic brain centers was reduced by afferent surgical denervation (dorsal rhizotomy, a procedure in which the dorsal roots from Th10-L2 were damaged).

The number of abovementioned evidence suggests that the kidneys are both recipients and generators of increased SNS activity (Fig. 19.1). To explain this, a short description of the function of the renal nerves should be given.

Kidneys are innervated by two types of fibers: (1) sensory afferent fibers leading from the central nervous system (axons of the neurons located in thoracic and lumbar sympathetic trunks) to the kidneys and (2) sympathetic efferent fibers which start in the kidneys and conduct nerve impulses to the central nervous system (cell bodies localized ipsilateral Th6-L4 trunks). Both types of fibers localized along the renal arteries in adventitia enter the kidneys at the hilum and extend to the vascular and tubular compartments.

Activation of the efferent fibers leads to blood pressure increase. Norepinephrine is released from nerve endings, and it activates β_1 adrenoreceptors located on renin-containing juxtaglomerular granular cells and α_1 receptors on the basolateral membrane of renal tubular epithelial cells in the proximal tubule and on the vascular smooth muscle cells of the intrarenal resistance vasculature. These receptor activations result in enhanced renin secretion (with subsequent RAS stimulation), increased renal tubular sodium reabsorption and renal vasoconstriction, reduced renal blood flow, and decreased glomerular filtration rate [5].

Afferent fibers are located in almost every part of human kidney, however at the highest density in renal pelvis. These fibers project to brain regions involved in cardiovascular control: the subfornical organs, the brainstem, and the hypothalamus [5]. Messages concerning hydrostatic pressure in renal pelvis are transmitted by mechanoreceptors. It was shown that afferent fibers are activated in response to pelvic wall tension increase. The afferent sensory nerves are stimulated also by chemoreceptors responding to ischemia and chemical changes in kidney interstitium. Probably, from the clinician point of view, the important factor causing sympathetic afferent sensory nerve stimulation in CKD patients is kidney ischemia. Experimental studies have shown that in rats, acute ischemia caused by renal artery stenosis activates SNS. Rise in blood pressure was abolished in these animals after renal denervation of stenotic kidneys. Another data indicate that in two-kidney, one-clip hypertension in rat, denervation is associated with decrease of SNS activity. In clinical study, it was shown that SNS activity is higher in patients with renovascular hypertension. It was also shown that renal blood flow increase as a result of successful angioplasty normalizes MSNA. Above-quoted results of both experimental and clinical studies suggest that afferent activation affects SNS centers in central nervous system and thereby increases central SNS activity and can cause hypertension.

As it was discussed above, SNS overactivity is present in CKD patients even with normal kidney function. However, magnitude of SNS activity increases with the CKD progression. Grassi et al. showed that the intensity of the SNS overactivation is inversely related to the glomerular filtration rate and parallels the severity of CKD [3].

What are the consequences of SNS overactivity in CKD patients? There are some lines of evidence that SNS overactivity may contribute to the pathogenesis of cardiovascular morbidity and mortality in these patients. Penne et al. assessed MSNA in 66 CKD stage 3–4 patients and followed them for 7 years. They showed that MSNA was significantly associated with the composite of all-cause mortality and nonfatal cardiovascular events [6].

Zoccali et al. studied the activity of SNS estimated by plasma norepinephrine concentration in 228 patients undergoing regular hemodialysis treatment for at least 6 months. During the 34 ± 15 months follow-up period, the cardiovascular events such as angina episodes documented with ECG, myocardial infarction, arrhythmia, or stroke were recorded. Plasma NE concentration was above the normal range in 45% of patients. It was also shown in this study that overactivity of SNS was associated with the number of fatal and nonfatal cardiovascular events [7]. In a study of

197 hemodialyzed patients with chronic kidney disease (with more than 6 months vintage of hemodialysis therapy), it has been shown that among subjects with NE plasma concentration located in third tertile, mean heart wall thickness was higher, and concentric left ventricular hypertrophy was more prevalent then in patients from two other tertiles. In these patients, plasma NE concentration was an independent cardiovascular risk factor. In another study, it has been shown that patients undergoing continuous ambulatory peritoneal dialysis (CAPD) have 3.5 times higher plasma NE concentration than in healthy subjects. It is also important to stress that in patients treated with CAPD, plasma NE concentration was 1.7 times higher than in hemodialysis patients.

Results of animal experiments suggest that SNS overactivity participates in CKD progression. Dorsal rhizotomy both in subtotally nephrectomized rats and in uninephrectomized Dahl salt-sensitive hypertensive rats prevents albuminuria and glomerulosclerosis.

Given the pathophysiological evidence described above, the reduction of SNS activity in CKD is a promising aim of therapy. In the recent years, two nonpharmacological interventional methods of such a treatment RDN and BAT were introduced.

Renal Denervation

The earliest invasive methods of hypertension treatment, introduced in 1920s, was surgical thoracolumbar sympathectomy (splanchnicectomy). The operation procedure leads to the section of sympathetic trunks along with removal great splanchnic nerves from the celiac ganglion to mid-thoracic levels. This surgical early experience of 1226 splanchnicectomies was summarized by Smithwick et al. [8]. This method reduced blood pressure and improved mortality but was characterized by high surgical risk and led to severe long-term complications (urine and fecal incontinence, erectile dysfunction, orthostatic hypotension) mainly due to extensive and nonselective damage of SNS nerves, and therefore the use of this antihypertensive treatment method was finally ceased. To avoid such complications, the methods of more selective ablation of renal SNS nerves were needed. Before current status of these methods will be described in this chapter, some data concerning anatomy of renal nerves in humans should be given.

Kidney sympathetic innervation begins in intermediolateral column of the spinal cord. Neuronal track leads from through pregangliotic fibers to sympathetic trunk which includes splanchnic ganglia and then aortorenal ganglia. Sympathetic fibers leave aortorenal ganglia as postgangliotic nerves run alongside with renal artery and reach the kidney at the hilus. From this point, nerve fibers are dividing simultaneously with the divisions of arteries. It should be mentioned that in case of additional renal arteries, the presence of parallel to these vessels sympathetic nerves was revealed. Sakakura et al. investigated distribution of periarterial sympathetic nerve fibers located around kidney arteries [9]. The autopsy studies showed that there were fewer nerves surrounding the renal arteries in the distal segments compared

Table 19.1 Methods of endovascular renal nerve ablation

Method of renal denervation	Product name	Type of catheter	Current experience
Radiofrequency ablation (RFA)	Symplicity RFA catheter	Single-electrode RFA catheter	Randomized clinical study
	EnligHTN RFA catheter	Multielectrode catheter	Nonrandomized clinical study
	ThermoCool RFA	Irrigated RFA catheter	Nonrandomized clinical study
Ultrasonic ablation	PARADISE ultrasonic catheter	Ultrasonic balloon catheter	Nonrandomized clinical study
	TIVUS ultrasonic catheter	Ultrasonic autoregulating balloon catheter	Proof-of-concept clinical study
Pharmacological ablation	Bullfrog microinfusion catheter	Microneedle-equipped balloon catheter	Experimental study

RFA radiofrequency ablation

with the proximal and middle segments and the mean distance from renal artery lumen to nerve location is the lowest in the distal segments. Additionally the higher total number of nerves in ventral region than in dorsal part of renal arteries was shown. Nevertheless, on average, more than 75% of nerves are placed within a distance of 4.3 mm from renal artery lumen. This anatomy of renal nerves (i.e., vicinity to renal arteries lumens) allowed to develop procedures of selective renal SNS nerve damages by applying different stimuli through devices placed in renal arteries, i.e., RDN.

Unfortunately currently, there are no clinically useful methods to precisely define the anatomical localization of renal SNS nerves in particular patient. The preferred segment of renal artery for the effective intervention is also unknown. It is unclear whether it is better to ablate renal SNS nerves in proximal segment (where bigger but fewer nerves are localized) or in distal segment (where smaller but more nerves are present).

Percutaneous, intravascular catheter-based procedures, described below, aimed to damage selectively renal nerves are still under development and investigations (Table 19.1). The agents used to damage renal arteries in experimental or clinical studies are radiofrequency energy (RF), ultrasound energy, and pharmacological ones (Table 19.1).

RF ablation is so far the most developed method of RDN. The procedure using RF generator enables to injury renal sympathetic nerves with controlled heat (45–70 °C). Systems using single electrode (e.g., Symplicity) need several application of energy in every renal artery. Multielectrode systems (like EnligHTN) are composed of a several-arm tip and deliver energy in a few positions at the same time. It results in shorter duration of the treatment and reduces the volume of contrast medium used in the procedure. The Celsius ThermoCool RFA catheter system uses a saline-irrigated catheter for RDN. Saline irrigation was used in this catheter to prevent the thrombus formation and endothelium damage during RF RDN at the ablation site. Furthermore, given the adventitial location of the renal SNS nerves, saline irrigation might project ablation lesions deeper within the tissue, which potentially may increase RDN effectiveness.

To date the most data concerning safety and effectiveness of RDN in treatment of resistant hypertension comes from the Symplicity HTN-1, HTN-2, and HTN-3 trials. In these studies, RDN were done with single RF electrode catheter Symplicity. Similar inclusion and exclusion criteria were used in all Symplicity trials, and these studies involved patients in whom despite at least triple antihypertensive therapy office systolic blood pressure (SBP) were not lower than 160 mmHg (150 mmHg in the presence of diabetes type 2). In Symplicity HTN-3 trial besides the abovementioned office blood pressure criteria, additionally systolic 24 h ambulatory blood pressure monitoring (ABPM) higher or equal 135 mmHg was required as inclusion criterium. Exclusion criteria included eGFR <45 ml/min/1.73 m^2, diabetes mellitus type I, secondary causes of hypertension, and renovascular anatomical abnormalities such as renal artery stenosis, previous angioplasty, or double and multiple renal arteries. The first of these studies (Symplicity HTN-1) was a nonrandomized "proof of concept" study [10]. In this study, 144 patients with resistant hypertension were observed after RDN. A reduction of SBP by 27 mmHg and diastolic blood pressure (DBP) by 17 mmHg at 6 months of follow-up was found. In the second study (Symplicity HTN-2), 106 patients with resistant hypertension were randomly allocated to RDN with previous treatment or to maintain previous treatment alone (control group) [11]. A SBP reduction of 32 and DBP reduction of 12 mmHg was observed after renal denervation compared with the control group (1 and 0 mmHg, respectively). Long-term data (36 months follow-up) from both abovementioned studies showed that antihypertensive effect was maintained and even became greater. Both these trials did not reveal any significant safety issues. However, there were concerns about the design of the Symplicity HTN-1 and HTN-2 studies (lack of ABPM and the unblinded design). To overcome these limitations, the prospective, single-blind, randomized, sham-controlled study was done (Symplicity HTN-3) [12]. In this study, 535 patients with resistant hypertension were randomly allocated to RDN or sham procedure (control group). Six months after procedure, there was significant office SBP reduction from baseline in both groups (14 vs 12 mmHg, respectively), but between the active and control group, both office and 24 h ABPM did not differ significantly.

Results of the Symplicity HTN-3 study are difficult to interpret due to the number of methodological issues. Further analysis of data from Symplicity HTN-3 has shown that only 19 patients (5%) had complete procedure of ablation that covered 360° of both renal arteries and only 68 patients complete procedure of ablation of one renal artery. It might be linked to the fact that 60 of 111 operators performed during the study only 1 or 2 renal denervation intervention. Office systolic BP in the group with complete RDN procedure of both arteries was reduced by 24 ± 23 mmHg in comparison to patients with incomplete RDN procedure where office SBP decreased only by 14 ± 24. In contrast to previous studies conducted in Europe, about 25% of patients in the Symplicity HTN-3 were African-Americans. There were racial differences in antihypertensive RDN effects. In a group of non-African-Americans, office systolic blood pressure was decreased by 15 mmHg after RDN and 9 mmHg after sham procedure (the difference was significant). No significant difference was observed in African-Americans between RDN and sham group (reduction in office SBP was 15 mmHg and 18 mmHg, respectively). Moreover in 39% of patients, changes in antihypertensive medication during the study period were noted. Symplicity HTN-3 study confirmed, however, that RDN seems to be safe.

Results of two randomized studies comparing RDN with intensified drug treatment in patients with resistant hypertension were recently published – DENER-HTN and PRAGUE-15 study. In the DENER-HTN study, 106 patients with resistant hypertension were randomly assigned to receive either RDN (with the use single RF electrode catheter Symplicity) together with standardized intensification of medical antihypertensive therapy or standardized intensification of medical antihypertensive therapy alone (control group). In this trial, blood pressure reduction after 6 months follow-up was significantly greater in the interventional than in the control group (systolic daytime and nighttime blood pressure differences between groups were 6/6 mmHg, respectively). Results of the study acknowledge superiority of renal denervation over the intensification of pharmacological treatment of resistant hypertension. In the PRAGUE-15 study, 106 patients with resistant hypertension were randomly assigned to receive either renal denervation (with the use single RF electrode catheter Symplicity) or to intensify pharmacological treatment including spironolactone (if tolerated) [13] . In this study, antihypertensive effect of RDN was similar to group with intensified medical treatment (significant reduction in 24 h ABPM SBP after 6 months 9 vs 8 mmHg, respectively).

Recently, Desch et al. published results of a randomized, sham-controlled study in patients with so-called mild resistant hypertension. In this study, 71 patients with mild resistant hypertension were randomly allocated to RDN (with Symplicity FLEX catheter) or sham procedure (control group). Six months after procedure, 24 h ABPM systolic blood pressure reduction was similar in studied groups (7 vs 4 mmHg, respectively) [14].

Despite whole spectrum of clinical studies (i.e., intervention vs control vs sham procedure vs standardized pharmacotherapy), effectiveness of RF RDN ablation in hypertensive patients is still a matter of debate and needs further studies.

Another agent used to induce renal nerve damage is ultrasound energy. Catheters in renal arteries emitting ultrasound energy generate heat resulting in degeneration of renal nerves. The systems PARADISE and TIVUS utilize such energy [15]. PARADISE (ReCor Percutaneous Renal Denervation System) catheter consists of self-centering ultrasonic wave generator and balloon. The ultrasonic sound waves emitted from the central core of the balloon produce frictional heating of soft tissues outside of the artery leading to circumferential ablation of renal SNS nerves, while the fluid-filled balloon cools the endoluminal surface of the artery. Therefore endothelium is protected by cooled fluid inside inflated balloon. Additionally, using ultrasound probe allows to eliminate contact between the device and vessel wall. Preliminary clinical data from 11 patients showed the reduction of office SBP of 36 and DBP of 17 mmHg 3 months after RDN done with this system. In the TIVUS (therapeutic intravascular ultrasound) system, the ultrasound beam, delivered by the ultrasonic wave generator, does not contact arterial wall directly and remote thermal energy delivery to the adventitia of arteries sparing intimal arteries layers. This system offers self-regulating safety technology that monitors local tissue temperature that prevents overtreatment if blood temperature becomes excessively elevated. In the TIVUS-I study, in 17 patients, SBP reduction of 26 mmHg and DBP reduction of 10 mmHg 3 months after treatment with the TIVUS system was found.

Another method of RDN relies on renal sympathetic nerve injury caused by neurotoxins. For this purpose, the Bullfrog microinfusion catheters with microneedle and protective balloon system was designed. The needle penetrates vessel wall and delivery sympatholytic neurotoxin guanethidine in the perivascular area of nearby SNS fibers causing nerve degeneration. Another proposed chemical agent for nerve injury is the alkaloid vincristine. These approaches so far were used in experimental studies only.

Currently under investigation, it is also the methods of noninvasive RDN. This method uses low-intensity focused ultrasound that avoids many of the challenges of invasive endovascular intervention. Kona Medical developed such a noninvasive method of external focused ultrasound aimed to destroy renal SNS nerves. The preliminary results of WAVE III study used noninvasive RDN with such a system showed in 22 patients with resistant hypertension a SBP reduction of 20 mmHg and DBP reduction of 6 mmHg at 3 months after procedure.

Renal Denervation in CKD

Taking into account the pathophysiological evidence described above (i.e., SNS overactivity in CKD and the role of renal SNS nerves in pathogenesis of hypertension), the use of RDN in the treatment of CKD patients may be proposed. The aim of RDN in CKD patients may be both renoprotection (measured by reduction of GFR decline and proteinuria lowering) and improved blood pressure control.

In experimental studies, the renoprotective effect of renal denervation has been showed. In Dahl salt-sensitive hypertensive rats after nephrectomy, RDN is associated with local inhibition of SNS within the kidney and prevention of glomerular sclerosis. In rats with aortic regurgitation (as a model of chronic heart failure), RDN and olmesartan lead to decrease of albuminuria and limit podocyte injury. In rats after 5/6 nephrectomy after dorsal rhizotomy, the reduction of creatinine serum concentration, blood pressure decrease, and less glomerulosclerosis was found. In another experimental study, it was shown that dorsal rhizotomy in rats after 5/6 nephrectomy also reduces albuminuria.

So far, in most of clinical studies evaluating RDN, CKD was an exclusion criterium. However, some data concerning the influence of RDN on kidney function comes from the studies involving hypertensive patients without overt kidney disease. Symplicity HTN-1 and HTN-2 trials revealed that renal function after RDN assessed by serum creatinine and cystatin C concentrations or eGFR was preserved during 1 year follow-up. Nevertheless in some patients, slight decrease of eGFR after RDN was observed. This worsening of renal function might be caused by procedure itself or was related to progression of hypertensive kidney disease. In Symplicity HTN-2 study, the decrease of urine albumin-to-creatinine ratio (UACR) 6 months after RDN was shown [11]. Similarly, in the other clinical studies, a significant decrease of albuminuria measured by UACR in resistant hypertension patients treated with RDN was found.

There are three preliminary clinical studies evaluating the effect of RDN on kidney function in CKD patients (Table 19.2). Hering et al. studied 15 patients with stage 3–4 CKD (eGFR 31 ml/min.) and resistant hypertension. Taking into account impaired kidney function in these studied patients, CO_2 angiography was performed. It was revealed that renal function after RDN in this group of patients was preserved during 1 year follow-up. In this study, RDN did not affect significantly proteinuria [16]. Ott et al. in other clinical study in a group of 27 patients with stage 3–4 CKD (eGFR 48 ml/min.) and resistant hypertension found that RDN slows decline of renal function. They found significant annual difference in eGFR changes before and 1 year after RDN (−5 vs +1.5 ml/min per 1.73 m^2 per year, respectively) [17]. Kiuchi et.al. had shown that patients with CKD stage 2-4, treated by renal denervation benefit not only by lowering the blood pressure but also improving kidney function. RDN in 24-month observation led to renal function (measured by mean eGFR) improvement by 42% and albuminuria decrease by 87% [18]. These promising results suggesting nephroprotective properties of RDN need to be however confirmed in larger studies.

Dörr et al. in resistant hypertension patients with preserved and slightly impaired kidney function (i.e., with eGFR <45 ml/min/1.73 m^2) analyzed the influence of RDN on acute kidney injury biomarkers (urinary concentrations of neutrophil gelatinase-associated lipocain, NGAL, and kidney injury molecule – KIM-1). In this study, no significant changes of eGFR and urinary NGAL and KIM-1 concentrations after RDN were found [19].

As SNS hyperactivity is one of the causes of blood pressure increase in CKD patients, it raises the question whether RDN might be an effective antihypertensive treatment in this group of patients. Hering et al. in already-quoted study had shown that RDN is an effective antihypertensive treatment in patients with CKD stage 3–4 and resistant hypertension (mean blood pressure reduction 1 year after RDN was 33/19 mmHg) (Table 19.2). Additionally in this study, it was found that RDN significantly decreased nighttime ABPM [16]. Similarly Ott et al. in other clinical study in patients with CKD stage 3–4 and resistant hypertension found that RDN leads to significant blood pressure reduction (1 year after RDN SBP reduction was 20 mmHg and DBP reduction was 8 mmHg) [17]. Case reports and results of small observational study (12 patients) showed that RDN leads to blood pressure reduction also in hemodialysis CKD patients.

Besides antihypertensive properties, SNS afferent nerve disruption by RDN may be advantageous in the case of renal pain control. In some patients with ADPKD, chronic and abdominal, flank, or back pain is present due to enlarged cystic kidneys

Table 19.2 Clinical studies on interventional treatments of resistant hypertension in chronic kidney disease patients

	Hering et al.		Ott et al.		Kiuchi et al.		Wallbach et al.	
Patients (n)	15		27		30		23	
Age (years)	61 ± 9		63 ± 9		55 ± 10		61 ± 10	
Number of antihypertensive drugs	5.6 ± 1.3		6.2 ± 1.1		4.6 ± 1.3		6.6 ± 1.6	
Method of intervention	RDN		RDN		RDN		BAT	
	Baseline	6 months after intervention	Baseline	12 months after intervention	Baseline	24 months after intervention	Baseline	6 months after intervention
Office SBP (mmHg)	174 ± 22	142***	156 ± 12	136 ± 19***	185 ± 18	131 ± 15***	161 ± 32	144 ± 32**
Office DBP (mmHg)	91 ± 16	76***	82 ± 13	74 ± 14**	107 ± 13	87 ± 9***	87 ± 15	77 ± 17**
eGFR (ml/min)	31 ± 9	29 ± 7	48 ± 12	49 ± 15	62 ± 23	88 ± 40***	54 ± 28	60 ± 26*
UACR (mg/g creatinine)	592 ± 955	355 ± 276	–	–	99	11***	48	45*
Proteinuria (mg/g creatinine)	–	–	–	–	–		284	136*

SBP systolic blood pressure, *DBP* diastolic blood pressure, *eGFR* estimated glomerular filtration rate, *RDN* renal denervation, *BAT* baroreflex activation therapy, *UACR* urinary albumin-to-creatinine ratio; *p<0.05; **p<0.01; ***p<0.001

stimulating nociceptive afferent SNS. There is also a case report describing the ADPKD patient in whom RDN leads to immediate resolution of 5-year chronic flank pain.

There are some limitations of the RDN use in CKD patients. In some patients with advanced CKD, atrophic renal arteries are characterized by too low diameter to perform RDN. Also the measures to prevent contrast media nephrotoxicity (mainly proper hydration) should be strictly applied before RDN in this group of patients. Alternatively carbon dioxide as contrast agent might be used [16].

Promising results from small clinical studies (presented in Table 19.2) and case reports may suggest that in CKD patients, RDN demonstrates nephroprotective effects. However the role of RDN in the long-term treatment of these patients needs to be confirmed by further clinical studies.

Baroreflex Activation Therapy

Another method of invasive nonpharmacological antihypertensive treatment, based mainly on SNS activity reduction, is BAT.

Baroreceptors participate in baroreceptor reflex, which is one of the crucial homeostatic mechanisms of maintenance the adequate blood pressure. Baroreceptors are mechanoreceptors located in aortic arch, carotid sinuses, and carotid arteries. Afferent nerves run from carotid sinus within glossopharyngeal nerve, and afferent nerves from aortic arch run along with the vagus nerve. Both abovementioned nerves terminate in nucleus of the tractus solitarius localized in the medulla oblongata. Efferent fibers are the part of both sympathetic and parasympathetic nervous system. Baroreceptors are activated by stretch of the vessel wall. Pressure induces excitation and generates signals transmitted to the central nervous system. Due to blood pressure increase, the further distension of the carotid sinuses and aortic arch is observed. The greater stretch increases baroreceptor signalization. With the baroreceptor activation, SNS is inhibited, and the parasympathetic nervous system is activated. Sympathetic restrain is associated with reduction of peripheral vascular resistance, while parasympathetic activation results in depression of the heart rate and contractility. Both actions result in blood pressure decrease.

Clinical studies have shown that baroreflex sensitivity is lower in the elderly subjects and hypertensive patients as well as CKD patients. Impaired baroreflex control of HR is directly correlated with the severity of CKD and is an independent risk factor of sudden cardiac death in people with CKD.

The first study concerning the effect of the baroreceptor stimulation on blood pressure was done in 1965. Bilgutay and Lillehei used implantable device attached to the carotid sinus in hypertensive dogs. The baroreceptors stimulation resulted in blood pressure decrease. Subsequently these authors used this technique in two hypertensive patients. It also resulted with the significant blood pressure reduction. More recently experimental studies confirmed these early observations. It was found that bilateral electric activation of carotid baroreflex in dogs lowered mean arterial pressure and reduced plasma norepinephrine concentration. Assessment of acute electric baroreflex activation was done in 11 patients undergoing elective carotid surgery. Significant voltage-dependent blood pressure reduction was observed (SBP was reduced by 18 mmHg and DBP by 8 mmHg).

For clinical use of BAT, the Rheos system was developed. This system is composed of implantable pulse generator with two electrodes attached bilaterally to carotid sinuses. The multicenter Rheos feasibility trial that included ten hypertensive patients [20] was designed to assess safety, device performance, and protocol parameters of the Rheos system in patients with resistant hypertension. The surgical procedure was successful in all cases. Generator discharge resulted in acute, energy dose-depended SBP decrease of 41 mmHg. No significant bradycardia was observed. BAT using Rheos system results not only in decreased blood pressure but also leads to the reduction of MSNA and both decrease of plasma norepinephrine and renin concentrations. Scheffers et al. confirmed short- and long-term antihypertensive effect of BAT. Forty-five patients with resistant hypertension were involved in the Device-Based Therapy Hypertension Trial (DEBuT-HT). Blood pressure decreased from SBP 179 to 158 mmHg and DBP from 105 to 93 mmHg after 3 months of BAT was found. Further reduction of blood pressure (SBP to 146 mmHg and DBP to 83 mmHg) was observed after 2 years of BAT. It should be stressed, however, that in this clinical study with Rheos system, eight patients experienced serious adverse effects related to the procedure or related to the device [21].

The double-blind, randomized, placebo-controlled Rheos Pivotal Trial involved 265 hypertensive patients [22]. Patients were randomized to Group A and Group B. The difference in the two groups was period of delayed device activation (1 month after the implantation in Group A and after 7 months in Group B). It was shown that 42% subjects from Group A and 24% subjects from Group B reached the target SBP ≤ 140 mmHg after 6 months BAT. The vast majority of subjects (~81%) benefits of SBP reduction over 10 mmHg.

The second-generation BAT systems is Barostim neo. The main differences between Barostim and previously used Rheos system are unilateral carotid sinus activation and largely reduced electrode size. The device consists of one lead electrode and pulse generator controlled with computer system via radiofrequency telemetry. The device was tested in a single-arm, open-label, nonrandomized study that included 30 patients with refractory hypertension. The blood pressure reduction observed during 6 months observation (SBP reduced by 26 mmHg and DBP by 12 mmHg) was comparable to those achieved previously with bilateral baroreflex activation. It is worth noted that this procedure and system seems to be safe. There were no related to the procedure or device adverse effects in 90% of subjects [23]. Recent research confirms the effectiveness of BAT for the treatment of resistant arterial hypertension [24].

Results of the abovementioned studies suggest that BAT with the use of Barostim neo is not only effective antihypertensive therapy but also seems to be safe procedure.

Baroreflex Activation Therapy in CKD

Based on the pathophysiological evidence described above (i.e., SNS overactivity and the impaired baroreflexes in CKD and the role of baroreflexes in blood pressure regulation), the use of BAT in the treatment of CKD patients is worth to study. The aim of BAT in CKD patients might be both renoprotection and improved blood pressure control.

There is only single preliminary clinical study evaluating the effect of BAT on kidney function in CKD patients (Table 19.2). Wallbach et al. studied prospectively 23 CKD patients with resistant hypertension. The evaluation of kidney function and proteinuria was done before and 6 months after Barostim system implantation. It was found that BAT improved renal function (eGFR increase from 54 to 60 ml/min) and reduced proteinuria (from 284 to 136 mg/g creatinine) [25]. These preliminary results showed a potentially nephroprotective effect of BAT in hypertensive CKD patients.

Two preliminary clinical studies evaluated the effect of BAT on blood pressure in CKD patients. Wallbach et al. in already-quoted study have shown that BAT is an effective antihypertensive treatment in hypertensive CKD (Table 19.2). The reduction of blood pressure in this study (mean BP was reduced from 117 to 104 mmHg) was comparable with the achieved in the already-quoted studies with non-CKD patients [25]. Recently, Beige et al. in preliminary clinical study demonstrated that BAT is well tolerated and effective nonpharmacological, interventional, antihypertensive therapy in hemodialysis CKD patients with resistant hypertension [26]. In this study in six hemodialysis patients, Barostim neo system was implanted. At the baseline, SBP was 194 mmHg and DBP 97 mmHg. Twelve months BAT leads to SBP reduction to 137 mmHg and DBP reduction to 73 mmHg.

Described above the promising results of preliminary clinical studies suggest that in CKD patients, BAT is characterized by some nephroprotective effect and that BAT is an effective antihypertensive treatment in this group of patients need to be confirmed in the further studies.

Conclusions

Patients with chronic kidney disease are characterized by sympathetic nervous system hyperactivity, which leads to hypertension and/or organ damage. Experimental and clinical studies have shown that reduction in sympathetic nervous system activity with pharmacological treatment, catheter-based renal denervation, or baroreceptor activation inhibits the progression of chronic kidney disease and improves renal function and survival. However, properly planned and performed randomized clinical trials are still needed in order to confirm the clinical value of this type of treatment.

References

1. Converse RL Jr, Jacobsen TN, Toto RD, Jost CM, Cosentino F, Fouad-Tarazi F, Victor RG. Sympathetic overactivity in patients with chronic renal failure. N Engl J Med. 1992;327:1912–8.
2. Hausberg M, Kosch M, Harmelink P, Barenbrock M, Hohage H, Kisters K, Dietl KH, Rahn KH. Sympathetic nerve activity in end-stage renal disease. Circulation. 2002;106:1974–9.
3. Grassi G, Quarti-Trevano F, Seravalle G, Arenare F, Volpe M, Furiani S, Dell'Oro R, Mancia G. Early sympathetic activation in the initial clinical stages of chronic renal failure. Hypertension. 2011;57:846–51.
4. Ye S, Zhong H, Yanamadala V, Campese VM. Renal injury caused by intrarenal injection of phenol increases afferent and efferent renal sympathetic nerve activity. Am J Hypertens. 2002;15:717–24.
5. Johns EJ, Abdulla MH. Renal nerves in blood pressure regulation. Curr Opin Nephrol Hypertens. 2013;22:504–10.
6. Penne EL, Neumann J, Klein IH, Oey PL, Bots ML, Blankestijn PJ. Sympathetic hyperactivity and clinical outcome in chronic kidney disease patients during standard treatment. J Nephrol. 2009;22:208–15.
7. Zoccali C, Mallamaci F, Parlongo S, Cutrupi S, Benedetto FA, Tripepi G, Bonanno G, Rapisarda F, Fatuzzo P, Seminara G, Cataliotti A, Stancanelli B, Malatino LS. Plasma norepinephrine predicts survival and incident cardiovascular events in patients with end-stage renal disease. Circulation. 2002;105:1354–9.
8. Smithwick RH, Thompson JE. Splanchnicectomy for essential hypertension; results in 1,266 cases. J Am Med Assoc. 1953;152:1501–4.
9. Sakakura K, Ladich E, Cheng Q, Otsuka F, Yahagi K, Fowler DR, Kolodgie FD, Virmani R, Joner M. Anatomic assessment of sympathetic peri-arterial renal nerves in man. J Am Coll Cardiol. 2014;640:635–43.
10. Krum H, Schlaich M, Whitbourn R, Sobotka PA, Sadowski J, Bartus K, Kapelak B, Walton A, Sievert H, Thambar S, Abraham WT, Esler M. Catheter-based renal sympathetic denervation for resistant hypertension: a multicentre safety and proof-of-principle cohort study. Lancet. 2009;373:1275–81.
11. Esler MD, Krum H, Sobotka PA, Schlaich MP, Schmieder RE, Böhm M. Renal sympathetic denervation in patients with treatment-resistant hypertension (the Symplicity HTN-2 trial): a randomised controlled trial. Symplicity HTN-2 investigators. Lancet. 2010;376:1903–9.
12. Bhatt DL, Kandzari DE, O'Neill WW, D'Agostino R, Flack JM, Katzen BT, Leon MB, Liu M, Mauri L, Negoita M, Cohen SA, Oparil S, Rocha-Singh K, Townsend RR. Bakris GL; SYMPLICITY HTN-3 investigators. A controlled trial of renal denervation for resistant hypertension. N Engl J Med. 2014;370:1393–401.
13. Rosa J, Widimsky P, Touek P, Petrak O, Curila K, Waldauf P, Bedna F, Zelinka T, Holaj R, Strauch B, Somloova Z, Taborsky M, Vaclavik J, Kocianova E, Branny M, Nykl I, Jiravsky O, Widimsky J. Randomized comparison of renal denervation versus intensified pharmacotherapy including spironolactone in true-resistant hypertension: six-month results from the Prague-15 study. Hypertension. 2015;65(2):407–13.
14. Desch S, Okon T, Heinemann D, Kulle K, Röhnert K, Sonnabend M, Petzold M, Müller U, Schuler G, Eitel I, Thiele H, Lurz P. Randomized sham-controlled trial of renal sympathetic denervation in mild resistant hypertension. Hypertension. 2015;65:1202–8.
15. Bunte MC, Infante de Oliveira E, Shishehbor MH. Endovascular treatment of resistant and uncontrolled hypertension: therapies on the horizon. JACC Cardiovasc Interv. 2013;6:1–9.
16. Hering D, Mahfoud F, Walton AS, Krum H, Lambert GW, Lambert EA, Sobotka PA, Böhm M, Cremers B, Esler MD, Schlaich MP. Renal denervation in moderate to severe CKD. J Am Soc Nephrol. 2012;23:1250–7.

17. Ott C, Mahfoud F, Schmid A, Toennes SW, Ewen S, Ditting T, Veelken R, Ukena C, Uder M, Böhm M, Schmieder RE. Renal denervation preserves renal function in patients with chronic kidney disease and resistant hypertension. J Hypertens. 2015;33:1261–6.
18. Kiuchi MG, Graciano ML, de Queiroz Carreira MAM, Kiuchi T, Chen S, Lugon JR. Long-term effects of renal sympathetic denervation on hypertensive patients with mild to moderate chronic kidney disease. J Clin Hypertens. 2016;18(3):190–6.
19. Dörr O, Liebetrau C, Möllmann H, Achenbach S, Sedding D, Szardien S, Willmer M, Rixe J, Troidl C, Elsässer A, Hamm C, Nef HM. Renal sympathetic denervation does not aggravate functional or structural renal damage. J Am Coll Cardiol. 2013;61:479–80.
20. Illig KA, Levy M, Sanchez L, Trachiotis GD, Shanley C, Irwin E, Pertile T, Kieval R, Cody R. An implantable carotid sinus stimulator for drug-resistant hypertension: surgical technique and short-term outcome from the multicenter phase II Rheos feasibility trial. J Vasc Surg. 2006;44:1213–8.
21. Scheffers IJ, Kroon AA, Schmidli J, Jordan J, Tordoir JJ, Mohaupt MG, Luft FC, Haller H, Menne J, Engeli S, Ceral J, Eckert S, Erglis A, Narkiewicz K, Philipp T, de Leeuw PW. Novel baroreflex activation therapy in resistant hypertension: results of a European multi-center feasibility study. J Am Coll Cardiol. 2010;56(15):1254–8.
22. Bisognano JD, Bakris G, Nadim MK, Sanchez L, Kroon AA, Schafer J, de Leeuw PW, Sica DA. Baroreflex activation therapy lowers blood pressure in patients with resistant hypertension: results from the double-blind, randomized, placebo-controlled rheos pivotal trial. J Am Coll Cardiol. 2011;58:765–73.
23. Hoppe UC, Brandt MC, Wachter R, Beige J, Rump LC, Kroon AA, Cates AW, Lovett EG, Haller H. Minimally invasive system for baroreflex activation therapy chronically lowers blood pressure with pacemaker-like safety profile: results from the Barostim neo trial. J Am Soc Hypertens. 2012;6:270–6.
24. Halbach M, Hickethier T, Madershahian N, Reuter H, Brandt MC, Hoppe UC, Müller-Ehmsen J. Acute on/off effects and chronic blood pressure reduction after long-term baroreflex activation therapy in resistant hypertension. J Hypertens. 2015;33:1697–703.
25. Wallbach M, Lehnig LY, Schroer C, Hasenfuss G, Müller GA, Wachter R, Koziolek MJ. Impact of baroreflex activation therapy on renal function-a pilot study. Am J Nephrol. 2014;40:371–80.
26. Beige J, Koziolek MJ, Hennig G, Hamza A, Wendt R, Müller GA, Wallbach M. Baroreflex activation therapy in patients with end-stage renal failure: proof of concept. J Hypertens. 2015;33:2344–9.

Chapter 20
The Effect of CPAP Therapy on Resistant Hypertension in Obstructive Sleep Apnea Syndrome Patients with Chronic Kidney Disease

Abdullah Özkök, Asiye Kanbay, and Oğuz Köktürk

Obstructive Sleep Apnea Syndrome (OSAS), Hypertension (HT) and Chronic Kidney Disease (CKD)

Obstructive sleep apnea syndrome (OSAS) is caused by repeated episodes of apnea-hypopnea due to upper airway obstruction leading to oxygen desaturation. OSAS is an independent risk factor for cardiovascular disease including hypertension, coronary artery disease, and stroke [1, 2]. OSAS is common affecting 5–20% of the general population, and it is still underdiagnosed in many cases [3, 4].

A strong relationship exists between OSAS and hypertension (HT). Approximately half of the patients with OSAS are hypertensive, and 30–40% of patients with HT have been reported to have OSAS [5, 6]. In a prospective study, patients with OSAS were found to have three times higher risk of HT [7]. Furthermore, a dose-response relationship between the severity of OSAS and HT was detected in this study. Confirming this finding, in Wisconsin Sleep Cohort Study, apnea-hypopnea index was found to be associated linearly with higher 24-h ambulatory blood pressure (BP) levels [8]. The important role of OSAS in hypertension has also been recognized by the Joint National Committee VII report [9], American Heart Association [10], and the European Society of Hypertension Guidelines [11].

OSAS may also be related to the development of incident HT in normotensive patients; however controversy exists in this issue. In the Wisconsin Sleep Cohort

A. Özkök
Istanbul Medeniyet University, Goztepe Education and Research Hospital, Section of Nephrology, Istanbul, Turkey

A. Kanbay (✉)
Istanbul Medeniyet University, Faculty of Medicine, Department of Pulmonary Medicine, Istanbul, Turkey
e-mail: kanbaydr@yahoo.com

O. Köktürk
Gazi University, Faculty of Medicine, Department of Pulmonary Medicine, Ankara, Turkey

© Springer International Publishing AG 2017
A. Covic et al. (eds.), *Resistant Hypertension in Chronic Kidney Disease*,
DOI 10.1007/978-3-319-56827-0_20

Study [7], patients with moderate-to-severe OSAS were found to have 3.2-fold increased odds of developing HT relative to subjects without OSAS in 4 years of follow-up period. In another large prospective cohort study, untreated OSAS patients including patients who were non-adherent to continuous positive airway pressure (CPAP) or refused CPAP treatment were all associated with increased risk for incident hypertension [12]. However, in contrary to these results, no increased risk of incident HT could be found in Sleep Heart Health Study at 5 years of follow-up period [13].

HT associated with OSAS tends to be resistant, nocturnal, and non-dipper [14, 15]. Prevalence of OSAS in patients with resistant hypertension (RH) has been reported to be around 64–83% [16, 17]. In a study performed on patients with RH, 96% of the male and 65% of the female patients had significant OSAS [16]. Indeed, OSAS has been regarded as the most common secondary cause of RH [17].

Non-dipping pattern of HT is associated with increased risk of cardiovascular events [18], end-organ damage, and less favorable outcomes [19]. Non-dipping HT is very frequent in patients with OSAS. In untreated patients with mild to severe OSAS, prevalence of non-dipping has been reported to be 84% [20].

OSAS, HT, and chronic kidney disease (CKD) are closely related to each other. HT is well established to be a major etiological factor for the development and progression of CKD [21]. Treatment of HT is shown to decrease the rate of kidney dysfunction [22]. In a study performed on CKD and non-CKD subjects, RH and severe OSAS were found to be more prevalent in patients with advanced kidney disease [23]. Furthermore, patients with end-stage renal disease with severe OSAS were found to have seven times higher risk to have RH. A direct reciprocal association between OSAS and CKD has also been hypothesized; CKD may increase the risk of OSAS and OSAS may accelerate the progression to end-stage renal disease (ESRD). OSAS was found to be present in 50–70% of patients with ESRD [24].

Pathophysiology of HT in OSAS

Many pathophysiological mechanisms have been proposed for the development of HT in patients with OSAS such as increased renin-angiotensin-aldosterone system (RAAS) activity, sympathetic nervous system (SNS) activity, increased inflammation and oxidative stress, increased endothelin release, endothelial dysfunction, and arterial stiffness.

RAAS is the principal pathway in the regulation of BP and thus the overactivity of RAAS is shown to be the main inciting event in HT. Patients with OSAS were shown to have increased serum aldosterone levels [25] and 24-h urinary excretion of aldosterone [26]. Furthermore, plasma aldosterone levels were found to be directly associated with the severity of OSAS in patients with resistant HT [25]. Aldosterone may contribute to the pathogenesis of OSAS by the way of renal sodium retention leading increased airway resistance due to parapharyngeal edema. Supporting this hypothesis, treatment with aldosterone antagonists has been shown to improve OSAS in patients with RH [27].

Patients with OSAS were also found to have increased plasma angiotensin II levels. Moreover, treatment of OSAS with CPAP significantly decreased plasma renin and angiotensin II levels in parallel to reductions in BP [28]. In several other studies, increased inflammation and oxidative stress were shown to reduce nitric oxide (NO) levels leading to impaired vasodilatation in patients with OSAS, and CPAP treatment reversed NO levels [29, 30]. In the other study, both serum endothelin levels and BP were significantly reduced after CPAP therapy [31].

Importance of SNS overactivity has been clearly shown in OSAS-induced HT. In animal experiments, chronic hypoxemia due to OSAS was shown to induce SNS activity which in turn activated RAAS and increased vascular resistance leading to hypertension [32]. However recent findings suggested that SNS overactivity could cause OSAS. In a renal denervation study, central SNS outflow and BP were significantly decreased and OSAS was improved with denervation treatment [33]. In another words, SNS overactivity might be the trigger for both RH and OSAS.

Increased arterial stiffness is a well-known risk factor for HT and it may also play a role in OSAS-induced HT [34, 35]. In several studies performed on patients with severe OSAS, CPAP treatment was found to significantly decrease arterial stiffness in 4 weeks [36, 37]. In contrary, in the study by Jones et al. [38], arterial stiffness was not affected after 12 weeks of CPAP treatment. However, in a recent meta-analysis, significant improvements were found in all parameters of arterial stiffness after CPAP treatment [39].

A part of the strong relationship between OSAS and HT may also be explained by common risk factors such as obesity. Obesity may induce HT by the way of RAAS activation, impaired sodium excretion, and increased SNS activity in patients with OSAS.

Role of Continuous Positive Airway Pressure (CPAP) for the Treatment of Hypertension (HT) in OSAS

The contributive effect of OSAS on HT has been clearly demonstrated in the previous studies. However, there are conflicting results about the role of CPAP on the treatment of hypertension. Controversies on these results may stem from multiple issues including differences in study designs, degree of OSAS and CPAP compliances, treatment durations and accuracy, and methods of BP measurements.

In a prospective, multicenter randomized controlled trial (RCT), 194 patients with OSAS and RH were randomized to two groups as CPAP group or no therapy group [40]. After a 12-week follow-up period, significant decrease in 24-h mean BP (3.1; 95% confidence interval, 0.6–5.6 mmHg) and 24-h diastolic BP (3.2; 95%confidence interval, 1.0–5.4) were observed in the CPAP group. Furthermore, nocturnal BP dip was evident in the CPAP group.

In another randomized prospective trial performed on patients with OSAS and RH with a 3-month follow-up period, CPAP treatment significantly reduced 24-h BP. Moreover number of patients with a dipping pattern significantly increased in the CPAP group. These positive findings were only observed in patients who used CPAP more than 5.8 h [41]. In the study by Dernaika et al., CPAP treatment resulted in de-escalation of antihypertensive treatment in 71% of subjects with RH [42].

In a study by Cantolla et al. [43] performed on patients with a new diagnosis of HT and OSAS, 12 weeks of CPAP treatment significantly decreased 24-h ambulatory BP of 2 mmHg and nocturnal systolic BP of 3.1 mmHg. Also percentage of patients with non-dipping HT was reduced in the CPAP group. Adherence to CPAP treatment is known to be important in effective treatment of OSAS-induced HT [13, 44]. Similarly in this study, the reduction in BP was higher in patients with a CPAP use of more than 3 h/night.

In the study by Pedrosa et al. [45], patients with confirmed RH and moderate to severe OSAS were randomized to medical therapy or to medical treatment plus CPAP for 6 months. The treatment of OSAS with CPAP significantly reduced daytime BP in patients with RH.

In the study by Muxfeldt et al. [46], 117 patients with RH and moderate to severe OSAS were randomized to 6 months of CPAP treatment or no therapy while maintaining antihypertensive treatments. CPAP treatment was not effective on clinic and ambulatory BP levels; however nighttime systolic and nocturnal BP levels might be affected favorably in patients with uncontrolled ambulatory BP levels.

In a large prospective multicenter RCT performed on 725 non-sleepy patients with OSAS, CPAP did not result in a statistically significant reduction in the incidence of HT or cardiovascular events during a median follow-up period of 4 years [47].

CPAP treatment may also be effective in patients with prehypertension and masked HT. In the randomized study by Drager et al. [48] performed on patients with severe OSAS, 3 months of effective treatment with CPAP significantly decreased BP and resulted in a 42% decrease in the frequency of prehypertension and an 87% decrease in the frequency of masked HT. Authors concluded that these results might suggest that OSAS might be a risk factor for both prehypertension and masked HT and that the early treatment of OSAS might prevent the development of sustained HT.

Summary of the meta-analyses about the role of CPAP on the treatment of HT is presented in Table 20.1. Accordingly, the overall treatment effects were modest but still significant except one meta-analysis by Alajmi et al. [49]. Even these moderate improvements in BP have been shown to reduce morbidity and mortality [50].

Importance of CPAP Adherence

The efficacy of CPAP as an antihypertensive treatment is significantly associated with the numbers of hours of adherence to CPAP. Each hour of CPAP use was found to be associated with a 1.3 mmHg reduction in mean BP in patients with OSAS and RH [40]. Similarly, in several other studies, at least 5 h of CPAP use/night was shown to significantly decrease BP [41, 44]. However, adherence to CPAP is usually low. Average CPAP use in clinical trials is usually around 4–5 h/night. Even if the

Table 20.1 Meta-analyses about the role of CPAP on the treatment of IIT in patients with OSAS

Study, reference, year	Number of studies	Sample size	Change in SBP, mmHg (95% CI)	Change in DBP, mmHg (95% CI)	Note
Bazzano et al. [58]	16	818	−2.46 (−4.31 to −0.62)	−1.83 (−3.05 to −0.61)	Net reductions in BP not statistically different between day- and nighttime
Haentjens et al. [59]	12	572	−1.64 (−2.67 to −0.60)	−1.48 (−2.18 to −0.78)	Better BP control with increasing OSAS severity and CPAP adherence
Alajmi et al. [49]	10	587	−1.38 (3.6 to −0.88)	−1.52 (3.1 to −0.07)	Nonsignificant
Montesi et al. [60]	28	1948	−2.58 (−3.57 to −1.59)	−2.01 (−2.84 to −1.18)	Significant reductions in BP seen in studies with sleepier patients with more severe OSAS and higher CPAP adherence
Hu et al. [61]	7	794	−2.32 (−3.65 to −1.00)	−1.98 (−2.82 to −1.14)	Better improvement in nocturnal SBP. Patients with resistant HT or receiving antihypertensives benefited most from CPAP
Liu et al. [62]	5	446	−4.78 (−7.95 to −1.61)	−2.95 (−5.37 to −0.53)	Included only the studies performed on patients with resistant HT. CPAP also associated with reductions in nocturnal DBP
Schein et al. [63]	16	1166	−4.92 (−8.70 to −1.14) (night-time)	−3.46 (−6.75 to −0.17) (24-h)	Significant reductions in mean 24 h BP [−3.56 mmHg (−6.79 to −0.33)]
Iftikhar et al. [64]	6	329	−7.21 (−9.04 to −5.38)	−4.99 (−6.01 to −3.96)	Included only the studies performed on patients with resistant HT
Fava et al. [65]	29	1820	−2.6 ± 0.6	−2.0 ± 0.4	Higher baseline AHI associated with greater mean decrease in systolic BP

Abbreviations: AHI apnea-hypopnea index, *CI* confidence interval, *DBP* diastolic blood pressure, *HT* hypertension, *SBP* systolic blood pressure

patients are adherent to CPAP treatment, BP control could not be established in nearly 30% of patients using CPAP treatment for more than 4 h/night [40, 47]. Until recently, no clinical or laboratory parameter has been known to predict the patients who will respond favorably to CPAP treatment. In a promising study by Torre et al. [51], a singular cluster of miRNAs associated with cardiovascular system appeared to specifically define the patients with RH and OSAS who responded to CPAP with favorable decreases in mean BP. The measurement of a specific cluster of miRNAs may enable generation of a predictive screening tool (HIPARCO Score) to predict the responders.

Possible Mechanisms of Action of CPAP Treatment on Blood Pressure Control

Mechanism of action of CPAP on the treatment of HT is not clearly known; however CPAP was shown to reduce RAAS [52] and SNS activity [53, 54]; decrease plasma noradrenaline levels [55], free-oxygen radicals, and inflammatory mediators [56, 57]; and improve the endothelial dysfunction [30] and arterial stiffness [36, 37] associated with OSAS.

Possible Role of CPAP in HT Treatment of CKD Patients

Although OSAS was found to be related to RH in patients with both CKD and kidney failure [23], no study has been designed to address the possible favorable effects of CPAP treatment on BP control in patients with both OSAS and CKD. Mainly three mechanisms have been proposed in the strong relationship between OSAS, RH, and CKD: hypervolemia, high RAAS, and SNS activity. Since treatment of OSAS with CPAP has been shown to reduce RAAS and SNS activity [52–54], CPAP is strongly expected to be effective in BP control also in CKD patients.

Arterial stiffness is common and exaggerated in CKD patients, and it plays an important role in HT of CKD. CPAP was shown to effectively improve arterial stiffness in non-CKD patients [39]; thus it may also be effective in this population in the treatment of arterial stiffness and HT.

In addition to favorable effects on BP control, CPAP may also increase renal survival by reducing glomerular hyperfiltration, intraglomerular HT, glomerulosclerosis, and renal fibrosis.

References

1. Peker Y, Kraiczi H, Hedner J, et al. An independent association between obstructive sleep apnoea and coronary artery disease. Eur Respir J. 1999;14:179–84.
2. Yaggi HK, Concato J, Kernan WN, et al. Obstructive sleep apnea as a risk factor for stroke and death. N Engl J Med. 2005;353:2034–41.
3. Young T, Peppard PE, Gottlieb DJ. Epidemiology of obstructive sleep apnea: a population health perspective. Am J Respir Crit Care Med. 2002;165:1217–39.
4. Young T, Palta M, Dempsey J, et al. The occurrence of sleepdisordered breathing among middle-aged adults. N Engl J Med. 1993;328:1230–5.
5. Fletcher ED, DeBehnke RD, Lovoi MS, et al. Undiagnosed sleep apnea in patients with essential hypertension. Ann Intern Med. 1985;103(2):190–5.
6. Lavie P, Ben-Yosef R, Rubin AE. Prevalence of sleep apnea syndrome among patients with essential hypertension. Am Heart J. 1984;108(2):373–6.

7. Peppard PE, Young T, Palta M, Skatrud J. Prospective study of the association between sleep-disordered breathing and hypertension. N Engl J Med. 2000;342:1378–84.
8. Hla KM, Young TB, Bidwell T, Palta M, Skatrud JB, Dempsey J. Sleep apnea and hypertension. A population-based study. Ann Intern Med. 1994;120(5):382–8.
9. Chobanian AV, Bakris GL, Black HR, Cushman WC, Green LA, Izzo JL Jr, et al. The seventh report of the Joint National Committee on prevention, detection, evaluation, and treatment of high blood pressure: the JNC 7 report. JAMA. 2003;289:2560–72.
10. Calhoun DA, Jones D, Textor S, Goff DC, Murphy TP, Toto RD, et al. Resistant hypertension: diagnosis, evaluation, and treatment. A scientific statement from the American Heart Association professional education Committee of the Council for high blood pressure research. Hypertension. 2008;51:1403–19.
11. Mancia G, Laurent S, Agabiti-Rosei E, Ambrosioni E, Burnier M, Caulfield MJ, et al. Reappraisal of European guidelines on hypertension management: a European Society of Hypertension Task Force document. Blood Press. 2009;18:308–47.
12. Marin JM, Agusti A, Villar I, Forner M, Nieto D, Carrizo SJ, et al. Association between treated and untreated obstructive sleep apnea and risk of hypertension. JAMA. 2012;307:2169–76.
13. O'Connor GT, Caffo B, Newman AB, et al. Prospective study of the association between sleep-disordered breathing and hypertension: the sleep Heart health study. Am J Respir Crit Care Med. 2009;179(12):1159–64.
14. Baguet JP, Hammer L, Levy P, Pierre H, Rossini E, Mouret S, Ormezzano O, Mallion JM, Pepin JL. Night-time and diastolic hypertension are common and underestimated conditions in newly diagnosed apnoeic patients. J Hypertens. 2005;23:521–7.
15. Hla KM, Young T, Finn L, Peppard PE, Szklo-Coxe M, Stubbs M. Longitudinal association of sleep-disordered breathing and nondipping of nocturnal blood pressure in the Wisconsin sleep cohort study. Sleep. 2008;31:795–800.
16. Logan AG, Perlikowski SM, Mente A, Tisler A, Tkacova R, Niroumand M, et al. High prevalence of unrecognized sleep apnoea in drug-resistant hypertension. J Hypertens. 2001;19:2271–7.
17. Pedrosa RP, Drager LF, Gonzaga CC, Sousa MG, de Paula LK, Amaro AC, et al. Obstructive sleep apnea: the most common secondary cause of hypertension associated with resistant hypertension. Hypertension. 2011;58:811–7.
18. Chobanian AV, Bakris GL, Black HR, Cushman WC, Green LA, Izzo JL, et al. Seventh report of the Joint National Committee on prevention, detection, evaluation, and treatment of high blood pressure. Hypertension. 2003;42:1206–52.
19. Mancia G, De Backer G, Dominiczak A, Cifkova R, Fagard R, Germano G, et al. 2007 guidelines for the Management of Arterial Hypertension: the task force for the management of arterial hypertension of the European Society of Hypertension and the European Society of Cardiology. J Hypertens. 2007;25:1105–87.
20. Loredo JS, Ancoli-Israel S, Dimsdale JE. Sleep quality and blood pressure dipping in obstructive sleep apnea. Am J Hypertens. 2001;14:887–92.
21. Yu HT. Progression of chronic renal failure. Arch Intern Med. 2003;163:1417–29.
22. Wright JT Jr, Bakris G, Greene T, et al. Effect of blood pressure lowering and antihypertensive drug class on progression of hypertensive kidney disease: results from the AASK trial. JAMA. 2002;288:2421–31.
23. Abdel-Kader K, Dohar S, Shah N, et al. Resistant hypertension and obstructive sleep apnea in the setting of kidney disease. J Hypertens. 2012;30:960–6.
24. Kraus MA, Hamburger RJ. Sleep apnea in renal failure. Adv Perit Dial. 1997;13:88–92.
25. Pratt-Ubunama MN, Nishizaka MK, Boedefeld RL, et al. Plasma aldosterone is related to severity of obstructive sleep apnea in subjects with resistant hypertension. Chest. 2007;131:453–9.
26. Calhoun DA, Nishizaka MK, Zaman MA, Harding SM. Aldosterone excretion among subjects with resistant hypertension and symptoms of sleep apnea. Chest. 2004;125(1):112–7.

27. Gaddam K, Pimenta E, Thomas SJ, et al. Spironolactone reduces severity of obstructive sleep apnoea in patients with resistant hypertension: a preliminary report. J Hum Hypertens. 2010;24:532–7.
28. Moller DS, Lind P, Strunge B, Pedersen EB. Abnormal vasoactive hormones and 24-hour blood pressure in obstruc- tive sleep apnea. Am J Hypertens. 2003;16:274–80.
29. Imadojemu VA, Gleeson K, Quraishi SA, Kunselman AR, Sinoway LI, Leuenberger UA. Impaired vasodilator responses in obstructive sleep apnea are improved with continuous positive airway pressure therapy. Am J Respir Crit Care Med. 2002;165:950–3.
30. Ip MS, Lam B, Chan LY, Zheng L, Tsang KW, Fung PC, et al. Circulating nitric oxide is suppressed in obstructive sleep apnea and is reversed by nasal continuous positive airway pressure. Am J Respir Crit Care Med. 2000;162:2166–71.
31. Phillips BG, Narkiewicz K, Pesek CA, Haynes WG, Dyken ME, Somers VK. Effects of obstructive sleep apnea on endothelin-1 and blood pressure. J Hypertens. 1999;17:61–6.
32. Dempsey JA, Veasey SC, Morgan BJ, O'Donnell CP. Pathophysiology of sleep apnea. Physiol Rev. 2010;90:47–112.
33. Witkowski A, Prejbisz A, Florczak E, et al. Effects of renal sympathetic denervation on blood pressure, sleep apnea course, and glycemic control in patients with resistant hypertension and sleep apnea. Hypertension. 2011;58:559–65.
34. O'Rourke MF, Nichols WW. Aortic diameter, aortic stiffness, and wave reflection increase with age and isolated systolic hypertension. Hypertension. 2005;45:652–8.
35. Doonan RJ, Scheffler P, Lalli M, Kimoff RJ, Petridou ET, Daskalopoulos ME, Daskalopoulou SS. Increased arterial stiffness in obstructive sleep apnea: a systematic review. Hypertens Res. 2011;34:23–32.
36. Kohler M, Pepperell JC, Casadei B, et al. CPAP and measures of cardiovascular risk in males with OSAS. Eur Respir J. 2008;32:1488–96.
37. Drager LF, Bortolotto LA, Figueiredo AC, et al. Effects of continuous positive airway pressure on early signs of atherosclerosis in obstructive sleep apnea. Am J Respir Crit Care Med. 2007;176:706–12.
38. Jones A, Vennelle M, Connell M, et al. The effect of continuous positive airway pressure therapy on arterial stiffness and endothelial function in obstructive sleep apnea: a randomized controlled trial in patients without cardiovascular disease. Sleep Med. 2013;14:1260–5.
39. Vlachantoni IT, Dikaiakou E, Antonopoulos CN, et al. Effects of continuous positive airway pressure (CPAP) treatment for obstructive sleep apnea in arterial stiffness: a meta-analysis. Sleep Med Rev. 2013;17:19–28.
40. Martinez-Garcia MA, Capote F, Campos-Rodriguez F, Lloberes P, Diaz de Atauri MJ, Somoza M, et al. Effect of CPAP on blood pressure in patients with obstructive sleep apnea and resistant hypertension: the HIPARCO randomized clinical trial. JAMA. 2013;310:2407–15.
41. Lozano L, Tovar JL, Sampol G, et al. Continuous positive airway pressure treatment in sleep apnea patients with resistant hypertension: a randomized, controlled trial. J Hypertens. 2010;28(10):2161–8.
42. Dernaika TA, Kinasewitz GT, Tawk MM. Effects of nocturnal continuous positive airway pressure therapy in patients with resistant hypertension and obstructive sleep apnea. J Clin Sleep Med. 2009;5(2):103–7.
43. Durán-Cantolla J, Aizpuru F, Montserrat JM, Ballester E, Terán-Santos J, Aguirregomoscorta JI, Gonzalez M, Lloberes P, Masa JF, De La Peña M, Carrizo S, Mayos M, Barbé F. Spanish sleep and breathing group. Continuous positive airway pressure as treatment for systemic hypertension in people with obstructive sleep apnoea: randomised controlled trial. BMJ. 2010;341:c5991.
44. Barbé F, Durán-Cantolla J, Capote F, De LPM, Chiner E, Masa JF, et al. Long-term effect of continuous positive airway pressure in hypertensive patients with sleep apnea. Am J Respir Crit Care Med. 2010;181:718–26.

45. Pedrosa RP, Drager LF, de Paula LK, Amaro AC, Bortolotto LA, Lorenzi-Filho G. Effects of OSA treatment on BP in patients with resistant hypertension: a randomized trial. Chest. 2013;144(5):1487–94.
46. Muxfeldt ES, Margallo V, Costa LM, Guimarães G, Cavalcante AH, Azevedo JC, de Souza F, Cardoso CR, Salles GF. Effects of continuous positive airway pressure treatment on clinic and ambulatory blood pressures in patients with obstructive sleep apnea and resistant hypertension: a randomized controlled trial. Hypertension. 2015;65(4):736–42.
47. Barbé F, Durán-Cantolla J, Sánchez-de-la-Torre M, Martínez-Alonso M, Carmona C, Barceló A, Chiner E, Masa JF, Gonzalez M, Marín JM, Garcia-Rio F, Diaz de Atauri J, Terán J, Mayos M, de la Peña M, Monasterio C, del Campo F, Montserrat JM. Spanish sleep and breathing network. Effect of continuous positive airway pressure on the incidence of hypertension and cardiovascular events in nonsleepy patients with obstructive sleep apnea: a randomized controlled trial. JAMA. 2012;307(20):2161–8.
48. Drager LF, Pedrosa RP, Diniz PM, Diegues-Silva L, Marcondes B, Couto RB, Giorgi DM, Krieger EM, Lorenzi-Filho G. The effects of continuous positive airway pressure on prehypertension and masked hypertension in men with severe obstructive sleep apnea. Hypertension. 2011;57(3):549–55.
49. Alajmi M, Mulgrew AT, Fox J, Davidson W, Schulzer M, Mak E, Ryan CF, Fleetham J, Choi P, Ayas NT. Impact of continuous positive airway pressure therapy on blood pressure in patients with obstructive sleep apnea hypopnea: a meta-analysis of randomized controlled trials. Lung. 2007;185(2):67–72.
50. Lewington S, Clarke R, Qizilbash N, Peto R, Collins R, Prospective Studies Collaboration. Age-specific relevance of usual blood pressure to vascular mortality: a meta-analysis of individual data for one million adults in 61 prospective studies. Lancet. 2002;360:1903–13.
51. Sánchez-de-la-Torre M, Khalyfa A, Sánchez-de-la-Torre A, Martinez-Alonso M, Martinez-García MÁ, Barceló A, Lloberes P, Campos-Rodriguez F, Capote F, Diaz-de-Atauri MJ, Somoza M, González M, Masa JF, Gozal D, Barbé F. Spanish sleep network. Precision Medicine in patients with resistant hypertension and obstructive sleep apnea: blood pressure response to continuous positive airway pressure treatment. J Am Coll Cardiol. 2015;66(9):1023–32.
52. Bradley TD, Floras JS. Obstructive sleep apnoea and its cardiovascular consequences. Lancet. 2009;373:82–93.
53. Hedner J, Darpo B, Ejnell H. Reduction in sympathetic activity after long-term CPAP treatment in sleep apnoea: cardiovascular implications. Eur Respir J. 1995;8:222–9.
54. Narkiewicz K, Kato M, Phillips BJ. Nocturnal continuous positive airway pressure decreases daytime sympathetic traffic in obstructive sleep apnea. Circulation. 1999;100:2332–5.
55. Heitmann J, Ehlenz K, Penzel T, Becker HF, Grote L, Voigt KH, et al. Sympathetic activity is reduced by nCPAP in hypertensive obstructive sleep apnoea patients. Eur Respir J. 2004;23:255–62.
56. Schulz R, Mahmoudi S, Hattar K. Enhanced release of super oxide from polymorphonuclear neutrophils in obstructive sleep apnea: impact of continuous positive airway pressure therapy. Am J Respir Crit Care Med. 2000;162:566–70.
57. Chin K, Nakamura T, Shimizu K. Effects of nasal continuous positive airway pressure on soluble cell adhesion molecules in patients with obstructive sleep apnea syndrome. Am J Med. 2000;109:562–7.
58. Bazzano LA, Khan Z, Reynolds K, He J. Effect of nocturnal nasal continuous positive airway pressure on blood pressure in obstructive sleep apnea. Hypertension. 2007;50(2):417–23.
59. Haentjens P, Van Meerhaeghe A, Moscariello A, De Weerdt S, Poppe K, Dupont A, Velkeniers B. The impact of continuous positive airway pressure on blood pressure in patients with obstructive sleep apnea syndrome: evidence from a meta-analysis of placebo-controlled randomized trials. Arch Intern Med. 2007;167(8):757–64.

60. Montesi SB, Edwards BA, Malhotra A, Bakker JP. The effect of continuous positive airway pressure treatment on blood pressure: a systematic review and meta-analysis of randomized controlled trials. J Clin Sleep Med. 2012;8(5):587–96.
61. Hu X, Fan J, Chen S, Yin Y, Zrenner B. The role of continuous positive airway pressure in blood pressure control for patients with obstructive sleep apnea and hypertension: a meta-analysis of randomized controlled trials. J Clin Hypertens (Greenwich). 2015;17(3):215–22.
62. Liu L, Cao Q, Guo Z, Dai Q. Continuous positive airway pressure in patients with obstructive sleep apnea and resistant hypertension: a meta-analysis of randomized controlled trials. J Clin Hypertens (Greenwich). 2015;18(2):153–8.
63. Schein AS, Kerkhoff AC, Coronel CC, Plentz RD, Sbruzzi G. Continuous positive airway pressure reduces blood pressure in patients with obstructive sleep apnea; a systematic review and meta-analysis with 1000 patients. J Hypertens. 2014;32(9):1762–73.
64. Iftikhar IH, Valentine CW, Bittencourt LR, Cohen DL, Fedson AC, Gíslason T, Penzel T, Phillips CL, Yu-sheng L, Pack AI, Magalang UJ. Effects of continuous positive airway pressure on blood pressure in patients with resistant hypertension and obstructive sleep apnea: a meta-analysis. J Hypertens. 2014;32(12):2341–50.
65. Fava C, Dorigoni S, Dalle Vedove F, Danese E, Montagnana M, Guidi GC, Narkiewicz K, Minuz P. Effect of CPAP on blood pressure in patients with OSA/hypopnea a systematic review and meta-analysis. Chest. 2014;145(4):762–71.

Chapter 21
Teaching Programmes

David Goldsmith and Silvia Badarau

The disease burden attributable to arterial hypertension is substantial, accounting for or contributing to 62% of all strokes and 49% of all cases of heart disease, culminating in an estimated 7.1 million deaths a year, equivalent to 13% of total worldwide deaths. Although most cases of hypertension can be effectively treated with lifestyle changes or drugs, or both, hidden within this population lies a cohort at the extreme end of the cardiovascular risk spectrum—those with hypertension that is truly resistant to treatment. Finding this relatively small but important group of patients is a diagnostic and practical challenge, even more so if the patient already has a significant pathology, such as severe left ventricular hypertrophy (LVH), heart failure or chronic kidney disease.

What is *resistant hypertension*? Resistant hypertension is defined in the 2008 American Heart Association scientific statement and the 2013 guidelines from the European Society of Hypertension and Cardiology (ESH/ESC) as blood pressure that remains above goal—typically seated clinic blood pressure > 140/90 mmHg—in spite of concurrent use of three antihypertensive agents of different classes (1, 2), one of which should be a diuretic, at optimal or maximally tolerated doses. The NICE guidance from 2012 suggests that resistant hypertension should be diagnosed only after confirming inadequate blood pressure control despite treatment, by the use of ambulatory blood pressure monitoring (i.e. mean daytime blood pressure > 135/85 mmHg), thereby excluding the so-called white coat hypertension. The optimal target blood pressure in patients treated for resistant hypertension is widely accepted to be < 140/90 mmHg though lower targets than this should be considered in both diabetes and chronic kidney disease (especially with proteinuria). Patients whose blood pressure is controlled to goal with four or more medications are considered to have resistant hypertension (1, 2).

D. Goldsmith (✉)
Guy's and St Thomas' Hospitals, London, UK
e-mail: david.goldsmith@gstt.nhs.uk

S. Badarau
Department of Nephrology, Gr. T. Popa University of Medicine and Pharmacy, Iaşi, Romania

© Springer International Publishing AG 2017   333
A. Covic et al. (eds.), *Resistant Hypertension in Chronic Kidney Disease*,
DOI 10.1007/978-3-319-56827-0_21

Patients with resistant hypertension are at high risk for adverse cardiovascular events and are more likely than those with controlled hypertension to have a secondary cause, which is usually at least in part reversible.

Typical Characteristics of Patients with Resistant Hypertension

- Older age; especially >75 years
- High baseline blood pressure and chronicity of uncontrolled hypertension
- Target organ damage (e.g. left ventricular hypertrophy, chronic kidney disease)
- Diabetes
- Obesity
- Atherosclerotic vascular disease
- Aortic stiffening—systolic > > diastolic BP elevation
- Female gender
- Black race
- Excessive dietary sodium intake

Biochemical Evaluation for Patients with Suspected Resistant Hypertension

Preliminary biochemical tests should be conducted before specialist referral. These can help to delineate a potential secondary cause of resistant hypertension whether unearthed by the patient's history and physical examination or not, signal the development of renal dysfunction and help monitor the response to and side effects from antihypertensive agents.

- Urea and electrolytes
- Estimated glomerular filtration rate
- Plasma glucose
- Plasma renin/aldosterone levels
- 24-hour urinary metanephrines or normetanephrines (for phaeochromocytoma)
- Urine analysis—microalbuminuria and macroalbuminuria, invisible haematuria

Factors Associated with Pseudo-Resistant Hypertension

Clinicians should first attempt to exclude pseudo-resistant hypertension. For this to happen, they have to actively consider, look for and eliminate the factors associated with pseudo-resistant hypertension before a diagnosis of true resistant hypertension is made. These factors can be patient or physician related.

Factors Associated with the Patient

- White coat effect.
- Severely calcified or arteriosclerotic arteries that are poorly compressible on palpation, giving rise to cuff-related artefact (especially in elderly patients). Plain X-ray of forearms and upper arms is usually sufficient to disclose heavily calcified upper limb arteries.
- Poor patient concordance with treatment/non-adherence to medications.
- Side effects of antihypertensive medication.
- Complicated dosing regimens.
- Inadequate patient education.
- Memory or psychiatric issues or poor cognition (especially in elderly patients).
- Difficult relationship between patient and doctor.
- Costs of drugs (in some healthcare systems).

Factors Associated with the Physician

- Poor office blood pressure measurement technique
- Clinical inertia
- Inadequate doses of antihypertensive drugs
- Inappropriate choice of antihypertensive combinations
- Poor communication and lack of time, or desire, to invest in patient education

It should be recognised that systolic BP elevation is much likelier, in older patients, to prove to be resistant, because of the natural age-related widening of aortic pulse pressure, due to progressive age-related arterial stiffening. Indeed, it is important to stress that overzealous efforts to 'crack' systolic elevation of BP might lead to inappropriate and potentially dangerous reductions in diastolic BP, upon which coronary arterial blood flow is heavily dependent.

Factors Contributing to Resistant Hypertension/Risk Factors for Resistant Hypertension

Lifestyle Factors

- Obesity
- Excess alcohol intake
- Excess dietary sodium

Drug-Related Causes (Short-Circuiting Pharmacological Actions, Sodium Retention and Others)

Patients themselves can be taking drugs, formally or informally, which can interfere with antihypertensive medications or be pressor (3).

- Non-steroidal anti-inflammatory drugs.
- Contraceptive hormones—combined oral contraceptives are more often associated with elevated blood pressure, whereas menopausal hormone therapy has minimal effects on blood pressure.
- Adrenal steroid hormones.
- Sympathomimetic agents (nasal decongestants, diet pills).
- Erythropoietin, cyclosporine and tacrolimus.
- Liquorice (suppresses the metabolism of cortisol).
- Herbal supplements (ephedra, bitter orange, etc.).
- Cocaine and amphetamines misuse.

Chronic Volume Overload

- Impaired, and declining, kidney function
- High salt intake
- Inadequate diuretic therapy

   Suboptimal therapy is usually represented by failure to use an adequate diuretic therapy and lack of properly selected drugs and dosage.

Secondary Causes of Resistant Hypertension and their Pertinent Features

- Primary hyperaldosteronism—Hypokalaemia, fatigue, low renin levels despite drug treatment that would be expected to elevate rennin levels (i.e. ACE inhibitor or angiotensin receptor blocker plus a calcium channel blocker and diuretic) and usually raised aldosterone levels
- Renal artery stenosis—Carotid, abdominal or femoral bruits; history of flash pulmonary oedema; young females (fibromuscular dysplasia); history of atherosclerotic disease
- Renal parenchymal disease—Albuminuria/proteinuria, or microscopic haematuria, reduced eGFR or formally measured renal function, nocturia and oedema

  - Renal cystic disease—classically ADPKD

- Obstructive sleep apnoea—Obesity, short neck, daytime somnolence, snoring, frequent night-time awakenings and witnessed apnoea
- Phaeochromocytoma—Episodic palpitations, labile BP, headaches and sweating.
- Thyroid diseases—Eye signs, weight loss or gain, heat or cold intolerance, heart failure, tachycardia, bradycardia and anxiety or fatigue.
- Cushing's syndrome—Centripetal obesity, moon facies, abdominal striae and interscapular fat deposition
- Coarctation of the aorta—Radio-radial or radio-femoral delay, diminished femoral pulses and rib notching on chest radiograph
- Intracranial tumours—Early morning headache and family history

  - Porphyria

In patients with true resistant hypertension, thiazide diuretics, particularly chlorthalidone, should be considered as one of the initial agents. The other two agents should include calcium channel blockers and angiotensin-converting enzyme inhibitors for cardiovascular protection. An increasing body of evidence has suggested benefits of mineralocorticoid receptor antagonists, such as spironolactone (grade 2B) and eplerenone, in improving blood pressure control in patients with resistant hypertension, regardless of circulating aldosterone levels. Thus, this class of drugs should be considered for patients whose blood pressure remains elevated after treatment with a three-drug regimen to maximal or near-maximal doses. Resistant hypertension may be associated with secondary causes of hypertension including obstructive sleep apnoea or primary aldosteronism. Treating these disorders can significantly improve blood pressure beyond medical therapy alone (4–6).

A number of new interventions and devices might help target truly refractory patients—these include renal sympathetic denervation, formation of a large proximal arteriovenous fistula, carotid sinus baroreflex stimulation and several other options (7–9).

Teaching and Disseminating Guidelines

In terms of teaching, and disseminating the guidelines that do exist, in a practical and pragmatic way, this is best done in three complementary ways:

(a) A referral system to a specialist centre which mandates the provision of 'check-list' information on the patient referral pathway screen or sheet. Links to explanations for the need to provide the information should be readily accessible, ideally prompted as the form is completed by the referring team. This will prompt referrers to recognise the features which are the most insightful in terms of making a correct diagnosis.

(b) In the patient evaluation and treatment recommendation report which the secondary or evaluating centre sends back to the referring physician or unit, a stylised check-list response should list the relevant questions selected from the whole investigation set, with an explanation as to why some tests were done (e.g. patient blood levels of measurable antihypertensive drugs, renal angiography, adrenal vein sampling) and why other tests were not done (e.g. adrenal gland imaging, cardiac MRI). Not all investigations will necessarily be needed to be repeated if they have been done before—if a coarctation of the aorta has previously been excluded by imaging, it is unlikely that repeat imaging to detect that condition will be diagnostically fruitful.

(c) A physical or video/VOIP linked complex case multidisciplinary meeting, to provide service needs but also to allow for teaching and training of juniors. Ideally, the patient history would be presented by the referring team, additional features then added by the attending physician team and then biochemical, radiological, haemodynamic, psychological, pharmacological, pathological and other relevant perspectives would be added in. This case presentation and the associated discussion and recommendations could easily be recorded as a file, and perhaps as a CD, and, with some anonymization, could act as an excellent teaching case to permit trainees and less experienced consultants learn the nuances and finer points of this challenging condition. Formalising a service of this type will help encourage and refine future referrals; help to coordinate future research, teaching and training initiatives; and allow for potential research study participation now and in the future.

Future Perspectives

Prospective epidemiological studies are required to delineate the true prevalence, incidence and prognostic implications of resistant hypertension, and a consensus between national and international professional bodies is required on a universal definition of resistant hypertension to allow robust comparisons between future studies.

Unanswered Questions

- Is there one class of drug that is commonly the most effective in resistant hypertension?
- What patient characteristics, if any, define which drug is likely to be the most effective?
- What are the ideal constituents of multidrug regimens in resistant hypertension? A prospective randomised controlled trial of different drug combinations is required
- Is there a role for routine plasma renin measurements to stratify drug treatment for resistant hypertension, and would this be cost-effective? Is there a role for renin profiling in the management of resistant hypertension?
- What is the future role of device therapies in resistant hypertension management? Do they have an additive effect to antihypertensive drugs?
- What strategies are most effective in supporting adherence to drug regimens and lifestyle factors?
- Are there system-based or team-based strategies that can organise the health system to better identify, monitor and treat resistant hypertension?

Ongoing Audit and Research

Audit

- Any specialist centre, or referral unit, should keep an ongoing audit of the number of patients needing three BP-reducing drugs, or more than three drugs, to achieve BP target, and also the number of patients on more than three BP-reducing drugs whose BP remains above target.
- Of those above, an ongoing audit should be kept of checks of accuracy of clinic, and home, BP, use of ambulatory BP, checks of compliance with BP medication (interview, pill counting, blood level measurement) and diagnostic effort undertaken to exclude underlying endocrine or renal causation for secondary hypertension.
- In patients sent to a specialist centre for further evaluation, diagnosis and treatment, an ongoing audit should be kept of the new perspectives, and findings, arising from a specialist referral, compared to assumptions or diagnoses made prior to referral. This would help to identify any clinical 'blind spots' in the referring units.

Research

- Studies of the effect of continuous positive airway pressure in patients with resistant hypertension secondary to obstructive sleep apnoea (ClinicalTrials.gov Identifiers: NCT01508754 and NCT00929175).
- The Resistant Arterial Hypertension Cohort Study (RAHyCo) (ClinicalTrials. gov Identifier NCT01083017) is investigating the epidemiology of resistant hypertension and evaluating the efficacy and feasibility of a standardised treatment regimen (including randomisation of two doses of chlortalidone). It is also studying two interventions in a group of non-compliant patients and will study environmental and genetic variables of individuals with resistant hypertension within a family design. It plans to enrol 200 patients and is due to complete in April 2018.

Teaching Points

- Resistant hypertension is the uncontrolled blood pressure despite treatment with at least three antihypertensive agents (one of which is a diuretic) at best tolerated doses.
- Patients with resistant hypertension are almost 50% more likely to experience an adverse cardiovascular event compared with patients with blood pressure controlled by three or fewer antihypertensive agents.
- The prevalence of resistant hypertension is 10–20% of the general hypertensive population.
- The diagnosis of true resistant hypertension should exclude apparent or pseudo-resistant hypertension has been undertaken.
- 5 to 10% of resistant hypertension patients have an underlying secondary cause for their elevated blood pressure.
- The best available evidence supports the use of spironolactone as the preferred fourth drug if the patient's blood potassium level is ≤ 4.5 mmol/L.
- Attention should be paid to SBP, PP and DBP to try to ensure a sensible and safe therapeutic outcome.

With higher blood potassium levels, intensification of thiazide-like diuretic therapy should be considered.

Recommended Reading

1. Calhoun DA, Jones D, Textor S, et al. Resistant hypertension: diagnosis, evaluation, and treatment a scientific statement from the American Heart Association professional education Committee of the Council for high blood pressure research. Hypertension. 2008;51:1403.
2. Calhoun DA, White WB. Effectiveness of the selective aldosterone blocker, eplerenone, in patients with resistant hypertension. J Am Soc Hypertens. 2008;2:462.
3. Grossman E, Messerli FH. Drug-induced hypertension: an unappreciated cause of secondary hypertension. Am J Med. 2012;125:14.
4. Mancia G, Fagard R, Narkiewicz K, Redón J, Zanchetti A, Böhm M, Task Force Members, et al. 2013 ESH/ESC guidelines for the management of arterial hypertension: the task force for the management of arterial hypertension of the European Society of Hypertension (ESH) and of the European Society of Cardiology (ESC). J Hypertens. 2013;31(7):1281.
5. Oxlund CS, Henriksen JE, Tarnow L, et al. Low dose spironolactone reduces blood pressure in patients with resistant hypertension and type 2 diabetes mellitus: a double blind randomized clinical trial. J Hypertens. 2013;31:2094.
6. Vongpatanasin W. Resistant hypertension: a review of diagnosis and management. JAMA. 2014;311:2216.
7. Williams B, MacDonald TM, Morant S, et al. Spironolactone versus placebo, bisoprolol, and doxazosin to determine the optimal treatment for drug-resistant hypertension (PATHWAY-2): a randomised, double-blind, crossover trial. Lancet. 2015;386:2059.

Chapter 22
Resistant Hypertension and the General Practitioner (Monitoring and Treatment)

Yalcin Solak

Patients with resistant hypertension (RH) deserve a special attention because RH is associated with higher absolute renal and cardiovascular risks, more health-care expenditure, and greater prevalence of secondary hypertension and target organ damage. This translates into more human suffering and health-care dollars compared with hypertension under control. Notably, the single and the most effective way of reducing this increased cardiovascular risk is just achieving sustained blood pressure (BP) control. Thus, this fundamental aim of hypertension management becomes more compelling and challenging in RT patients [1].

RH is quite common. Although its prevalence varies from study to study owing to differences in definition of RH and population characteristic, it has been reported somewhere between 10 and 30%. Some clinical settings are associated with much higher prevalence rates; De Nicola et al. [2] reported that approximately 38% of the patients in a chronic kidney disease clinic had fulfilled the definition of RH. Considering that hypertension is the most common disease worldwide and the increasing share of RH among hypertensive patients, it's likely that general practitioners (GPs) will encounter patients with RH in their routine practice. Thus, GPs should have the essential knowledge of monitoring and treatment of RH.

In this chapter the author will review the fundamental components of follow-up and treatment of RH from a GP point of view.

Y. Solak (✉)
Division of Nephrology, Department of Internal Medicine, Sakarya University Training and Research Hospital, Sakarya, Turkey
e-mail: yalcinsolakmd@gmail.com

© Springer International Publishing AG 2017   343
A. Covic et al. (eds.), *Resistant Hypertension in Chronic Kidney Disease*,
DOI 10.1007/978-3-319-56827-0_22

Monitoring of the Patient with Resistant Hypertension

Since the scope of this chapter is monitoring and treatment issues, we assume that the patient with RH has been assessed in terms of pseudoresistance to antihypertensive therapy. At this point, recognition of causes of pseudoresistance should be investigated one-by-one in a patient who fulfills the definition of RH. Since many patients in Western health-care systems first see their GP and attend GP clinics more frequently than specialized ones, GPs have the unique advantage of monitoring their patients more closely and generally have more data regarding their patients' compliance with treatment. GPs can also more frequently see their patients and track their progress with antihypertensive treatment.

Perhaps, the most important aim of the management of a patient with RH is the sustained achievement of BP goals. To this end, GPs first determine the way with which they monitor BP goals. These means of monitoring include office BP measurements, ambulatory BP monitoring (ABPM), and home BP monitoring (HBPM).

Ambulatory Blood Pressure Monitoring

Office measurements of blood pressure offer some readily available data, but they cannot provide as many measurements as attained with ABPM or home blood pressure monitoring (HBPM). Moreover, office BP measurements cannot rule out white-coat effect as a cause of resistant hypertension.

ABPM is an important component of both the diagnosis and monitoring of RH. The technique allows the physician to correctly diagnose RH while excluding white-coat hypertension. In addition, in a previously diagnosed patient with RH, ABPM this time may be required to rule out white-coat effect as a potential cause of RH. The American Heart Association recommends the use of ABPM in patients with RH to rule out white-coat effect in a position statement [3]. Some other authors also implemented ABPM in the diagnosis and monitoring of RH [4].

In a cross-sectional study, Muxfeldt et al. [5] evaluated 286 patients with RH. Based on results of ABPM measurements, 161 of these patients were diagnosed as "true" RH, whereas 125 (43.7%) were white-coat RH. As can be seen with the results of this study, ABPM can also provide additional data such as dipping pattern and early morning surge, which are independent predictors of future cardiovascular risk. If a patient is diagnosed as white-coat RH, then treatment decisions should not be based on office BP measurements; instead ABPM data should be used to achieve BP targets.

ABPM can predict fatal and nonfatal cardiovascular outcomes more accurately in patients with RH compared to office blood pressure measurements. Magnanini et al. [6] studied 328 women with RH. Patients with true RH had a higher cardiovascular event rate compared to patients with white-coat RH after a follow-up of approximately 4 years. Daytime ambulatory BP was a significant predictor of cardiovascular events, while office BP measurements were not. Salles et al. [7] also demonstrated that in patients with RH, one standard deviation increase in ambulatory night time SBP and DBP was associated with 38 and 36% higher risk of future cardiovascular events, respectively. These authors also demonstrated that office BP results were not associated with adverse cardiovascular events.

One additional benefit of implementing ABPM in the diagnosis and management of RH is recognition of masked hypertension (MH). MH is fairly common (up to 20% of the population) and is associated with adverse cardiovascular outcomes [8]. Unfortunately, there is no way to diagnose MH solely with office BP measurements, because ABPM is not generally ordered in patients who are found to be normotensive in the office.

The role of ABPM in the diagnosis and monitoring of RH is much less studied in patients with kidney disease. In a study of 156 patients with chronic kidney disease (CKD) and RH, prevalence of white-coat RH, MH, and true RH were 29.5, 5.8 and 58.3%, respectively. Thus, if ABPM had not been performed, one in every three patients would be managed inappropriately just based on office blood pressure measurements. Then, this would lead to increased cost and adverse events owing to inappropriate management of RH [9]. A larger and more recent study conducted on patients with stages 1–5 chronic kidney disease found that misclassification of BP control at the office was observed in one out of three patients with hypertension. Thus, this latter study reinforces the importance of implementation of ABPM in monitoring of hypertensive patients as well [10].

ABPM takes on greater importance in patients with CKD and hypertension, because high-risk features which can only be identified by ABPM such as MH and nondipping status are more common in patients with CKD [11]. Better prognostic role of ABPM has also been shown in CKD patients compared to office BP measurements [12].

Routine use of ABPM in the diagnosis of hypertension is still an active matter of debate. Only British guidelines recommend routine use of ABPM to exclude white-coat hypertension while making a diagnosis of hypertension [13]. Only some countries have included ABPM in reimbursement plans and in limited settings [14]. Thus, there is still some time ahead for implementation of ABPM as a standard diagnostic and monitoring tool of hypertension in the general practice (also in the evaluation of RH). In the meantime, home blood pressure monitoring (HBPM) seems a reasonable alternative.

Home Blood Pressure Monitoring

HBPM, if the measurement device is appropriate and calibrated, can provide multiple daytime measurements. However, HBPM is prone to errors owing to greater role of the patient in the process and cannot offer data during sleep, which is important prognostically. In a very recent study, Muxfeldt et al. [15] evaluated 240 patients who provided ABPM and 5-day HBPM results. The authors found a good agreement between ABPM and HBPM results. In another study of 73 subjects with RH, HBPM was found to be a reliable alternative to ABPM in the diagnosis of true RH [16]. Although HBPM cannot provide blood pressure data during sleep, nevertheless it allows the detection of white-coat hypertension, masked hypertension, and blood pressure pattern during the day and the awake night [17].

In summary, general practitioners should monitor antihypertensive therapy preferentially with multiple blood pressure measurements. Office blood pressure measurements must be fully in compliance with best practice guidelines. GPs should be knowledgeable about advantage and disadvantages of ABPM and HBPM techniques. They should be aware of the high prevalence of pseudoresistant hypertension (mainly owing to white-coat RH) and the ability of ABPM and HBPM to exclude pseudoresistance before undertaking further costly investigations for the true causes of RH.

Important Factors Related to Resistance and the Role of the GP

Nonadherence

Once the true nature of RH is confirmed, GP should investigate whether the nonadherence is at play in the RH patient. Nonadherence to prescribed medications is more common in primary care compared to tertiary centers [18]. Several factors are related to nonadherence such as adverse effects of the drugs, pill number and complexity of the antihypertensive regimen, education level, and cultural issues. Number of the pills is particularly relevant in RH because as the definition implies, these patients simultaneously use at least three medications from different classes. A study by Jung et al. [19] showed that out of 108 patients with RH, 40 patients were nonadherent based on toxicological urine analysis.

Nonadherence may be a more challenging problem in CKD population because of increased number of the elderly patients, polypharmacy, and decreased cognitive function. Thus, GPs should look for possible adherence problems when they encounter with a CKD patient who has RH. Education, prescribing combined pharmaceutical forms (two drugs in one pill), frequent review of possible adverse effects of medications, and close follow-up may help reducing nonadherence.

Salt Intake

Salt restriction can reduce blood pressure both in the hypertensive and normotensive subjects. This blood pressure reducing capacity is particularly prominent in patients with RH [20]. CKD, particularly in advanced stages, is a salt-retaining disease.

Pressure natriuresis tries to compensate decreased salt excretion at the expense of elevated systemic blood pressures. Increased salt intake also have detrimental effects on vascular wall and kidney independent of its effects resulting from blood pressure elevation [21]. Moreover, CKD renders individuals to be more salt sensitive even if they were salt nonsensitive before the beginning of hypertension [11].

Owing to reasons specified above, salt restriction and volume control are crucial points of management in an individual CKD patient with RH. GP should emphasize the importance of salt restriction in the diet and monitor adherence of the patient to salt-restricted diet.

General Approach to RH from a GP Perspective

Primary care physicians may have the chance to encounter both a patient who was already diagnosed as RH at a tertiary referral center and a naïve patient whose RH has been diagnosed by the GP. At both situations, a good communication with hypertension specialists is a prerequisite for comprehensive and uninterrupted care for the RH patient.

After diagnosing true RH and ruling out white-coat RH and nonadherence, the GP also address the issue of salt intake as a potential cause and propagator of RH in a CKD patient. If the GP excluded white-coat RH, and nonadherence, and confirmed correct combination of antihypertensive medications at maximally tolerated doses, then he or she should look for secondary causes of RH. The prevalence of resistant hypertension in patients with CKD is over 50% [22], and CKD is among the causes of secondary hypertension. Investigation of all secondary causes nonselectively may not be prudent and feasible in a primary care setting; thus, referral of the patient for a specialized hypertension clinic for this reason may be required. CKD perhaps is the most apparent cause of secondary hypertension owing to nearly universal testing of serum creatinine and urinalysis in every patient with hypertension. Nevertheless, considering the high prevalence of CKD in the general population, a patient might have both CKD and another underlying cause for his/her RH. Thus, in the presence of specific laboratory and/or physical examination findings suggestive of a specific cause of secondary hypertension, the presence of CKD should not preclude investigation of these likely causes. Unlike the progressive and mostly irreversible nature of CKD, many causes of secondary hypertension are amenable to treatment and lead to cure or amelioration of hypertension.

Another responsibility of the GP at this point is to assess the overall risk of the patient with RH in terms of total cardiovascular risk. And, as the holistic caregiver of the patient, all other detected risk factors for CV disease such as diabetes and dyslipidemia should be treated according to most current guideline recommendations. Every effort should be exerted to halt the progression of CKD. Because CKD both is a cause and a consequence of elevated blood pressure, slowing the progression of CKD may be allowed to manage RH more effectively.

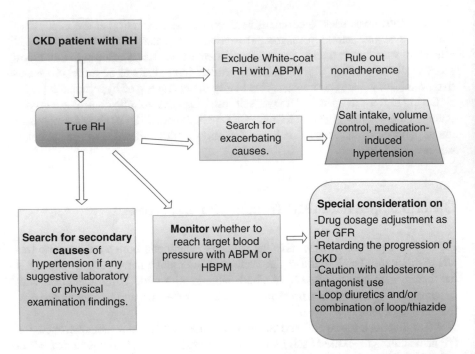

Fig. 22.1 General approach to resistant hypertension from a GP viewpoint. GPs should be in a close contact with hypertension specialists and nephrologists. *CKD* chronic kidney disease, *RH* resistant hypertension, *ABPM* ambulatory blood pressure monitoring, *HBPM* home blood pressure monitoring, *GFR* glomerular filtration rate

The general approach of the GP to a CKD patient with RH is summarized in Fig. 22.1.

Special Considerations of CKD as a Cause of RH and Implications for the GP

Some features of a patient with hypertension seem independent risk factors for the refractoriness of hypertension. In a recent study, Modolo and colleagues [23] found that white-coat effect, black race, and left ventricular mass index were independent predictors of resistant hypertension. In an analysis of Framingham study cohort [24], older age, presence of left ventricular hypertrophy, and obesity were determined as the strongest predictors of the lack of systolic blood pressure control.

Chronic kidney disease is much more common in the elderly, because glomerular filtration rate decreases as part of normal aging and comorbid conditions such as diabetes mellitus, hypertension, and atherosclerosis are common among elderly patients. Left ventricular hypertrophy is very frequent in patients with CKD. Renovascular disease, both macro- and microvascular, is also very prevalent in this patient population. One of the increasingly recognized causes of treatment resistant hypertension, obstructive sleep apnea syndrome, is also reported to be frequent among patients with CKD [25]. Most of these risk factors and comorbid conditions occurring in patients with CKD also lead to further deterioration of kidney function. Additional decline in GFR in turn makes the control of blood pressure more challenging. For instance, CKD was detected in 30% of patients with sleep apnea syndrome [26]. Thus, CKD patient presents with factors which renders them resistant to antihypertensive agents.

Thus, CKD patient with resistant hypertension is not just hypertensive due to diminished GFR. In fact, these patients can harbor a number of concomitant disorders simultaneously. Thus, detection and treatment or amelioration of these disorders should be undertaken to achieve optimal blood pressure targets and retard the progression of chronic kidney disease. GPs should carefully evaluate these patients as part of the global cardiovascular risk assessment. For example, the presence of obesity and snoring should prompt the GP to test for obstructive sleep apnea. Once detected, specific expert recommendations should be sought for these disorders to take the blood pressure under control as well as improving cardiovascular prognosis. In this regard, elderly patients with CKD and resistant hypertension may sometimes be very difficult to manage, and a team of special experts including a nephrologist, a cardiologist, an endocrinologist, and a dietician may be needed to optimize the care of the patient. However, GPs should be at the core of this team to coordinate the recommendations of different disciplines, which may at times complicate the others. GPs as the primary physicians of these patients should not only be in a close cooperation with other specialists of the patients but also be familiar with living environment of the patient and close relatives.

Treatment of RH in CKD from a General Practice Perspective

General principles of hypertension treatment also apply to the treatment of RH. Since treatment of RH has been comprehensively evaluated in previous chapters, in this chapter we will discuss the topic with a special emphasis on a general practice setting to avoid redundancy. GPs should be knowledgeable about correct combinations of antihypertensive medication classes in general. Sometimes, physician-induced or iatrogenic pseudoresistant hypertension can be seen simply because of the use of inadequate doses or wrong combinations of antihypertensive medications. Physician inertia can be described as reluctance to maximize drug therapy, either by adding antihypertensive drugs or by switching drug category, in order to achieve blood pressure goals. Studies have shown that physician inertia is an important cause of resistant hypertension [27]. This may be a significant concern especially in patients with CKD when GP themselves feels uncomfortable with the complexity of the patient or reluctant to change antihypertensive treatment regimen with fear of potential adverse effects. GPs should aim to reach maximally tolerated doses of proper antihypertensive combinations apparently in a patient with RH keeping the following points in mind.

A few points deserve special focus in the pharmacologic management of RH patients with CKD:

1. Salt restriction and volume regulation are central parts of the management of RH in patients with CKD. As a part of the definition of RH, diuretics are sine qua non of therapeutic armamentarium in hypertension. While thiazide and thiazide-type diuretics constitute the mainstay of diuretic therapy used in hypertension, patients with CKD differs in this regard. Efficacy of thiazides diminishes once the creatinine clearance value falls below 50 ml/min [28]. Thus, loop diuretics are the diuretic of choice in patients with stages 3–5 CKD (when GFR <30 ml/min). GPs should be aware of this shift of diuretic choice in patients with CKD and should be able to change thiazide to furosemide or other loop diuretics timely in patients with deteriorating kidney function. Continuous monitoring of weight changes and edema formation in advanced stages of CKD may help adjusting the dose of the loop diuretics.

    Contrary to the classical belief, some evidence, albeit limited, has shown that thiazide diuretics may be as effective as furosemide in stages 4–5 CKD [29]. Combination of the latter two may even be a more effective way to lower blood pressure, particularly in hypervolemic patients [30].

2. Some antihypertensive medications require dose adjustment according to creatinine clearance. Failure to do so may lead to appearance of adverse effects and nonadherence. Most ACE inhibitors are renally excreted and consequently require dosage adjustment in case of diminished GFR with exceptions of dually excreted ACE inhibitors, fosinopril and trandolapril. When aiming maximally tolerated doses of ACE inhibitors, this condition should be kept in mind by the GP. In contrast to ACE inhibitors, angiotensin receptor blockers undergo considerable hepatic elimination, rendering their use less problematic in the patient with reduced clearance. Some beta-blockers including acebutolol, atenolol, betaxolol, and bisoprolol accumulate in renal patients and require dose adjustment as well.

3. Spironolactone has been shown to be an effective adjunct in the patient with RH [31]. Since primary aldosteronism forms up to 20% of cases of RH in some series, spironolactone is an important and frequently used agent in these patients [32]. However, when a patient has reduced GFR, the most dangerous adverse effect of spironolactone emerges, hyperkalemia. Patients with stages 3–5 CKD are prone to hyperkalemia; thus, addition of spironolactone to the antihypertensive regimen of these patients increases the risk of life-threatening severe hyperkalemia [33]. When prescribed to the patient with GFR values >30 ml/min, close follow-up is the rule. Type 2 diabetes mellitus and concomitant use of ACE inhibitors or ARBs increase the risk of hyperkalemia further. GPs should closely follow these patients and instruct them not to have a diet rich in fruit and vegetables. Same principles apply to the more specific aldosterone antagonist, eplerenone, as well.

4. Some medications used for other reasons in renal patients may transform hypertension into RH (not a true RH). Cyclosporine, steroids (in renal transplant recipients) and erythropoietin (in patients with renal anemia) are examples. GPs should be aware of these and other drugs used in this highly comorbid patient population. Over the counter medications, NSAIDs, antidepressants, oral contraceptive pills, and a host of other potential culprits should be elucidated in patients with RH.

5. While struggling to achieve target BP levels in patients with RH, GPs should also aim at retarding the progression of kidney disease when selecting antihypertensive medications. In this respect, rugs which have been shown to reduce proteinuria and slow the progression of kidney disease such as ACE inhibitors and ARBs should be constant components of the antihypertensive regimen. Nondihydropyridine calcium channel blockers (CCB) should be chosen over dihydropyridine CCBs owing to their more favorable effects on proteinuria [34]. Combined use of ACE inhibitor and ARB should be avoided particularly in patients with moderate to severe renal disease.

References

1. Chobanian AV, Bakris GL, Black HR, Cushman WC, Green LA, Izzo JL Jr, et al. Seventh report of the joint National Committee on prevention, detection, evaluation, and treatment of high blood pressure. Hypertension. 2003;42(6):1206–52.
2. De Nicola L, Borrelli S, Gabbai FB, Chiodini P, Zamboli P, Iodice C, et al. Burden of resistant hypertension in hypertensive patients with non-dialysis chronic kidney disease. Kidney Blood Press Res. 2011;34(1):58–67.
3. Calhoun DA, Jones D, Textor S, Goff DC, Murphy TP, Toto RD, et al. Resistant hypertension: diagnosis, evaluation, and treatment. A scientific statement from the American Heart Association professional education Committee of the Council for high blood pressure research. Hypertension. 2008;51(6):1403–19.
4. Muxfeldt ES, de Souza F, Salles GF. Resistant hypertension: a practical clinical approach. J Hum Hypertens. 2013;27(11):657–62.
5. Muxfeldt ES, Bloch KV, Nogueira AR, Salles GF. Twenty-four hour ambulatory blood pressure monitoring pattern of resistant hypertension. Blood Press Monit. 2003;8(5):181–5.
6. Magnanini MM, Nogueira Ada R, Carvalho MS, Bloch KV. Ambulatory blood pressure monitoring and cardiovascular risk in resistant hypertensive women. Arq Bras Cardiol. 2009;92(6): 448–53, 467–72, 484–9.
7. Salles GF, Cardoso CR, Muxfeldt ES. Prognostic influence of office and ambulatory blood pressures in resistant hypertension. Arch Intern Med. 2008;168(21):2340–6.
8. Burnier M, Wuerzner G. Ambulatory blood pressure and adherence monitoring: diagnosing pseudoresistant hypertension. Semin Nephrol. 2014;34(5):498–505.
9. Shafi S, Sarac E, Tran H. Ambulatory blood pressure monitoring in patients with chronic kidney disease and resistant hypertension. J Clin Hypertens (Greenwich). 2012;14(9):611–7.
10. Gorostidi M, Sarafidis PA, de la Sierra A, Segura J, de la Cruz JJ, Banegas JR, et al. Differences between office and 24-hour blood pressure control in hypertensive patients with CKD: a 5,693-patient cross-sectional analysis from Spain. Am J Kidney Dis. 2013;62(2):285–94.
11. Drexler YR, Bomback AS. Definition, identification and treatment of resistant hypertension in chronic kidney disease patients. Nephrol Dial Transplant. 2014;29(7):1327–35.

12. Minutolo R, Agarwal R, Borrelli S, Chiodini P, Bellizzi V, Nappi F, et al. Prognostic role of ambulatory blood pressure measurement in patients with nondialysis chronic kidney disease. Arch Intern Med. 2011;171(12):1090–8.

13. National Institute for Health and Clinical Excellence. Hypertension: clinical management of hypertension in adults [clinical guideline 127]. London: NICE; 2011.

14. O'Brien E, Parati G, Stergiou G, Asmar R, Beilin L, Bilo G, et al. European Society of Hypertension position paper on ambulatory blood pressure monitoring. J Hypertens. 2013;31(9):1731–68.

15. Muxfeldt ES, Barros GS, Viegas BB, Carlos FO, Salles GF. Is home blood pressure monitoring useful in the management of patients with resistant hypertension? Am J Hypertens. 2015;28(2):190–9.

16. Nasothimiou EG, Tzamouranis D, Roussias LG, Stergiou GS. Home versus ambulatory blood pressure monitoring in the diagnosis of clinic resistant and true resistant hypertension. J Hum Hypertens. 2012;26(12):696–700.

17. Ruiz-Hurtado G, Gorostidi M, Waeber B, Ruilope LM. Ambulatory and home blood pressure monitoring in people with chronic kidney disease. Time to abandon clinic blood pressure measurements? Curr Opin Nephrol Hypertens. 2015;24(6):488–91.

18. Yakovlevitch M, Black HR. Resistant hypertension in a tertiary care clinic. Arch Intern Med. 1991;151(9):1786–92.

19. Jung O, Gechter JL, Wunder C, Paulke A, Bartel C, Geiger H, et al. Resistant hypertension? Assessment of adherence by toxicological urine analysis. J Hypertens. 2013;31(4):766–74.

20. Pimenta E, Gaddam KK, Oparil S, Aban I, Husain S, Dell'Italia LJ, et al. Effects of dietary sodium reduction on blood pressure in subjects with resistant hypertension: results from a randomized trial. Hypertension. 2009;54(3):475–81.

21. Kanbay M, Chen Y, Solak Y, Sanders PW. Mechanisms and consequences of salt sensitivity and dietary salt intake. Curr Opin Nephrol Hypertens. 2011;20(1):37–43.

22. Kaplan NM. Resistant hypertension. J Hypertens. 2005;23(8):1441–4.

23. Modolo R, de Faria AP, Sabbatini AR, Barbaro NR, Ritter AM, Moreno H. Refractory and resistant hypertension: characteristics and differences observed in a specialized clinic. J Am Soc Hypertens. 2015;9(5):397–402.

24. Lloyd-Jones DM, Evans JC, Larson MG, O'Donnell CJ, Roccella EJ, Levy D. Differential control of systolic and diastolic blood pressure: factors associated with lack of blood pressure control in the community. Hypertension. 2000;36(4):594–9.

25. Abuyassin B, Sharma K, Ayas NT, Laher I. Obstructive sleep apnea and kidney disease: a potential bidirectional relationship? J Clin Sleep Med. 2015;11(8):915–24.

26. Iseki K, Tohyama K, Matsumoto T, Nakamura H. High prevalence of chronic kidney disease among patients with sleep related breathing disorder (SRBD). Hypertens Res. 2008;31(2):249–55.

27. Hyman DJ, Pavlik VN. Self-reported hypertension treatment practices among primary care physicians: blood pressure thresholds, drug choices, and the role of guidelines and evidence-based medicine. Arch Intern Med. 2000;160(15):2281–6.

28. Agarwal R, Sinha AD. Thiazide diuretics in advanced chronic kidney disease. J Am Soc Hypertens. 2012;6(5):299–308.

29. Dussol B, Moussi-Frances J, Morange S, Somma-Delpero C, Mundler O, Berland Y. A pilot study comparing furosemide and hydrochlorothiazide in patients with hypertension and stage 4 or 5 chronic kidney disease. J Clin Hypertens (Greenwich). 2012;14(1):32–7.

30. Judd E, Calhoun DA. Management of hypertension in CKD: beyond the guidelines. Adv Chronic Kidney Dis. 2015;22(2):116–22.

31. Chapman N, Dobson J, Wilson S, Dahlof B, Sever PS, Wedel H, et al. Effect of spironolactone on blood pressure in subjects with resistant hypertension. Hypertension. 2007;49(4):839–45.

32. Rossi GP, Bernini G, Caliumi C, Desideri G, Fabris B, Ferri C, et al. A prospective study of the prevalence of primary aldosteronism in 1,125 hypertensive patients. J Am Coll Cardiol. 2006;48(11):2293–300.

33. Sica DA. Pharmacologic issues in treating hypertension in CKD. Adv Chronic Kidney Dis. 2011;18(1):42–7.
34. Toto RD. Proteinuria reduction: mandatory consideration or option when selecting an antihypertensive agent? Curr Hypertens Rep. 2005;7(5):374–8.

Index

A
ACE/ARB inhibition, 225
Activated renin-angiotensin-aldosterone
    system, 199
Adiponectin, 115
Adrenaline hypothesis, 92
Adrenal steroid hormones, 336
Adverse effects, 191
Afferent fibers, 309
Afferent renal nerve activity (ARNA), 94
African American Study of Kidney Disease
    and Hypertension (AASK) study,
    41, 45
Afro-American/Asian patients, 42
Aging, 183
Albumin/creatinine ratio (ACR), 145
Albuminuria, 33, 261
Aldosterone, 131
Aldosterone blockage
    mineralocorticoid receptor antagonists,
        222–223
    spironolactone, 223
Aldosterone escape pathway, 98
Aldosterone homeostasis, 98
Aliskiren in the Evaluation of Proteinuria in
    Diabetes (AVOID) trial, 293
ALLHAT study, 80
Alpha-adrenergic blockers, 295
Alpha-agonists, 295
Alpha-blockers, 299
Ambulatory arterial stiffness index (AASI), 143
Ambulatory blood pressure monitoring
    (ABPM), 15, 39, 60, 80, 143, 145,
    312, 344, 345
    altered BP profiles, 42–45

altered circadian profile, 44, 45
BP measurements, 39
catheter-based radiofrequency, 52
diuretic therapy, 53
and HBPM, 41
masked hypertension, 39
neurohumoral activity, 52
nocturnal BP, 40
office blood pressure, 40
pseudoresistance, 46–48
resistant hypertension, 45–51
RH in CKD, 49–52
role, 345
WCH, 39
American Heart Association (AHA), 59, 69,
    77, 234, 285, 344
American Heart Association Scientific
    Statement, 73
American Society of Hypertension (ASH), 233
Amphetamines, 46
Analgesic nephropathy (AN), 20
Angiotensin converting enzyme (ACE), 152
Angiotensin converting enzyme inhibitors
    (ACEi), 174
Angiotensin II type 2 receptor (AT2R),
    97, 263
Angiotensin receptor blockers (ARBs), 26,
    174, 240, 268
Angiotensin type 1 receptor (AT1R), 100
Angiotensin-converting enzyme inhibitors
    (ACE-I), 97, 268
Antihypertensive agents, 334
Antihypertensive-based strategy, 266
Antihypertensive drug groups, 284–285
Antihypertensive drugs, 42, 45

© Springer International Publishing AG 2017
A. Covic et al. (eds.), *Resistant Hypertension in Chronic Kidney Disease*,
DOI 10.1007/978-3-319-56827-0

Printed in the United States
By Bookmasters